23.99

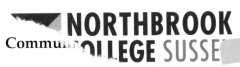

NORTHBROOK
Commu...**COLLEGE** SUSSE...
...r Education

KT-471-892

E140465

Community Health Care Nursing

THIRD EDITION

David Sines
Frances Appleby
Marion Frost

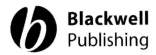
Blackwell
Publishing

© 1995, 2001 by Blackwell Science Ltd for first and second editions
© 2005 by Blackwell Publishing Ltd for third edition

Editorial offices:
Blackwell Publishing Ltd, 9600 Garsington Road, Oxford OX4 2DQ, UK
 Tel: +44 (0)1865 776868
Blackwell Publishing Inc., 350 Main Street, Malden, MA 02148-5020, USA
 Tel: +1 781 388 8250
Blackwell Publishing Asia Pty Ltd, 550 Swanston Street, Carlton, Victoria 3053, Australia
 Tel: +61 (0)3 8359 1011

The right of the Author to be identified as the Author of this Work has been asserted in accordance with the
Copyright, Designs and Patents Act 1988.

All rights reserved. No part of this publication may be reproduced, stored in a retrieval system, or transmitted,
in any form or by any means, electronic, mechanical, photocopying, recording or otherwise, except as permitted
by the UK Copyright, Designs and Patents Act 1988, without the prior permission of the publisher.

First edition published 1995 by Blackwell Science Ltd
Second edition published 2001
Third edition published 2005 by Blackwell Publishing Ltd
2   2006

Library of Congress Cataloging-in-Publication Data
Community health care nursing / [edited by] David Sines, Frances Appleby, Marion Frost. — 3rd ed.
    p. ; cm.
  Includes bibliographical references and index.
  ISBN-10: 1–4051–2748–1 (pbk. : alk. paper)
  ISBN-13: 978–1–4051–2748–6 (pbk. : alk. paper)
  1. Community health nursing—Great Britain.   2. Primary health care—Great Britain.   [DNLM: 1. Community
Health Nursing—Great Britain.   2. Primary Health Care—Great Britain.   WY 106 C7342 2005]   I. Sines, David.
II. Appleby, Frances M.   III. Frost, Marion.

  RT98.C6315 2005
  610.73′43—dc22
  2004029552

ISBN-13: 978–14051–2748–6
ISBN-10: 1–4051–2748–1

A catalogue record for this title is available from the British Library

Set in 9.5/12pt Palatino
by Integra Software Services Pvt. Ltd, Pondicherry, India
Printed and bound in Singapore
by Markono Print Media Pte Ltd

NORTHBROOK COLLEGE DESIGN + TECHNOLOGY	
140465	Class No 615.73 SiN
MACAULAY	10 Oct 2007
Location. 2399	WE BW HO

The publisher's policy is to use permanent paper from mills that operate a sustainable forestry policy,
and which has been manufactured from pulp processed using acid-free and elementary chlorine-free practices.
Furthermore, the publisher ensures that the text paper and cover board used have met acceptable environmental
accreditation standards.

For further information on Blackwell Publishing, visit our website:
www.blackwellnursing.com

Crown copyright. Crown copyright material is reproduced with the permission of the controller of HMSO.

Contents

Contributors

Anne Akamo   *School Nurse Team Leader, Lambeth Primary Care NHS Trust, Lower Marsh, Waterloo, London, SE1 7NT*

Frances Appleby   *Principal Lecturer in Health Visiting & Community Health Care Nursing, Faculty of Health & Social Care, London South Bank University, 103 Borough Road, London, SE1 0AA*

Owen Barr   *Senior Lecturer in Nursing & Learning Disabilities, School of Nursing, University of Ulster, Magee Campus, Co Londonderry, Northern Ireland, BTH8 7JL*

Julie Bliss   *Lecturer, School of Health & Life Sciences, King's College, James Clerk Maxwell Building, 57 Waterloo Road, London, SE1 8WA*

Sue Boran   *Senior Lecturer in Community Health Care Nursing, Faculty of Health & Social Care, London South Bank University, 103 Borough Road, London, SE1 0AA*

Linda Burke   *Deputy Director of Academic Development, Kingston University, Kingston upon Thames, Surrey, KT1 1LQ*

Ann Clarridge   *Principal Lecturer in Non-Medical Prescribing and Community Health Care Nursing, Faculty of Health & Social Care, London South Bank University, 103 Borough Road, London, SE1 0AA*

Pat Colliety   *Director of Studies, European Institute of Health & Medical Sciences, University of Surrey, Guildford, Surrey, GU2 7TE*

Ami David   *Director of Nursing, Dartford, Gravesham and Swanley NHS Primary Care Trust, Livingstone Hospital, Dartford, Kent, DA1 1SA*

David Dickson   *Senior Lecturer, School of Communication & Behavioural Sciences, University of Ulster at Jordanstown, Newtownabbey, Co Antrim, Northern Ireland, BT37 OQB*

Dita Engová   *Senior Lecturer in Non Medical Prescribing/Pharmacology, Faculty of Health & Social Care, London South Bank University, 103 Borough Road, London, SE1 0AA*

Marion Frost   *Principal Lecturer in Specialist Community Public Health Nursing, Faculty of Health & Social Care, London South Bank University, 103 Borough Road, London, SE1 0AA*

Ben Gray   *School of Education, Anglia Polytechnic University, Chelmsford, Essex*

Anne Harriss   *Reader in Educational Development, Faculty of Health & Social Care, London South Bank University, 103 Borough Road, London, SE1 0AA*

Ann Long   *Former Senior Lecturer in Community Health Care Nursing, University of Ulster at Jordanstown, Newtownabbey, Co Antrim, Northern Ireland*

Patrick McCartan   *Lecturer in Nursing, School of Nursing & Midwifery, Queens University Belfast*

Elizabeth Porter   *Programme Leader, Specialist Practice, Department of Nursing, Southampton University, Highfield, Southampton, SO17 1BJ*

Elizabeth A. Raymond   *Former Principal Lecturer in Health Visiting & Community Health Care Nursing, Faculty of Health & Social Care, London South Bank University, 103 Borough Road, London, SE1 0AA*

Anne Robotham   *Former Principal Lecturer in Community Health, School of Health Sciences,*

University of Wolverhampton, Wulfiuna Street, Wolverhampton, WV1 1SB

Mary Saunders *Principal Lecturer in General Practice Nursing, Faculty of Health & Social Care, London South Bank University, 103 Borough Road, London, SE1 OAA*

Karol Selvey *Clinical Manager/Specialist Nurse Practitioner, The Old Court House Surgery, Sutton, Surrey*

David Sines *Executive Dean, Faculty of Health & Social Care, London South Bank University, 103 Borough Road, London, SE1 OAA*

Pam Smith *Research Professor, European Institute of Health for Medical Sciences, University of Surrey, Duke of Kent Building, Stag Hill, Surrey, GU2 7TE*

Stephanie Stanwick *Chief Executive, Dartford, Gravesham and Swanley NHS Primary Care Trust, Livingstone Hospital, Dartford, Kent, DA1 1SA*

Ann Taket *Professor and Director of the Institute of Primary Care and Public Health, Faculty of Health & Social Care, London South Bank University, 103 Borough Road, London, SE1 OAA*

Val Thurtle *Senior Lecturer in Community Health Care Nursing, Faculty of Health & Social Care, London South Bank University, 103 Borough Road, London, SE1 OAA*

Vasso Vydelingum *Director of Studies/Senior Clinical Lecturer, European Institute of Health & Medical Sciences, University of Surrey, Guildford, Surrey, GU2 7TE*

Mark Whiting *Consultant Nurse of Children with Complex Health Needs, Hertfordshire Partnership NHS Trust, 99 Waverley Road, St Albans, Hertfordshire, AL3 5TL*

Jane Wills *Reader in Public Health, Faculty of Health & Social Care, London South Bank University, 103 Borough Road, London, SE1 OAA*

Preface

Welcome to the third edition of *Community Health Care Nursing*. The past eight years have been characterised by significant change and investment in the development of responsive services for patients and clients in the community. Parallel investment has been witnessed in the design and commissioning of new workforce solutions that have demanded major revision to the way in which we prepare community nurses to work in primary care settings.

At the heart of these changes has been the Government's commitment to establish community health care/primary care nursing as the focus for promoting health gain for the population and its constituent neighbourhoods. Associated with these changes has been a major refocusing on, 'shifting' emphasis within the NHS to embrace a, 'health-enabling' philosophy, rather than on a service that, 'majors' on responding to illness. Thus this book aims to change the focus of practitioner responses from 'treatment' to 'prevention' and 'expert practice'.

Government investment in the design of a new infrastructure to support primary care and public health initiatives has further strengthened the need for the nursing and health visiting professions to review the standard, kind and content of the education and practice base of community health care nursing. Other challenges have been the implementation of clinical governance, underpinned by the desire to promote clinical excellence and evidence-based practice and the need to systematically measure and 'performance measure' the quality of service delivery. In addition, priority has been given to the emergence of innovative solutions and practices designed to manage chronic disease and to place renewed attention on public health. Hence, a new professional part of the Nursing and Midwifery Council (NMC) register has been created to respond to public health and health protection, accompanied by a new practitioner – the specialist community public health nurse. For other community nurses the significance of case management, single case assessment and 'First Contact' programmes will demand skill enhancement and transaction.

This text acknowledges the changing face of community health care nursing in the UK and firmly places its academic base within a scientific framework that is underpinned and influenced by contemporary changes in social and economic policy.

There is no doubt that the pace of change involved in designing and developing a new culture of community health care nursing has required a radical and sometimes traumatic revision of personal attitudes and customised care and managerial practices. In their place we are now witnessing the advent and creation of new structures, processes and service systems, many of which have been developed and implemented by nurses working in the many constituent parts of the family of 'community health care nursing'.

This book considers some of the main issues to be addressed in the design and introduction of the profession of community health care nursing. Its roots are firmly established in the evolutionary nature of professional development and recognise the innovative, adaptable and flexible nature of the practitioners themselves. Consequently, the book contains examples of these changes and traces their origins and potential contribution to the implementation of community care and public health nursing. Lessons have been learnt from experimentation and research design and from experimental learning, and in so doing there will be, inevitably, some overlap between individual contributions and the solutions they propose for the delivery of effective community nursing care and specialist community public health nursing.

It is suggested that there is no one solution or 'blue-print' for local service design for any client group. The nature of our communities is as varied as the sub-cultural influences that shape them. No standard model has been prescribed and, wherever possible, contributors have deliberately avoided the inclusion of specific solutions. However, the book presents many ideas, examples and suggestions for the introduction and implementation of sound infrastructures for community health care nursing delivery that may be adapted to suit local conditions and requirements.

Within any attempt to describe the basis for comprehensive service design and implementation there will always be a temptation to capitalise on the experiences of others who have pioneered excellence in local services. This, in essence, is the business of community health care nursing. Contributors to this text have once again been selected for their own knowledge, experience and evidence of providing excellence in service delivery and education. Many who have realised the introduction of innovative practice in their localities will recognise common elements as they read this book that relate to their own experience, and this is of course the intention.

It is our contention that the realisation of excellence, in the design and delivery of community health care nursing services, relies upon the principle that the public, service users, carers and nurses require (and deserve) mutual recognition as key stakeholders in the development and implementation of future policy imperatives that aim to shape and influence the nature of our neighbourhood and nursing services. Some may challenge the 'realism' of our suggestions and recommendations, but there is one statement that cannot be challenged – they are all feasible – and evidence exists to suggest that further investment in the community nursing workforce will result in effective health gain for our population.

David Sines

Chapter 1 **The Context of Community Health Care Nursing**

David Sines

The context of service provision

In 2000 the Government launched the NHS plan that was supported by the introduction of new NHS structures including the inauguration of primary care trusts. The Health Act 1999 built on the principles of community/primary care enshrined within the NHS and Community Care Act 1990, which presented the strategic framework for the provision of all health and social care services in the UK. Current frameworks for the design and delivery of responsive primary care services are built on the principle of ensuring the 'existence of clear, national standards, supported by consistent evidence-based guidance to raise the quality of care provided by the health and social care services' (*The NHS Plan* 2000b). The NHS Plan sets out the rationale for the introduction of improvements in the way in which care is provided throughout the NHS and identifies the need for decisions relating to primary care to be made on the basis of the best evidence- and research-based practice. The details of the proposals for new locally designed services were further outlined by the Government in a major paper entitled *Shifting the Balance of Power* (DoH 2001), which included emphasis on the implementation of consultation with users of services and empowered front line staff to identify robust indicators of personal performance whilst obtaining greater access to control over the allocation and management of the resources required to deliver services. Throughout these papers has been a quest to 'break down' organisational barriers and to forge stronger links with local authorities, thus placing the needs of the patient/client at the centre of the care process. In so doing, a new foundation has been laid upon which to unite the principles of seamless care delivery. In practice this will require the provision of new inter-sectoral solutions to ensure that care is delivered between health and social service agencies through the development of positive partnerships and single case assessment between statutory agencies, consumers, their representatives and with the voluntary and independent sectors to provide a positive choice in the provision of services. Emphasis on primary care has been reaffirmed in that, wherever possible, care should be provided as close to the person's home as possible.

The enactment of this policy has reduced patient/client dependency on in-patient or long-stay residential care in favour of seeking the development of a range of options based on local need, which will be flexible enough to meet the demands of service provision required by local people in their neighbourhoods.

Tackling Health Inequalities: A programme for action (DoH 2003a) also reaffirmed the importance of investing in health improvement by requiring strategic health authorities and primary care trusts to assess and respond to the overall and specific needs of the indigenous population, reflecting social and environmental factors and individual behavioural responses. Emphasis has again been placed on the importance of developing partnerships between consumers and care providers to ensure that all UK citizens receive equal access to health care services. At the same time, Government is determined to remove competitive aspects of care provision in favour of promoting an open economy in care provision based on the principle of excellence and user involvement.

The NHS now requires all strategic health authorities to secure significant improvements in the way in which services are delivered to the population, emphasising the promotion of positive health and the promotion of high quality care in the community. In order to provide these services strategic health authorities must demonstrate that they provide a range of services to their clients and families as equal participants whenever decisions that will affect their lives are involved. Such principles now underpin the NHS philosophy and form the basis of the Government's health and social care strategy.

One major issue for primary care practitioners was the Government's issue of a mandate for the creation of new primary care trusts (DoH 1999b), which replaced the previous concept of GP fundholding. The 1999 Health Act made provision for the inauguration of primary care trust status in England. Such trusts now populate all regions of England and account for, and are monitored by, local strategic health authorities. The primary responsibility of the PCTs will be to assess and provide effective health care to a locally defined population in accordance with user wishes. This role and function requires that each primary care trust gathers intelligence data or information to advise on the actual health care needs of the local population and to demonstrate inter-professional and inter-agency collaboration (e.g. the formation of seamless links with local authority social service and housing departments). In partnership with central government, targets for health care delivery (which reflect national trends on health care) will be set by NHS strategic health authorities and these must be reflected in local service delivery plans and audit processes.

NHS providers must also determine the role that they are going to play, with local authority social service departments, in making their contribution to a range of comprehensive service developments for clients. The Health Act 1999 also demands that planning agreements should be reached between health and social service departments, which clearly identify which services will be provided by each agency and which identify the processes to be adopted in assessing the needs of individuals in their care. The principle of effective alliance building between the NHS and social services has been further clarified by the role of workforce development directorates located within strategic health authorities in England. Such directorates outline requirements

for health and social care services to work together to encourage the joint design, training and education of staff from both agencies in order to provide a workforce with the necessary capacity, skills and diversity to meet the needs of the local population.

The importance of working together in partnership is a requisite goal if the health of local communities is to be enhanced. For example, the Chief Medical Officer at the Department of Health confirmed his decision to develop the public health function of local health and social care providers – *Saving Lives, Our Healthier Nation* (DoH 1999a). In his report the CMO advised that public health was the responsibility of all health care practitioners and called for the implementation of a new 'public health practitioner'. The principles outlined in this paper placed a requirement on each government department to demonstrate emphasis on public health as a central concept within their business plan. For the health service, charged with responsibility to enact new National Service Frameworks and to produce integrated Health Improvement Plans for local communities, a fundamental review was required to assess local public health capacity and capability. The latter demanded an associated objective review of boundary issues between health and social care agencies (and the staff that they employ) in order to ensure that patients and clients have access to an integrated system of care, not constrained by outdated organisational disputes or territorial boundaries. Such principles were further confirmed in the Government's White Paper *Choosing Health* (DoH 2004b).

Emphasis has justly been placed on the promotion of health and alliance building between professionals and users of services. The focus of care is clearly placed within the community with an expectation that resources will be deployed to meet identified health and social care needs through the provision of integrated, peripatetic support from a range of professionals who will include doctors, community health care nurses, community specialist public health nurses, social workers, clinical psychologists, physiotherapists, speech therapists and occupational therapists (supported by an efficient and appropriately funded intermediate/acute sector, in-patient service). The acute sector will in turn complement the work of local primary health care workers who will continue to provide the first point of contact for clients and their families through the provision of effective intermediate and ambulatory treatment/assessment services. In turn such services will be supported by the implementation of primary care led 'walk in centres and treatment centres', thus providing a range of 'seamless' assessment, diagnostic and treatment services.

The context for primary care

Since 1999, the UK Government offices have produced a number of action plans and targets (e.g. *Saving Lives: Our Healthier Nation*, DoH 1999a; *The Wanless Report*, DoH 2004; *Choosing Health*, DoH 2004b), to ensure that the provision of primary health care and the provision of excellent public health becomes a priority in respect of the delivery of local health care services.

The following factors have influenced the pattern of primary care in the United Kingdom:

- In the Declaration of Alma Ata (1978) the World Health Organization stated that their aim of 'Health for All' by the year 2000 should be realised through the introduction of a range of targets for the promotion of health (and the prevention of ill health) for the population. The Government has adopted this aim, within resource constraints, as part of a Eurostrategy and, as a consequence, primary care/public health nursing students must be provided with opportunities throughout their education to acquire competence as 'knowledgeable practitioners' who are well prepared to enhance and advance public health and respond to client needs in the community.
- The publication of the 1999 Health Act, and its associated implementation strategies, emphasises the importance of caring for people in the community accompanied by reduced dependency on secondary health care service provision. The 1999 Department of Health strategy for nursing, midwifery

and health visiting *Making a Difference* (DoH 1999b) confirmed the essential role that community nurses and health visitors play in the transaction of the health care agenda. The strategy also noted that community nursing practitioners are ideally placed to respond quickly to the needs of individuals and families.

- Furthermore, the Department of Health issued further guidance relating to the contribution that primary care nurses can make to this agenda in a key document entitled *Liberating the Talents* (DoH 2002). Three key roles were identified for primary care practitioners:
  — First contact care/acute assessment, diagnosis, care, treatment and referral
  — Continuing care, case management, chronic disease management and delivering care within the context of the National Service Frameworks
  — Preventive/public health programmes to improve health and reduce inequalities such as smoking cessation, reducing teenage pregnancies, child health promotion, preventing falls in older people etc.
- The growth of consumerism and non-statutory sector care in the mixed economy of service provision suggests a demand for more equal relationships with clients/patients and health care professionals. There is also a growing expectation that individuals will assume responsibility for their own health and lifestyles.
- Changes in social policy have increasingly placed continuing care responsibilities on informal carers in the home. Demographic changes and economic demands are changing the nature of the family's caring role that may be influenced by the number of women entering the labour market. Similarly, the projected increase in the number of elderly persons requiring community care has also demanded additional nursing/public health resources.
- Rapid technological and pharmacological developments, nurse prescribing, genetics, the emergence of new patterns of disease and

disability, and the emergence of life threatening diseases, such as HIV infection, indicate a need for nurses who are flexible and able to respond to change.

- The full implementation of primary care trusts (and their associated primary health care teams) has also provided an impetus for change. The importance of inter-professional teamwork and inter-agency cooperation is emphasised. Primary care nursing teams have a major contribution to make in the assessment of individual and community health needs and priorities for their localities. Nurses must therefore be prepared to identify, communicate, influence and evaluate the development of local care plans to ensure the provision of access to a range of support services for clients and their families.
- The implementation of primary care trusts within the UK has influenced the purchase and provision of a range of differentiated primary care nursing services. Skill-mix reviews and increased attention on the provision of cost-effective packages of care will influence the deployment profile of primary care nurses in the future who must be able to provide flexible and holistic care to clients and carers (DoH 2002).
- The Government's investment in quality and standards will significantly influence the health care environment within which primary care nurses function. In particular, the emphasis on clinical governance and clinical effectiveness will demand the design and implementation of new models of role and functional accountability for primary care practitioners.

These influences have affected (and in many cases confirmed) the status of the primary care nurse as the 'lynchpin' within the context of a multi-disciplinary team of specialist health care practitioners. Their work has also been directed by the advent of consumerism that has placed new demands for new competencies amongst the workforce with an emphasis on therapeutic skills and care management (this concept will be discussed later in this text). In summary, this will require that primary care

nurses must be able to respond to the health needs, health gain requirements and expressed demands of their client so as to:

- Stimulate a healthy life-style and self-care
- Further educate families, informal carers, the community and other care workers
- Solve or assist in the solution of both individual and community health problems
- Orient their own as well as community efforts for health promotion and for the prevention of diseases, unnecessary suffering, disability and death
- Work in, and with, inter-professional teams, and participate in the development and leadership of such teams
- Participate in the enhancement and delivery of primary health care in a multi-disciplinary care context

Finally, in this section, the importance of public health is emphasised. The Nursing and Midwifery Council (NMC) have responded to the public health challenge by dedicating a new register to community specialist public health nurses. In so doing the NMC have advised that:

> 'The NMC have decided to set up part of the register for specialist public health nurses because it took the view that this form of practice has distinct characteristics that require public protection. These include the responsibility to work with both individuals and a population, which may mean taking decisions on behalf of a community or population.'

> (NMC 2004, p. 1)

In discharging this new role practitioners will be engaged in:

- Monitoring and profiling the health of their community/practice area
- Ensuring that public health issues are identified and reported to managers and commissioners
- Monitoring health outcomes of their interventions
- Improving the effectiveness of their activities

- Developing local health strategies and building healthy alliances necessary to implement these
- Developing and maintaining partnerships with clients, informal carers, other community members, and other professionals
- Collaborating with local authorities and other agencies to monitor and control health related issues considered to be hazardous to the well-being of the community
- Informing the public about public health issues; engaging in health promotion programmes
- Ensuring that members of the community have access to appropriate public health advice

The changing focus of primary care

Societal change moulds the institutions that are created to respond to the needs of the population. Demands change over time and in so doing socio-demographic factors drive the process of change that in turn requires the National Health Service to adapt its operational base. Examples of such changes relate to the needs of an increasingly ageing population, a reduction in the number of available informal carers, advances in scientific knowledge and technological innovation, and a heightened awareness of ethical challenges (such as genetics, embryology and euthanasia). Changes in Government policy and ideology also shape the health care agenda, and the reduced reliance upon the long-stay hospital for mental health and learning disability care provide clear examples of the need for the re-focusing of care in the community.

The impact of change, stimulated by a growing demand for flexible, high quality services provided within local communities will inevitably re-mould the NHS of the future. Resources have already been shifted to the community (although at a pace that is all too often criticised as being grossly inadequate to meet client need) and commissioners and providers are now required to demonstrate that the care they purchase and deliver is effective and responsive to consumer need (DoH 2001).

The *NHS Improvement Plan* (DoH 2004a) noted that the context of care is changing to secure the engagement of service users to maximise their potential for positive health gain. The focus of the provision of a 'health service' (as opposed to a 'sickness service') is emphasised in this report. Key features of our contemporary society suggest that such a focus on health promotion and public health is required since:

- People are living longer and healthier lives and are better informed about their needs and expectations of the health service
- Advising and supporting patients to make positive choices about their health status is prominent with particular regard to promoting self-management
- Demand to enable people to remain at home is rising thus placing emphasis on integrated care, chronic disease management and supporting healthy lifestyle choices and self care in the community (supported by robust, integrated case management principles)
- Significant emphasis has been placed on increasing social inclusion and valuing diversity for socially excluded groups i.e. those least likely to access health care
- Geographical diversity demands local adaptation of national health care solutions (particularly within the context of devolved government to the four countries of the UK)
- Consumers and practitioners are becoming increasingly dependent on new technological solutions e.g. tele-medicine, NHS Direct and web-based information systems

The DoH *Liberating the Talents* document (2002) confirms the role that primary care nurses are expected to play in this change process:

'Nurses, midwives and health visitors are the largest group of professionals involved and will therefore have a significant impact on patient led and community centred services. Like any profession their role cannot be described in isolation, and as the environment becomes more complex and uncertain, they will rely increasingly on a combination of developing their core skills (both general and specialist) and membership of multidisciplinary teams and networks. Their key attribute will be their ability to fit their skills with a wide range of others in a way that best meets the needs of the individual patient or group. They will play to the strengths of their professional role in integrating the medical and social aspects of health care, promoting self care and crossing organisational boundaries to maximize continuity of patient care and health improvement.' (Preface)

The next decade will be therefore be characterised by the development of highly focused primary care services that will respond to the needs of local practice populations. In this model, much of the activity currently carried out by the district general hospitals could be transferred to general local care units managed by primary care trusts. Such units will increasingly undertake minor and invasive surgery, routine diagnostic testing, support for cases requiring observation and most outpatient activity. Centralised hospital facilities will continue to deal with severely ill people and provide for major surgery. Older people and those with mental health needs or learning disabilities will also continue to be cared for (almost exclusively) in community care settings.

Progress towards achieving this vision for the future may be measured against a series of indicators outlined in *The New NHS Modern and Dependable* (DoH 1998) with regard to the following areas or 'domains' (and which were reinforced in *The NHS Plan* (DoH 2000):

- Targeted health improvement
  — The overall health status of populations, reflecting social and environmental factors and individual behaviour as well as care provided by the NHS and other care agencies
- Fair access
  — Access to elective surgery
  — Access to family planning services
  — Access to dentists
  — Access to health promotion
  — Access to community services

- Effective delivery of appropriate health care
  — Health promotion and disease prevention
  — Appropriateness of surgery
  — Primary care management (including care management, mental health in primary care and prescribing)
  — Compliance with standards (including discharge planning)
- Efficiency
  — Maximising use of resources e.g. day case rate and length of hospital stay
- Patient/carer experience
  — Choice
  — Accessibility
  — Co-ordination and communication
  — Waiting times
- Health outcomes of NHS care
  — NHS success in reducing risk
  — NHS success in reducing level of disease, impairment and complication of treatment
  — NHS success in optimising function and improving quality of life for patients and carers
  — NHS success in reducing premature death

There is little doubt that these indicators provide the primary care nursing profession with a range of major challenges that must be addressed if the balance of care is to shift, according to government policy, to the community. One specific question must relate to the future education and training that will be required to equip practitioners with the necessary skills, knowledge and value base to be able to function effectively in the community. In reality, there is also likely to be a re-allocation of tasks between nurses and others, including informal carers and other professionals. Primary care nurses must therefore be prepared to develop and change, drawing upon the very best of their past experience and becoming increasingly reliant upon the production of research evidence to inform their future practice.

This section has proposed that the most effective way to meet the health needs of the local population is to focus primary health care services within the very heart of naturally occurring communities and neighbourhoods. In so doing (using the general practice population of the focus and locus for care) opportunities for the further improvement of multi-disciplinary teamwork and improved communication systems with clients (and others) would be provided. In order to transact effective care, the potential role that primary care nurses can undertake to fulfil the new NHS mandate must be acknowledged.

The scope of primary care nursing practice within the context of a changing workforce

Current government policy provides considerable opportunities for the development of innovative care solutions within which nurses, often in partnership with social workers and other support staff, will be able to provide responsive services to clients in response to their identified needs. As agency boundaries break down between primary, intermediate, secondary and tertiary care sectors, and professional skills transcend previously defended frontiers, service users will have freer access to nursing skills. The way in which access is negotiated for nursing skills will, in the future, be through single case assessment and care management or contractual processes which should make nursing skills more easily accessible to the general practice population. Their understanding (often acquired from many years of experience and proven competence in the delivery of care to their clients) has placed primary care nurses in an ideal position within the new NHS to respond more flexibly to locally identified health related needs.

In April 2000, the Department of Health published a consultation paper entitled *A Health Service of all the Talents: Developing the NHS workforce* (DoH 2000). The paper noted the need for 'transformation' within the NHS workforce in order to ensure that it was 'fit for purpose' in delivering the proposed health care agenda. The paper confirmed that emphasis should be placed on:

- Team working across professional and organisational boundaries
- Flexible working to make best use of the range of skills and knowledge that staff possess
- Streamlined workforce planning and development which stems from the needs of patients, not professionals
- Maximising the contribution of all staff to patient care, doing away with barriers which say only doctors or nurses can provide particular types of care
- Modernising education and training to ensure staff are equipped with the skills they need to work in a complex, changing NHS
- Developing new, more flexible, careers for staff of all professions and grades
- Expanding the workforce to meet future demands

The direct impact of such proposals for primary care nurses has required practitioners to engage in life-long learning with the aim of continuously seeking to enhance their skills and knowledge in accordance with evidence-based practice for the benefit of their clients and patients. In addition, new flexible roles and responsibilities will demand that primary care nurses seek to validate their skills and practices through the process of peer review and to share learning/education with other professionals. Increased emphasis will also be placed on competence-based education and the generation of new career structures.

In order to respond to the demands of a new flexible workforce, primary care services will need to create, implement, share and explore key issues in relation to the local distribution, sustainability and transferability of innovative 'new role' solutions in primary and intermediate care in order to inform the competencies, practice, education and learning requirements of such new roles.

This will include:

- Agreeing actions arising from local and national discussion relating to the key practice, education/training and regulation issues that need to be addressed to enable sustainability and spread of new 'fit for purpose' primary care practitioners whose roles are designed to meet the demands of evolving and complex inter-professional health and social care workstreams

- Ensuring that universities and their associated partner trusts/social service departments, engage in the design and implementation of new education programmes that are informed by the standards of practice that will be identified through the national changing workforce programmes and other 'modernisation' imperatives
- Agreeing a framework for the development of competencies and associated regulation for new emergent roles in order to maximise opportunities for new ways of working within the NHS career framework
- Undertaking operational research and evaluation that are designed to measure the effectiveness and impact of such new roles and competencies

If these aims are to be achieved then there is a need to ensure that the primary, social and intermediate care workforce is not developed in isolation, but set within the context of national and local workforce requirements, supported by education frameworks developed in partnership with local practitioners. Links will also need to be made with first contact programmes and associated new advanced practitioner roles. Such 'new ways of working' have highlighted the challenges that the introduction of new roles present to employees, employers, regulators and educationalists.

New programmes of education will be required to support the emergent primary care workforce that reflect/include:

- Diversity to provide flexible entry and progression points for new roles
- Career/competence development within the context of *Agenda for Change* (DoH 2003b), and competence mapping
- The design and delivery of coherent educational packages to ensure coherent implementation of changing workforce requirements. Professional development for

nurses undertaking specialist roles, e.g. heart failure/chronic obstructive pulmonary disease, reducing readmission etc.

- The development of key leadership skills in primary care led services
- Embedding and mainstreaming new roles and new ways of working for a range of practitioners from assistant to advanced practitioners
- Designing innovative work-based practice assessment methods to ensure staff are 'fit for purpose' and safe and effective practitioners (thereby affording public protection)
- The design of virtual learning environment/ distance learning through the use of new learning and teaching methodologies
- The development of common learning with GPs, social workers and all members of the health care team (including intermediate care professionals)
- Determining and 'piloting' a range of new competencies for such new roles
- The development and implementation of a new 'role map' for a new inter-professional and multi–agency workforce
- Ensuring that the introduction of these new roles is underpinned by a short, medium and long-term strategic plan in order to ensure flexibility, transferability and sustainability, and to encourage recruitment and retention of staff working in these new evolving roles
- Recognition of key policy drivers impacting on service provision (particularly in relation to chronic disease management, single case assessment, care/case management, unscheduled care/out of hours provision and the new GMS contract), which require expediency in the introduction of these roles
- Ensuring that local delivery plans facilitate the ability to change workforce profiles; current and future workforce profiles should focus on matching local need with national policy
- The provision of flexible commissioning arrangements for education programmes in and across strategic health/social care economies
- Supporting effective educational provision through the creation of 'fit for purpose'

building design and knowledge transfer environments

- Celebrating, recognising and disseminating good practice

In addition proficient primary care practitioners will need to ensure that:

(1) They provide essential services to the community. These services are needed by a range of care groups with differing needs delivered in a variety of settings. Whatever the title, employer or setting there are, amongst others, core functions that our staff will need to provide: first contact, continuing care and the delivery of effective prevention/public health programmes.

(2) Their services are based on robust assessment of needs of individuals and populations and the skills required to meet those needs. These functions should be provided across all age and social groups according to need and designed around the journey that the patient/client takes. In order to safeguard vulnerable people the local population requires high quality generalist as well as specialist service responses.

(3) Patients, clients and communities are involved actively in service changes and provided with greater choice – services will therefore need to respond to the people who use and fund them.

(4) A significant number of the primary care nursing profession assume advanced and specialist roles across a range of core functions but in particular to:
   — Improve access to general practice services, as the role of nurses in assessing and managing conditions (previously seen to be the remit of GPs) is increasingly recognised
   — Provide more secondary care in the community (including care of people with chronic diseases, ambulatory and palliative care needs)
   — Lead and deliver priority public health interventions

(5) They engage in partnership with the wider health and social care team. As such there will be more generic working with practitioners working across settings, providing a wider range of care to individuals, families and communities. Support workers and qualified staff will become more integrated within the primary/social care workforce.

(6) They become more understanding of the commonality of roles across health and social care and hospitals and primary/community care with more joint posts and less anxiety about protecting professional roles when responding to patient and community needs

(7) Front line practitioners have greater freedom to innovate and make decisions about services and the care that they provide. This will need to be matched with greater accountability for individual professional judgement and the use of best available evidence.

(8) Effective leadership is evidenced if our services are to take on new roles, work differently and deliver the NHS plan improvements for patients, clients and communities. This will demand greater understanding of team development and the management capability to use human and financial resources creatively and to assess and manage risks accordingly within the parameters of 'safe practice'.

The workforce of the future will also prepare and deploy a range of competent assistant practitioners who will work in direct support of the professionally qualified primary care team. New roles are now emerging to support assistant practitioners to acquire a range of competencies that have been designed to enable them to respond to the needs of the local health/social care economy. Such roles interface with the development and implementation of new foundation degree programmes, informed by key health and social care imperatives including *Agenda for Change* (DoH 2003b), and the *Knowledge and Skills Framework* (DoH 2003c), and new emergent educational models supported and endorsed by the NHS.

As the scope of primary health care widens, opportunities for appropriately skilled and experienced primary care nurses to develop as advanced practitioners and nurse consultants will be provided. The challenge for the nurses themselves must be for them to articulate their skills, advance their practice (underpinned by evidence-based enquiry skills), and to market their contribution effectively to both their clients/patients and to commissioners of health/social care services.

New practice developments must emerge to fulfil patient and provider agency expectations as increasingly complex care packages are transferred from the hospital sector to the primary health care service. In order to ensure that nurses provide effective care to their clients, practitioners must ensure that they are effectively supervised in all areas of their practice and 'keep touch' with the aims and objectives of their clients and senior managers. There are many ways in achieving this objective and perhaps the most successful has been the provision of clinical supervision and positive feedback from line managers. Clinical supervision has been recommended in various forms by the NMC for all of its nurses with the aim of providing staff with a framework within which to receive positive feedback on their performance and to share their own perceptions of how effective they consider their contribution to client care to be (NMC 2002).

The main professional challenges for primary care nurses may be summarised as the need to:

- Maintain and develop specialist/advanced diagnostic, clinical/therapeutic skills and competence
- Expand knowledge and skills and to act upon research evidence
- Recognise and accept personal accountability for nursing actions
- Pursue continuing education to enhance competence and patient safety
- Market skills to an increasingly diverse range of health and social care commissioners

- Promote public health/protection and assist in the development and maintenance of 'healthy communities'
- Engage in effective clinical supervision
- Exercise strategic leadership skills
- Constantly evaluate personal and collective performance

International influences on the health care agenda

The organisation of health care delivery and nursing activity in the UK is also influenced by a number of international agreements and agendas that are negotiated within the World Health Organization and within the European Community.

For example, the Public Health chapter of the EC Treaty of Economic Union (European Parliament Committee Report on the Environment (The Maastricht Treaty) 1993), requires all European countries to contribute to the promotion of health awareness and health protection by encouraging the design and implementation of local health initiatives and community health programmes. Such activities are directed towards action that prevents the incidence of major diseases, including drug dependence, by promoting research into their causes and means of transmission, as well as health information and education. Health has also been afforded enhanced status as a standing item on the European Parliament agenda in Brussels. Article 153 of the Treaty of Amsterdam 1999, commits the EU to achieving 'a high level of human health protection'.

European influences also regulate the movement of nurses between member states; systems and directives have also been agreed to enable European countries to ascribe mutual recognition to their pre-qualifying systems of nurse education. These systems have been designed to facilitate mutual harmonisation and recognition between countries in the EC and provide a shared framework for the preparation of nurse specialists throughout the region.

Within the wider context, the World Health Organization also sets targets for health gain and health promotion. For example, in 1987

(WHO 1987) targets were published with the aim of improving the quality of health care delivery and surveillance for all world citizens. These targets have assisted in shaping the health care agenda in the UK and have facilitated the introduction of common standards for primary health services throughout the world. Other policy matters relate to the design of global health and nursing strategies based on the following principles:

- Equity – thus reducing the existence of inequalities between countries and within countries
- Health promotion – providing for the development of personal self-reliance and the acquisition of a positive sense of health
- Participation – requiring the active participation of world citizens in informing themselves (and others) about health matters
- Multi-sectoral cooperation – promoting international agreements on health targets, polices and strategies
- Primary health care – focusing attention on the importance of primary care delivery as the health care system closest to where clients live and work
- International cooperation – recognising that health problems cross international frontiers e.g. pollution

Conclusion

This chapter has considered the rapidly changing context within which the unified discipline of primary health care nursing operates. The chapter has outlined the challenges that face health care providers and commissioners and has demonstrated the nursing profession's commitment to furthering the role and function of the primary care practitioner within the public health agenda.

The Government's emphasis on primary care and public health will challenge traditional boundaries and working practices for all staff and demand the deconstruction of previously defended allegiances to uni-disciplinary patterns of working and professional titles. The latter will require re-definition as new opportunities

develop within a new seamless culture of inter-agency care provision. Such developments offer exciting opportunities for nurses and their clients/patients and provide the basis for infinite experiment in the design and implementation of new patterns of care delivery.

Therefore, the context within which health care is delivered in the UK influences the strategic and operational objectives that determine its standards and applications. The ideology or philosophy adopted by government health departments determine the nature of our health and social care systems and directs the structures and processes that we employ to meet the needs of our citizens.

During the past ten years the UK has witnessed a re-examination of personal and public values, thus reinforcing the need for clients to assume personal responsibility for their own social and health care needs. The reduction in dependency upon in-patient care in our hospitals has assisted in the transfer of care to the community and to our naturally occurring neighbourhood support systems. Care in the community and investment in public health/primary care strategy will become an increasing feature of our health care philosophy and, in partnership with a rationalised (and smaller) acute sector, will provide the context for our health care system for the foreseeable future.

The significant role that our primary care trusts, strategic health authorities and social service departments play further reinforce the Government's commitment to primary care. The importance of leadership for primary care nursing must be acknowledged and responsive systems put in place to facilitate the emergence of innovative practice in local practice settings. Nurses must also continue to advocate for their clients, families and communities and engage in raising health related issues for inclusion in local and government policy agendas. Above all they must demonstrate confidence and competence to assess risks and to practise safely in accordance with their professional code of practice (NMC 2002).

This chapter concludes with the following extract from the Department of Health (2002) publication *Liberating the Talents*:

'Nursing, Midwifery and Health Visiting make up the largest workforce in the NHS. They play a central role in a person's journey across sickness and health, home and hospital, birth and death. Like general practice, nursing in primary care has a long and proud tradition – providing expert care to individuals, families and communities in their homes, workplaces and schools, and in surgeries. They provide the full spectrum of care from primary prevention through to specialist disease management and palliative care. Primary care services are delivered in the real everyday world where life is lived, where health is shaped and where the majority of care takes place. Primary Care Trusts can ill afford not to harness and develop the skills of the workforce'. (p. 3).

The present book has been designed to examine and explore many of the key issues raised in this introductory chapter.

References

Department of Health (1998) *The New NHS Modern and Dependable: A National Framework for Assessing Performance*. DoH, London.

Department of Health (1999a) *Saving Lives, Our Healthier Nation*. DoH, London.

Department of Health (1999b) *Making a Difference – Strengthening the nursing, midwifery and health visiting contribution to health and healthcare*. DoH, London.

Department of Health (2000a) *A Health Service of all the talents: Developing the NHS workforce*. DoH, London.

Department of Health (2000b) *The NHS Plan: A plan for Investment, a Plan for Reform*. DoH, London.

Department of Health (2001) *Shifting the Balance of Power within the NHS*. DoH, London.

Department of Health (2002) *Liberating the Talents – Helping Primary Care Trusts and Nurses to Deliver the NHS Plan*. DoH, London.

Department of Health (2003a) *Tackling Health Inequalities: A Programme for Action 2003 – three year plan to tackle health inequalities*. DoH, London.

Department of Health (2003b) *Agenda for Change – Modernising the NHS Pay System*. DoH, London.

Department of Health (2003c) *The Knowledge and Skills Framework*. DoH, London.

Department of Health (2004a) *The NHS Improvement Plan, Putting People at the Heart of Public Services*. DoH, London.

Department of Health (2004b) *Choosing Health – The Choice Overview*. www.dh.gov.uk/policy and Guidance/Patient Choice.

European Parliament Committee on the Environment, Public Health and Consumer Protection (1993) *Draft Report on Public Health Policy After Maastricht*. PE 205.804 Or, EN. European Parliament, Brussels.

European Parliament (1999) *Treaty of Amsterdam, Article 153*, Brussels.

Nursing and Midwifery Council (2002) *The Code of Professional Conduct*. NMC, London.

Nursing and Midwifery Council (2004) *Standards for Specialist Community Public Health Nursing*, (C/04/57). NMC, London.

Standing Committee of Nurses of the EU (1994) *Public Health after Maastricht*. European Parliament, Brussels.

The NHS and Community Care Act 1990. HMSO, London.

The Health Act 1999. HMSO, London.

WHO (1978) *International Conference on Primary Health Care*, Alma Ata, Geneva.

WHO (1987) *Health for All. Declaration of WHO conference on Primary Health Care*, Alma Ata, Geneva.

Wanless, D. (2004) *Securing Good Health for the Whole Population – focus on prevention and the wider determinants of health*. The Stationery Office, London.

Chapter 2 **Social Policy in Public Health and Primary Care**

Linda Burke

Introduction

The last 15 years have seen unprecedented change in health and social care policy, all of which have had an impact on community nurses. Not least of these changes has been the radical shift towards a primary care led NHS. In the past, it appeared as if community nurses had been largely overlooked by policy makers (Walsh & Gough 2000) but with the election of the Labour Government in 1997, this all changed. It was emphatically stated by the Labour Government that nurses would be guaranteed a seat at the decision making table. Successive policy documents (DoH 1997, DoH 1998, DoH 1999, DoH 2000) have reinforced the message that nurses, midwives and health visitors have a crucial role in carrying out the government's plans for a new NHS.

Undoubtedly, nurses can make a unique and valuable contribution to policy development because of their knowledge and experience of working so closely with patients. However, whether nurses will make the most of this opportunity remains to be seen. Historically, nurses have been absent from the policy-making arena (Maslin-Prothero & Masterson 1998) for reasons which may be related to the nursing profession's relatively low position of power in the hierarchy of health and social care organisations (J. Robinson 1992). Hennessy (2000) asserts that it is also partly because nurses themselves have not taken responsibility for having a role within policy-making, probably because they do not believe they have enough knowledge of the policy process.

It is essential that nurses learn about and develop an understanding of social policy because the health of the patients and clients they interact with is affected by the many policies that are implemented in health and also in areas such as housing, employment, education, taxation, social security and the environment. Furthermore, it is only by having knowledge of policy that nurses will be able to influence and take on a more active role in policy-making and implementation.

The aim of this chapter is to provide community nurses with a broad understanding of the key developments in policy that have occurred within the health care sector. The chapter will concentrate on:

- The policy-making and implementation process
- Health care before 1948 and the evolution of the NHS
- Health policy under the Conservative Government from 1979–1997
- Current and future health care policy under the Labour Government

This chapter focuses particularly on health policy because it has the most immediate relevance for community nursing. However, it is important to recognise that other areas of social policy will also have a considerable impact on the health and well-being of clients.

The policy-making and implementation process

What is policy?

There are many different views about what constitutes a policy. Guba (1984) asserts that all policies fall into one or more of the following categories:

- Assertion of goals
- Standing decisions of a governing body
- Central guide to action
- Strategies to solve a problem
- Behaviours that have been sanctioned by a formal decision

- Norms of conduct
- Outputs of the policy-making system

There are two broad types of policy – universal and selective. Universal policies provide services or resources to everyone within a broad category, whereas selective policies focus on a clearly defined group (Gormley 1999). Universal policies can be seen to be more wasteful of resources but are more equitable, that is they attempt to provide an equal resource or service to everybody, whereas selective policies are based on the principle of equity, which means they target money at those perceived to be in the most need.

Social policies are generally considered as policies that provide a guide to organising the nation's resources for the perceived benefit of society. For example, Hennessy (2000) describes health policies as courses of action that are advantageous or expedient within the resources available to maintain or improve health. However, it is important to appreciate that just because something is labelled as social policy does not mean that it is necessarily beneficial for all of those on the receiving end. Policies are made within the prevailing ideological context of the government of the time which means they will reflect a particular view about what constitutes a good society and who is the most deserving of help (Titmus 1979).

Policies almost always suggest a course of action (Owen & Rogers 1999) but rarely prescribe what that action should be. Therefore, while policy includes the explicit decisions made by governments and their advisers, it also refers to the decisions and non-decisions made by managers and professionals, including nurses (Green & Thorogood 1998). This means that community nurses can play a significant part in shaping policy at all levels of health and social care organisations.

Who makes policy?

In order to set policy, groups manoeuvre to wield power, influence and control over each other. Such power is never equally shared and varies in each area of policy.

There are different theories of the distribution of power within society. They include pluralism, elitism, Marxism and corporate theorism. Pluralists believe power is widely and equally distributed among different interest groups who organise themselves around an issue, with the state acting as a referee in the bargaining process. Elitists assert that power is disproportionately concentrated in the hands of a limited number of functional or occupational elite groups who acquire their power through control of economic resources. Marxists' fundamental beliefs are based on the perception that the state is an agent for domination by the capital owning class over the working class. Finally, corporatist theory embraces the idea of the state working in conjunction with big business and other corporations such as trade unions to ensure private control of the means of production alongside public control.

While there is widespread agreement that, as in other fields of social welfare provision, the power of decision making is not equally distributed in health care (Harrison *et al.* 1990), there is considerable debate about where the power of policy-making lies. Ham (1992) warns that it is important not to overemphasise the influence of political parties on policy-making, as ideology is often overruled by pragmatism. However, there is no doubt that the government does control the most important factor in making the policy a reality – the resources. This is done in a number of ways, by cash limiting the NHS budget, ring-fencing money for specific causes, wage control and capital spending limits.

Additionally, the question of how much power is devolved to a local level within the NHS is debated. In the UK, once a political party is elected to power with a sufficient majority, it has almost entire control of policy. Furthermore, many commentators believe that the NHS is too politically sensitive an issue for the government to release its control over decision making (Klein 1989).

Conversely, it can be argued that although ministers come and go, civil servants are here to stay. Their understanding of the system is far greater than that of the ministers they serve and Ham (1992) argues it is they, not the government, who hold the real power. In addition to the civil service, the 1980s saw a growth in the number of quangos (quasi-autonomous non governmental organisations). These are non-elected bodies made up of individuals usually appointed by the government. Mullard (1995) asserted that in 1993 quangos had responsibility for spending over 30% of the nation's income without any form of public accountability.

There are also professional advisers, including representatives from nursing, allied health professionals and doctors. Medical influence within the NHS has long been recognised as the dominating power as doctors not only influence policy at the centre but also at the periphery through clinical decision making. It can be argued that the real power behind any health policy comes directly from the medical profession. However, since the introduction of general management into the NHS in 1984 (DHSS 1984) there has been an expansion in the power and influence of the manager and although the Labour Government has stated its commitment to increasing the power of professionals in policy-making there is a view that this is more rhetoric than reality (Ferlie & Fitzgerald 2002).

Finally, big business also has widespread influence on policy-making. Its power is largely related to control over resources for investment and its ability to gain access to the centre of power. Such influence is still evident, for example, lobbying by the tobacco industry against a ban on smoking in public places and the efforts of the food industry to continue to target advertising at children.

Consumer power is evident in pressure group activity, although there are concerns that such interest groups may exert influence on policy beyond their numbers. In addition, successive governments have given consumers a voice in local decision making for health care – currently this is through the patient advocacy and liaison service (DoH 2000). Also, the most powerful voice of the consumer could be said to be in the process of voting itself, although there are doubts about how representative the democratic process is because of in-built inequalities within the state, such as wealth, education, the availability of information and the electoral and political system.

Policy-making, therefore, depends on the interplay of different voices and interests competing for priority. There is usually considerable interdependence of professional, political, managerial and public influences in decision making. Nevertheless, it must be remembered that policy can be made with no consultation at all and often is.

How policy is made

In order to understand the complex process of policy development, theorists have used a number of different models; the rational comprehensive model, the incremental model and the bottom-up approach to policy development. Policy-making and implementation are sometimes viewed as separate processes but it can be argued that the distinction between construction and implementation of policy is unrealistic because often it is impossible to see where policy-making stops and implementation begins (Flynn 1997). Policy is often made and remade in the process of local implementation by the action of individuals and is the cumulative outcome of many decisions and responses by such individuals (Hogwood & Gunn 1984). Policy continues to evolve and change in the implementation phase (Ham & Hill 1993).

Rational model

The rational model owes much to the work of Pressman and Wildavsky (1973) who see the main value of this model in its potential as a radical model for implementing change and as a vehicle for strategic planning. Clear and achievable goals, a tendency towards centralised decision making and the importance of achieving specified outcomes are the fundamental principles of this model. Policy, it is asserted, comes in at the top of the organisation and is successfully passed down to the operatives at the bottom who execute it in its pure form. Implementers are merely agents for those who have initiated the policy. This is associated with hierarchical concepts of organisation and has an emphasis on control, compliance and consent from the individuals within the organisation.

Criticisms of this model include the difficulty of agreeing values and goals and the fact that such goals will usually become distorted and modified once they are implemented. Furthermore, the reality that policy often comes from the bottom-up does not fit into this model. Finally, the lack of negotiation inherent in this structure is questionable.

Incremental model

The incremental model focuses on the principles of negotiation, interaction and agreement in decision making, trial and error, pluralism and diffused authority, and limited reliance on theory and ideology. Its main proponent is Charles Lindblom (Lindblom & Woodhouse 1993) who argues that policy is often made this way and that democracy is best achieved through this process. However, criticisms include its lack of analysis and long-term planning, the belief that all views are compromised and an over rosy view of the status quo.

Bottom-up model

The third model is the bottom-up model of policy implementation used by Barrett and Fudge (1981). The principle underpinning this model is that policy implementation is an interactive, iterative, evolutionary process. Policy implementation is a continuous process of action and interaction between a changing policy and implementing actors and agencies who are inherently difficult to control. Its central focus is on what is done, the activities and behaviour of groups and individuals, exploring the way action relates to policy rather than assuming it follows from policy. At any one time it may not be clear whether policy is influencing action or action influencing policy. To understand actions and responses there is a need to look at the actors involved, the agencies in which they operate and the factors which influence their behaviour (Barrett & Fudge 1981). The main critique of the bottom-up approach to policy implementation is that it overestimates the discretion of individuals to implement policy and pays too little attention to the legal, financial and structural constraints which set limits on their ability to act (Hogwood & Gunn 1984).

Policy-making can rarely be seen as fitting any theory completely. It is an untidy process of considerable complexity and rarely proceeds in an orderly, rational fashion. More often it consists of a web of decisions evolving over a period of time and throughout the implementation process.

Policy implementation depends on a number of key factors. First, the policy itself and the political context and ideology of the time. Second, the organisational culture, including the way the organisation is structured, how hierarchical it is, and the style of the leader or manager, is important, as are the amount of discretion which individuals are allowed to interpret policy in the way they deem most appropriate, and good communication channels within the organisation. The role of individuals is critical as they may share the goals and values of the policy-makers, and the organisation, or have different priorities. Individuals or groups may have virtually autonomous power to shape the direction of policy, or at least to stand in the way of its effectiveness. This is particularly true of professional groups. Therefore, it is vital that the individual feels motivated and has the competence to implement the policy.

Another major issue to consider when implementing policy is the number of external constraints, for example, demographic change and new technology. Such factors may be out of the control of either policy-makers or implementers, but may have considerable impact on policy in practice.

Clearly policy implementation is a complex process in which factors as diverse as the individual, the resources, the organisation, the political context and, of course, the policy itself must be considered.

The evolution of the NHS

Pre 1948

By World War II a consensus was beginning to emerge that nationally co-ordinated health care provision was needed because health care was not comprehensive or of good enough quality (Klein 1989).

Before 1948, some national insurance and hospital, personal and domiciliary services had been introduced to address health and social care problems. However, the most significant change had been in public health services. The growth of industrialisation had led to over-crowding both in housing and in the workplace in factories. In such unsanitary conditions diseases such as cholera and typhoid had been able to spread. In 1848 the government introduced the Public Health Act to ensure the adequate supply of water and sewerage systems and set up a Board of Health (Gormley 1999). Over the years legislation was introduced in housing and education, which also impacted upon the general health of the population. This culminated in the work of William Beveridge whose report in 1942 set out a plan to tackle the effects of what he described as the five giants; want, idleness, ignorance, squalor and disease.

Another aspect of health policy related to sickness insurance. In 1911 insurance coverage had been introduced to assist low-wage workers when they were sick and to pay for GP services. Over the years this had been extended, but by 1939 there were still gaps in coverage, for example, the unemployed, self-employed and some women not in paid employment. Awareness was growing that provision needed to be available for all people.

Health care was provided in the home by GPs and district nurses. However GPs charged fees to many and tended to be located in wealthier areas. District nurse services had been set up in the nineteenth century and health visitors were registered from 1907. They were organised by voluntary or charitable associations and, although the care was generally good, provision was far from uniform. The 1946 NHS Act had a big impact on district nursing as it obliged local authorities to provide a free home nursing service and enabled local authorities to set up health centres (Walsh & Gough 2000).

Hospital care was delivered by a mixture of voluntary and public, or municipal, institutions. Municipal hospitals began to be established in the 1860s and were available to those who could not afford to pay. However, some had developed from the old workhouses, which meant local people were often reluctant to use them. Voluntary hospitals were supported mainly by charitable donations and the contributions of wealthy people who were treated there. While they were respected institutions in the main, they had a number of problems. Those who could not afford to pay were expected to bring a letter of recommendation from a hospital subscriber and they provided very selective services, for example infectious disease and maternity care was often not available.

Two major problems of hospital provision were brought to a head by World War II. Distribution of hospital beds was haphazard. Often there were more beds in wealthy areas where need was less and this led to competition between municipal and voluntary hospitals, particularly after 1930 when the running of workhouse hospitals had been taken over by local authorities. In addition, voluntary hospitals were experiencing severe financial problems as the demand for hospital care outstripped the resources available.

The NHS

After World War II a Labour government was elected under Clement Attlee with an expectation that there would be considerable social reform. Plans for a national health service were underway before the war, but it was the arrival of Aneurin Bevan at the Ministry of Health that accelerated the process of reform. The NHS was established on 5 July 1948 and had a number of key aims:

- The health of the whole population would be covered
- All services would be free at the point of delivery
- Provision would be comprehensive
- All services would be supplied and financed by the state
- The quality of the service would be improved to provide a good standard for all
- Services would be integrated, planned and distributed more effectively (Fatchett 1998).

The structure was tripartite. GPs were self-employed, independent contractors and were funded directly from central government on a capitation and fee for service basis organised through family practitioner committees. Hospitals were run by hospital boards and organised by 14 new regional health boards reporting to the Department of Health. The third strand comprised the local authorities. Their power with respect to health care provision was reduced in that they no longer had responsibility for hospitals (Gormley 1999), but they now had a role in health promotion and prevention of ill health which included health visiting, district nursing and environmental health. It is interesting that this role was seen as residual to the real business of health care, reflecting the ongoing view that health promotion was of secondary importance and effectively defining the NHS as an ill-health service. The tripartite structure was to cause problems for health care in the years to come in that it separated health and social care and gave the government very little power over the gatekeepers to the NHS – the GPs.

Health care under the Conservative Government 1979–1997

1979–1989

In 1979 a Conservative Government was elected under Margaret Thatcher and committed to reducing public expenditure. Conservative social policy at that time reflected two strands of ideology – the neo-liberal and the neo-conservative. Neo-conservatives focused on the family as the centre of social life, the importance of traditional moral values and strong law and order. Neo-liberalism, or 'new right' thinking, was more concerned with rolling back the frontiers of the state, the necessity of competition and the market, and the importance of introducing a business ethos into the public sector. New right thinking had had its place within Conservative Party policy for some time (Friedman 1962; Hayek 1982), but until the 1970s its effect was limited. From 1979 the influence of radical right think-tanks, such as the Adam Smith Institute, the Institute for Economic Affairs and the No Turning Back Group, was in the ascendency.

Policy towards the NHS from 1979 to 1989 did not reflect the principles of the new right as much as policy in other areas of welfare provision except in three areas. The first of these was an attempt to increase value for money in the NHS through general management, tighter monitoring and the pursuit of greater efficiency. Of these the introduction in 1983 of general managers at regional, district and unit level, was the most controversial as it was said to undermine clinical judgement and professional power (Harrison 1988). The Government asserted that it would lead to better decision making, tighter financial control and a clearer line of accountability to the Secretary of State.

Alongside this came cost control initiatives adopted from successful businesses, such as the use of performance indicators and the introduction of clinical budgeting (Appleby 1992). These measures met with some success. There was a rise in day cases, average length of stay reduced from 9.4 days in 1978 to 7.3 in 1986 and the number of patients treated increased. Clinical staff became increasingly aware of the cost of treatment (Timmins 1995). Hospitals were also permitted to gain income from the sale of assets and from 1983 to 1989, asset sales in England totalled £271 m, equal to 30% of the capital allocation of that year (Appleby 1992). Income generation was also encouraged, although the money earned in this way was relatively small.

The second policy thrust was stimulation of the private sector. Contracting out of ancillary services was compulsory from 1983, private nursing home sector use was encouraged and charges for prescriptions, dental and ophthalmic services increased. Alongside this, the percentage of people covered by some sort of private insurance increased from 3% of the population to 10% from 1979 to 1989 (Butler 1992).

Finally, the Government attempted to control spending on the NHS, but with limited success. Although spending as a proportion of gross national product started to drop, it followed a trend which began in the mid 1970s under the Labour Government. Conversely, nurses experienced their best pay rises to date under the Conservatives and the Pay Review Body was introduced. Administrative reorganisation in 1979 and 1984 proved costly and the number of administrators rose threefold. Growth in the number of private nursing homes was matched by an increase in those qualifying for financial help, proving expensive to the Treasury, as did increases in prescription costs, where income raised was offset by the rising costs of those exempt from paying. Private contracting had to be made compulsory before it was widely adopted and, even then, fewer than 20% of contracts were awarded to outside contractors. Additionally, the social cost was high with many staff made redundant. Even income generation, lauded by the Government as a large success, added resources of less than 0.3% to the NHS funds.

Overall, the thrust of health policy up to 1989 was somewhat incoherent and lacking in commitment to New Right principles. However, in 1989 all that was to change.

The internal market 1989–1997
In 1989 the Prime Minister, Margaret Thatcher, announced a cabinet level review of the NHS which resulted in the publication of the White Paper *Working for Patients* (DoH 1989). The government was influenced by the ideas of the American, Alan Enthoven (1985) and the new right, which included more use of the private sector, greater management input, and the introduction of the internal market. A key area where neo-liberal ideas were ignored was regarding resources, as funding still primarily came from general taxation and there was no fundamental change to the basic principle of a free service at the point of delivery.

The most significant change, which still remains, was the introduction of the internal market to the NHS. A division was created between those agencies responsible for purchasing health care and those who were providers of services. Health authorities were main purchasers of health care, purchasing services on behalf of GPs plus all emergency treatment required by their population. They were supported by newly formed GP fundholders who could purchase on their own behalf. Services could be purchased from any suppliers including the private sector and newly created NHS trust hospitals.

In theory, contracts were awarded on the basis of the best value for money, therefore knowledge of the price and quality of services was essential. To ensure this, managers were given much greater control over finances. Attention was given to performance indicators and the Family Health Services Authority gained a monitoring role over GPs. Additionally, incentives were introduced to the system, with money following the patient. Finally, to diversify supply and increase competition, the use of the private sector was developed through tax relief on private insurance for the over 65s.

It is highly debatable whether a truly 'free' market was actually created within the NHS as the market was effectively managed in that trusts were told they must provide core services such as accident and emergency departments, and education costs were removed from pricing decisions. Hospitals were not allowed free rein over their finances – borrowing and disposing of assets were only permissible within limits, and if deemed not against the public interest by the secretary of state (R. Robinson 1992).

The question of whether the introduction of competition increased efficiency and saved money was curiously ignored, as were indications from the USA that competition actually increased costs (R. Robinson 1992). Therefore, policies aimed at decreasing public spending and increasing the power of the market were potentially in conflict.

The Conservative Government claimed that power was devolved from the centre to the periphery as suppliers of health care could act independently of health authority control. However, it soon became apparent that the government was not prepared to decrease its control of such a politically sensitive institution as the NHS. Although the policy-making and operational arms of health policy were separated by the creation of a policy board, which determined policy, and the National Health Service Management Executive (NHSME) dealing with implementation, the NHSME was directly accountable to the government and its control was increased by the replacement of the regional health authorities with regional offices of the NHSME staffed by civil servants. The government also created a direct line of accountability, from top to bottom of the NHS, by the introduction of government appointments at all tiers of the NHS (Flynn 1992). Consumer and professional representation was also decreased. Formal powers of the community health council were limited to consultation and lay representation on health authorities was reduced. Professional representation was also cut as some professional groups, notably nurses, were no longer automatically represented on health authorities and the role of doctors was substantially reduced. The Chief Medical Officer and Chief Nursing Officer were also excluded from membership of the NHSME (Butler 1992).

Problems of Conservative party health care policy

There was some evidence that patients of GP fundholders received more choice of treatment. However, the problem was that, within a cash limited budget, this treatment was provided at the expense of patients of non-fundholding GPs, resulting, it was claimed, in a two-tier system and debates emerged whether fundholders were receiving an appropriate budget for the population they served. These issues had to be weighed against the alleged improved efficiency of fundholders in reaching screening targets, receiving better information about hospital follow-up appointments, negotiating the patients' drugs on discharge and speeding up the process of receiving laboratory test results (Robinson & Scheuer 1992).

The implementation of competition also proved expensive. Costs included:

- Employment of management consultants
- The expense of tax relief for the elderly
- The loss of economies of scale
- Administrative costs (which reached up to £300 m a year as the number of administrators trebled)
- Management costs

Furthermore, contracting had inherent inefficiencies inbuilt in that it limited sharing of good practice and inhibited long-term planning and innovation. One-year contracts proved an administrative nightmare because of the number

of purchasers – over 100 health authorities and more than 3500 fundholders (DoH 1997). One health authority reported issuing 60 000 invoices in one year!

Lack of professional representation, the increase of secrecy clauses for staff and the invisibility of the patient in decision making were also seen as major problems of the internal market (DoH 1997). Therefore, in 1997, when the Labour Government was elected, they vowed to address these problems and create a 'new NHS'.

Labour Government health care policy

The New NHS: Modern, Dependable (DoH 1997), describing the Labour Government's strategy for the NHS, was produced in November 1997. These intentions were further articulated in *The NHS Plan* (DoH 2000) and *The NHS Improvement Plan* (DoH 2004a). Within the NHS Plan the key principles of the new NHS are outlined as:

- The NHS will provide a universal service for all based on clinical need, not ability to pay
- The NHS will provide a comprehensive range of services
- The NHS will shape its services around the needs and preferences of individual patients, their families and their carers
- The NHS will respond to needs of different populations
- The NHS will work continuously to improve the quality of services and to minimise errors
- The NHS will support and value its staff
- Public funds for health care will be devoted solely to NHS patients
- The NHS will work together with others to ensure a seamless service for patients
- The NHS will help keep people healthy and work to reduce health inequalities
- The NHS will respect confidentiality of individual patients and provide open access to information about services, treatment and performance

Major changes have since been introduced and most significant amongst these for community nursing are:

- Changes to the organisation of the delivery of health care, notably the establishment of primary care trusts (PCTs)
- A statutory duty for the quality of care provision
- A stronger focus on public health
- Greater emphasis on the role of the patient
- An emphasis on the importance of the NHS as a model employer offering a model career to staff

Community nurses, midwives and health visitors are seen as central to the government's plans for developing this 'new NHS' and in transforming the rhetoric of the policy into the reality of practice.

Organisational change

The main thrust of Labour policy has been an espoused move towards decentralisation and ensuring that the structures within the NHS enable easier access to services for patients (DOH 2001a). To achieve this, organisational structures have been changed and new ones established.

First, regional offices have been closed down and the Department of Health is being reduced in size with an increasingly narrow core function of 'promoting effective stewardship of the nation's health' (DoH 2004a, p. 76). Strategic health authorities (SHAs) have been established which no longer have responsibility for commissioning health care. Their role is to lead the strategic development of local health services and per-formance monitor PCTs and NHS trusts, with the health authority Chief Executive answerable to the Secretary of State.

Primary care trusts are seen as the lead organisation within the NHS. They bring together general practitioners, community nurses and other agencies involved in health and social care, in each geographical area, to work together to improve the health of local people (DoH 2001a). Their main functions are to assess need, plan and secure all health services and improve the health of the local population. They are also responsible for engaging local communities in decision making and devolving power to front-line staff – notably community nurses. They are expected to work in partnership with other agencies to do this, in particular with other PCTs and with local authorities, and some may form care trusts to meet the needs of particular client groups. Significantly, PCTs have responsibility for the management, integration and development of all primary care services and it is anticipated that the new General Medical Services contract will assist PCTs in fulfilling this role, as this new national contract for GPs is flexible and outcomes based and gives PCTs the ability to shape services and increase primary care capacity to meet local needs (DoH 2004b). In order to meet these aims, PCTs need to have a strong infrastructure. Community nurses are identified as essential members of PCTs and this is undoubtedly an opportunity for nurses and health visitors to work as equal partners with other members of the health care team.

There is some question as to whether PCTs are all able to take on this role effectively. Concerns have been raised whether members of PCTs work together effectively and whether PCT members work for the organisation or represent professional interests (Burke & Harris 1999). The number of GP PCT members in relation to nurses is much higher, therefore nurses are worried that their views are ignored (McIntosh 1999). The need for consultation with each practice before decisions are made has implica-tions for the speed with which the PCT agenda can move forward. The main issue of concern however is the extent to which decentralisation is really taking place as SHAs have been reported as exerting undue pressure on PCTs under the guise of performance management. Although the government has talked about a supporting relationship and partnerships between SHAs and PCTs, there are some queries about the extent to which that will be possible if SHAs are accountable for PCT performance. Equally, Ferlie and Fitgerald (2002) argue that central control is unlikely to diminish as monitoring, regulation and performance management con-tinue to develop.

NHS trusts are still responsible for the delivery of most health care but a relatively new develop-ment is the introduction of foundation trusts. Foundation trusts have a number of freedoms that NHS trusts do not have, for example, to borrow money and invest in new services, plus they are no longer performance managed by the DoH but by an independent regulator. Their accountability is to local people, PCTs and this regulator rather than to the DoH. It is anticipated that all trusts will have foundation status within five years.

The government intends that a further supplier of health care will be the independent sector. Use of the independent sector is therefore encouraged and the development of independent sector treatment centres is currently taking place.

Quality assurance

The government is committed to putting quality at the forefront of the NHS and that nurses should play a key role in this process. Quality assurance or 'clinical governance' involves all those working in the NHS, plus patient representatives. The aim is to make clinical practice evidence-based and to disseminate best practice throughout the health service.

The structure for quality comprises five national initiatives, all of which should include nurses:

(1) The National Performance Framework, which develops indicators for health improvement, outcomes, efficiency, effective and appropriate care and fair access
(2) National Service Frameworks, to establish evidence-based pathways of care for major care or disease groups
(3) The National Institute for Clinical Excellence, which draws up guidelines on best practice and on clinical audit
(4) The Healthcare Commission, which monitors and reports on quality of commissioning and clinical services across the NHS and the private sector
(5) The Commission for Social Care Inspection, which performs similar functions for social care commissioners and providers

For the first time, national standards for health care will be used on which to base judgements about the quality of health care (DoH 2004c). The Department of Health has now published these

and it is the responsibility of the Healthcare Commission to develop the criteria which underpin these.

These systems will only work if the professionals closest to the patients – the nurses – are able to understand and maintain standards. Community nurses need to be involved from the start to make sure that realistic and practicable systems and standards are devised that are as appropriate to primary care as to acute services. They then must ensure that they are involved in the reviews, both as reviewers and when the reviews are taking place within their organisations to ensure that these are as effective as possible in improving the quality of patient care.

Increased focus on public health

From the early days of the Labour Government it was asserted that there needed to be a greater emphasis on public health (DoH 1997). This manifested itself in schemes such as Healthy Living Centres and the Sure Start programme, which aimed to help the development of services and improve health in disadvantaged areas. However, it is in *The NHS Improvement Plan* (DoH 2004a) that public health is most explicitly highlighted as an issue for future development. This may be because the Wanless Report (2002) indicated that the health of the population in England is not as good as that of other comparable countries. Poverty is a significant factor in determining life expectancy and inequalities are still considerable between social classes in England. In addition, England has relatively high levels of smoking, obesity and teenage pregnancy.

The NHS Improvement Plan (DoH 2004a) asserts that the NHS will become more of a health service than just a sickness service. As well as introducing a number of new targets for improving health and reducing death rates a number of ideas are proposed to facilitate this. A key proposal is the introduction of a new type of specialist clinician, most likely a nurse, called a 'community matron' who will work with patients with complex long-term conditions. In addition, much more investment in services closer to home for people with chronic illness is promised. An interesting development that may have an impact in making sure that public health is on the agenda of health care providers is that the Healthcare Commission has a new remit to review the delivery of health improvement, reduction of inequalities, public health delivery within PCTs and progress made against smoking cessation and sexual health targets (Walker 2004). Public health is also the seventh domain in the Department of Health's *Standards for Better Health* (DoH 2004c), against which the Healthcare Commission will be making judgements about quality.

The new public health White Paper *Choosing Health: making health choices easier* (DoH 2004d) suggests more detailed proposals for taking the public health agenda forward. However, it remains to be seen what the centre's decision will be regarding banning smoking in public places and addressing the relationship between advertising and childhood obesity.

Public health is the area in which community nurses are ideally placed to become leaders within the field. They can offer input not only in delivering public health care but also in developing standards for public health. As the practitioners who work closest to the patient it can be argued that they are ideally placed to make a unique contribution at a local and national level to ensure that public health policy developed is sensitive and responsive to patients' needs.

Patient involvement

From the start the Labour government determined to embrace a spirit of openness in the NHS and to involve patients more in policy and decision making. To facilitate this, a number of initiatives have taken place, including:

- Patient Advocacy and Liaison Services – which have been established in every NHS trust and PCT to provide support and advice to patients.
- Patients' representatives sitting on PCTs and NHS trusts are obliged to collect regular feedback from patients.
- The development of 'expert' patient programmes.

- Large scale surveys of public views of the NHS.
- Opening up trust and health authority meetings to the public.

There is some scepticism about this partnership approach, which was exacerbated with the decision to disband community health councils. There is also debate about how much particular individuals can be representative of the wider public and that there might be excessive influence of vocal groups over the direction in which the health service moves. It is still not known how much patients wish to be involved in making decisions about their care and whether they would rather leave these to the professionals. Nonetheless, the government is firmly committed to making this happen.

The NHS as a model employer offering a model career to staff

Within the NHS Plan there was a commitment to ensuring that the NHS should be a model employer (DoH 2002). Offering lifelong learning to staff was seen as essential to realising this aim. To achieve this the DoH publication *Working together, learning together – a framework for lifelong learning for the NHS* (2001b) established a programme for modernising learning and development. This is underpinned by the 'Skills Escalator', which is a strategy for recruiting a more diverse range of people to the NHS and for enabling new and existing staff to continuously develop their skills and take on new roles. The NHS university was set up as a 'corporate' university to develop learning programmes tailored to meet the immediate and urgent needs of all staff within the NHS.

Alongside this are initiatives to create more flexible working environments, improve childcare and tackle violence at work. Most significant is the introduction of a new national framework for pay – *Agenda for Change* (DoH 2003). All staff (except doctors and dentists) will be placed on a common pay spine rather than the hundreds there were before. NHS jobs will be assessed against a national job evaluation framework and there should be rewards for knowledge and skills rather than time served. This should provide incentives for staff to take on new responsibilities, change patterns of working and create new roles that cross boundaries.

Community nurses are well placed to make the most of the opportunities offered in 'HR in the NHS Plan' (DoH 2002). Their roles are suited to flexible working arrangements and the increased responsibilities that many now have should enable them to position themselves well on the new pay spine. It remains to be seen, however, whether staff within primary care will be willing to review current roles and ways of working.

Conclusion

There are indications that the changes and the extra resources allocated by the Labour government to health care are beginning to have an effect as maximum waiting times for operations has fallen from 18 months to nine months and staff numbers have increased by more than 20% (DoH 2004a). However, the government shows no sign of slowing down the pace of change in health care policy and policy developments are taking place at an equally fast rate in other parts of the welfare state including education, housing, social services, employment and matters within the remit of the Home Office.

In order to fulfil their roles effectively, community nurses will need to be aware of the changes that are happening in social policy and their potential impact on the profession and, more importantly, on clients. The nursing profession must ensure that community nurses have the knowledge and skills to enable them to influence policy development and implementation and grasp the opportunities available for them within the NHS. This has implications for the education and continuing professional development of community nurses. It is therefore essential that community nurses engage in lifelong learning and develop further their own unique knowledge base so that they can continue to provide high quality care to their clients and help shape the NHS of the future.

References

Appleby, J. (1992) *Financing Health Care in the 1990s.* Open University Press, Buckingham.

Barrett, S. & Fudge, C. (1981) *Policy and Action: Essays on the Implementation of Public Policy.* Methuen, London.

Burke, L.M. & Harris, D. (1999) Education for practice. In: *Specialists in Community Nursing: Current Issues in Community Nursing and Primary Health Care in Practice,* (ed. J. Littlewood), pp. 251–278. Churchill Livingstone, Edinburgh.

Butler, J. (1992) *Policies and Politics: Before and After Working for Patients.* Open University Press, Buckingham.

DHSS (1984) *Implementation of the NHS Management Inquiry Report.* The Stationery Office, London.

DoH (1989) *Working For Patients.* Department of Health, London.

DoH (1997) *The New NHS, Modern, Dependable.* Department of Health, London.

DoH (1998) *A First Class Service: Quality in the New NHS.* HSC 1998/113. Department of Health, London.

DoH (1999) *Making a Difference: Strengthening the Nursing, Midwifery and Health Visiting Contribution to Health and Healthcare.* Department of Health, London.

DoH (2000) *The NHS Plan: A Plan for Investment, A Plan for Reform.* Department of Health, London.

DoH (2001a) *Shifting the Balance of Power Within the NHS.* Department of Health, London.

DoH (2001b) *Working Together – Learning Together, a Framework for Lifelong Learning for the NHS.* Department of Health, London.

DoH (2002) *HR in the NHS Plan.* Department of Health, London.

DoH (2003) *Agenda for Change – Modernising the NHS Pay System.* Department of Health, London.

DoH (2004a) *The NHS Improvement Plan.* Department of Health, London.

DoH (2004b) *Delivering Investment in General Practice: Implementing the new GMS Contract.* Department of Health, London.

DoH (2004c) *Standards for Better Health: Health Care Standards for Services Under the NHS.* Department of Health, London.

DoH (2004d) *Choosing Health: Making Health Choices Easier.* Department of Health, London.

Enthoven, A. (1985) National Health Service market reform. *Health Affairs,* **10** (3), 60–70.

Fatchett, A. (1998) *Nursing in the New NHS, Modern, Dependable.* Bailliere Tindall, London.

Ferlie, E. & Fitzgerald, L. (2002) The sustainability of the new public management in the UK. In: *New Public Management, Current Trends and Future Prospects* (eds. K. McLaughlin, S.P. Osborne & E. Ferlie), pp. 341–353. Routledge, London.

Flynn, R. (1992) *Structures of Control in Health Management*. Routledge, London.

Flynn, N. (1997) *Public Sector Management*, 3rd edn. Prentice Hall, London.

Friedman, M. (1962) *Capitalism and Freedom*. University of Chicago Press, Chicago.

Gormley, K. (1999) The development of health and social care services. In: *Social Policy and Health Care*, (ed. K. Gormley), pp. 13–28. Harcourt Brace, London.

Green, J. & Thorogood, N. (1998) *Analysing Health Policy*. Longman, London.

Guba, E.G. (1984) Cited in: Owen, J.M. & Rogers, J. (1999) *Program Evaluation: Forms and Approaches*. Sage Publications, London.

Ham, C. (1992) *Health Policy in Britain: The Politics and Organisation of the NHS*, 3rd edn. Macmillan, London.

Ham, C. & Hill, M. (1993) *The Policy Process in the Modern Capitalist State*, 2nd edn. Wheatsheaf Books, Sussex.

Harrison, S. (1988) *Managing the NHS, Shifting the Frontier*. Chapman and Hall, London.

Harrison, S., Hunter, D. & Pollit, C. (1990) *The Dynamics of British Health Policy*. Routledge, London.

Hayek, F.A. (1982) *The Constitution of Liberty*. Routledge and Kegan Paul, London.

Hennessy, D. (2000) The emerging themes. In: *Health Policy and Nursing: Influence, Development and Impact*, (eds D. Hennessy & P. Spurgeon), pp. 1–38. Macmillan, Basingstoke.

Hogwood, B.W. & Gunn, L.A. (1984) *Policy Analysis for the Real World*. Oxford University Press, Oxford.

Klein, R. (1989) *The Politics of the NHS*. Longman, London.

Lindblom, C. & Woodhouse, E.J. (1993) *The Policy Making Process*, 3rd edn. Simon and Schuster, Englewood Cliffs, New Jersey.

Maslin-Prothero, S. & Masterson, A. (1998) Continuing care: developing a policy analysis for nursing. *Journal of Advanced Nursing*, **28** (3), 548–53.

McIntosh, K. (1999) Only two PCG chairs to be held by nurses. *Health Service Journal*, 25 Feb, 7.

Mullard, M. (1995) Introduction. In: *Policy Making in Britain: an Introduction* (ed M. Mullard), pp. 1–9. Routledge, London.

Owen, J.M. & Rogers, J. (1999) *Program Evaluation: Forms and Approaches*. Sage Publications, London.

Pressman, J. & Wildavsky, A. (1973) *Implementation*. University of California Press, Berkeley.

Robinson, J. (1992) Introduction: beginning the study of nursing policy. In: *Policy Issues in Nursing Education* (eds J. Robinson, A. Gray & R. Elkan), pp. 1–8. Open University Press, Milton Keynes.

Robinson R. (1992) *Competition and Health Care: A Comparative Analysis of UK Planning and US Experience*. King's Fund, London.

Robinson, R. & Scheuer, M. (1992) A footnote for fundholding. *Health Service Journal*, 13 Feb, 19–20.

Timmins, N. (1995) *The Five Giants: a Biography of the Welfare State*. Fontana Press, London.

Titmus, R. (1979) *Commitment to Welfare*. Allen and Unwin, London.

Walker, A. (2004) Raise a Glass to Public Health. *Health Service Journal*, 17 June, 16–18.

Walsh, N. & Gough, P. (2000) In: *Health Policy and Nursing: Influence, Development and Impact* (eds D. Hennessy & P. Spurgeon), pp. 1–38. Macmillan Press Ltd, Basingstoke.

Wanless, D. (2002) *Securing our Future Health – Taking a Long-term View*. The Stationery Office, London.

Chapter 3 **Primary Health Care in the Community**

Ann Taket

Introduction

This chapter begins by exploring the concept of primary health care (PHC), linking this to relevant international and national policy documents, and introducing the concept of PHC developed by the World Health Organization. The chapter then focuses on the UK. It explains how PHC is not just found within the NHS, reviews the different sectors involved in PHC, and then discusses the current structure of PHC in the NHS. Key concepts, including the primary health care team, primary care trusts and integrated heath and social care trusts, and the relevant current UK policy documents are introduced.

The chapter then moves on to discuss four important issues in the provision of primary health care in the community: health promotion; tackling health inequalities; health and regeneration; and tackling domestic violence. The subsection on each of these will explain why the issue is of particular significance and review briefly a number of studies/projects that illustrate what is happening/can be done; this will introduce a range of current research. The chapter then concludes with a short review of challenges for the future, emphasising the important role that the nursing profession has to play in meeting these challenges.

Primary health care – the concept

Providing a definition of PHC is not an easy matter. At its simplest, it is often understood as non-specialised health services, or alternatively as first-line health services. Thus, PHC is mainly provided outside hospitals to people who are living in the community. So far, so good. Matters become more complicated when the importance of the protection and promotion of health in

communities as well as the provision of health care to those who are ill is acknowledged, and also when trying to itemise the type of services and activities that are included within PHC. This section introduces the concept of PHC that is central to the work of the World Health Organization (WHO) and to international health policies to which the UK government is a signatory; a brief chronology is provided in Box 3.1. This understanding of PHC is reflected in the rhetoric of current UK health policy, although as will be seen later on, there are some tensions between policy statements and the reality of policy implementation.

The basis for WHO's health policy is the objective enshrined in the WHO constitution: 'the attainment by all peoples of the highest possible level of health'. This provided the basis for a key resolution passed in 1977 by the World Health Assembly (the governing body of WHO), stating that the main social target of governments and WHO should be the attainment, 'by all the people of the world by the year 2000, of a level of health that will permit them to lead a socially and economically productive life'. The resolution become popularly known as 'health for all by the year 2000' (after the phrase 'health for all' originated by the then Director General of WHO, Halfdan Mahler) and later abbreviated as HFA2000 or HFA.

Although the concept of PHC had existed for some time, it was only during the late 1960s and early 1970s that international health policy began to stress its particular importance. This arose out of concerns about the rising cost of health services and the lack of effectiveness of existing hospital oriented health service systems in tackling priority health problems, together with the realisation that the services particularly

Box 3.1	Health policy and PHC – a brief chronology
May 1977	World Health Assembly of the World Health Organization first adopted the 'Health for All' policy goal HFA or HFA2000: 'the main social target of governments and WHO in the following decades should be for all citizens of the world to attain by the year 2000 a level of health which will permit them to lead a socially and economically productive life'
1978	Alma Ata declaration on PHC (WHO/UNICEF 1978)
1979	Resolution in support of formulation of global, regional and national Health for All strategies adopted by World Health Assembly
1980	Adoption of regional strategies for Health for All
1981	Adoption of global Health for All strategy
1984	First set of European Health for All targets agreed (WHO/EURO 1985)
1986	Start of 'Healthy Cities' project Use of local level targets
1990–91	Revisions of European targets
1991	Adoption of second set of European targets – the common European health policy (WHO/EURO 1993)
1993	Adoption of EU Maastricht Treaty which contains a specific health component in terms of a new chapter on 'Public Health'
1997	EU Amsterdam Treaty strengthens public health provisions, introducing a requirement for a high level of human health protection to be assured in *all* Community policies and activities
1998	World Health Declaration adopted by World Health Assembly, Health for All policy for the 21st century, reaffirms commitment to PHC as defined in Alma Ata declaration Health 21 – the health for all policy framework for the WHO European Region adopted by the European Regional Committee
1999	Health 21 – the health for all policy framework for the WHO European Region published (WHO/EURO 1999)

needed in low income countries were not specialised hospital based care, but much more basic and less technically complex forms of care, with an emphasis on accessibility. Analysis of the failure of vertical disease control programmes (i.e. programmes focused on a single discrete disease and characterised by hierarchical organisation), such as WHO's global malaria campaign, contributed to the formulation of the PHC concept as the basic international strategy for health improvement (Gish 1992).

It was also argued that achieving 'health for all' would only be possible through a re-orientation of services towards the promotion and protection of health rather than an emphasis on the cure or care of those in ill-health. Thus a strengthening of community based services, where protection and promotion can take place, began to be seen as essential. This increased emphasis on PHC applied equally to all countries (low or high income), and so the predominant concern became the re-organisation of *all* health services with the aim of prioritising PHC. This represented a radical change from the earlier attitude which could be caricatured as: 'How can we continue to develop high technology medicine without spiralling costs and how can this be made available to poorer countries?'

A key event in the recognition of the importance of PHC was the 1978 conference held in Alma Ata, in the former USSR. This was sponsored by WHO and UNICEF (the United Nations Children's Fund), and attended by delegations from 134 governments and 67 UN organisations, specialised agencies and NGOs (non-governmental organisations) in official relations with WHO, including countries from all different stages of development. This conference reaffirmed health care as a fundamental right and reiterated that the inequalities that existed, both between and within countries, were unacceptable. Alma Ata was called at the time a 'historic collective expression of political will in the spirit of social equity' (WHO/UNICEF 1978).

The conference was also important for its development of an improved understanding of the content of PHC, key features of which are summarised in Box 3.2.

One tension within Europe has been between the role and influence of WHO and the European Union (EU) in health policy matters. The EU has dealt with health issues for four decades, initially with a very restricted health mandate, which was widened considerably by the Maastricht Treaty 1993 and the Amsterdam Treaty 1997. The Maastricht Treaty gave the Community a new objective of making 'a contribution to the attainment of a high level of health protection' which is applicable to all Community policies. Article 129 of the treaty sets out a framework for Community public health activities in pursuit of this objective. The Article provides for the adoption of incentive measures, excluding any harmonisation of member states' legislation, and recommendations. Finally, it stipulates that health protection

---

Box 3.2   The Alma Ata concept

Eight essential elements in the PHC sector

- Education about prevailing health problems and methods of prevention and control
- Promotion of food supply and proper nutrition
- Adequate supply of safe water and basic sanitation
- Maternal and child health services, including family planning
- Immunisation against major infectious diseases (diphtheria, tetanus, whooping cough, measles, polio, TB)
- Prevention and control of locally endemic diseases
- Appropriate treatment of common diseases and injuries
- Provision of essential drugs

Key features of PHC-based health services

- Service provision in relation to needs of population, available and accessible to all in the community
- Should cover promotive, preventive, curative and rehabilitative services (with prominence given to promotion and prevention)
- Community participation, individually and collectively, in planning and implementation of health care
- Multisectoral approach, multifactoral causation of ill-health and the importance of social and environmental factors should be recognised; coordinated action of health, education, agricultural, housing, sanitation, industry sectors is necessary
- Appropriate technology, (low cost, high quality essential drugs, self reliance and affordability, in keeping with local culture i.e. 'acceptable')
- Integration of different types of medical practitioners (non-allopathic and allopathic)
- Use of paramedics and community-based health workers

requirements shall form a constituent part of other Community policies.

The legal basis of the Community's public health activities was further extended in the Amsterdam Treaty, reflecting the evolving consensus on the importance of Community action in this field. With the continuing growth in membership of the EU, and its growth in concern with health matters through the Maastricht and Amsterdam treaties, an increased influence of the EU on health policy and health systems is clearly a real possibility. The mandate that the EU now possesses for health could be utilised to support the development of PHC. In practice it remains to be seen how this mandate will be used. Kokkonen and Kekomäki (1993) argue that there is considerable potential for legal and economic measures affecting health. Others conclude, however, that an expansion of the EU's role in health-related policies is likely to proceed only erratically. They argue that incrementalism, bargaining and compromises (Bomberg & Peterson 1993) dominate the process of policy formulation in the EU. Recent years have seen some closer links developing between the EU and WHO, but it remains to be seen how this will proceed with the European Regional Office of WHO under the leadership of the new Regional Director, Dr Marc Danzon, who took up office in February 2000. Some commentators (for example: Pannenborg 1991; Godlee 1995) have questioned the relevance of maintaining a WHO Regional Office in Europe with the increased health mandate of the EU.

Primary health care and the NHS

It should be obvious that, given the concept of PHC set out in the previous section, PHC is not just found within the NHS. This section begins with a review of different relevant actors in the UK context, and then moves on to a discussion of the current structure of PHC in the NHS. This introduces primary health care teams, the 'primary care led NHS', PCTs, integrated health and social care trusts, and Local Strategic Partnerships.

Primary health care – multiple sectors and services

The Alma Ata conceptualisation of PHC was noticeable for its wide concern with factors supporting health, not limiting itself purely to health services. There is explicit mention of water supplies, basic sanitation, education and the food supply, as well as recognition of the multifactoral causation of ill-health, including the importance of social and environmental factors. Achieving the promotion and protection of health, and successfully tackling health inequalities, requires action in *all* sectors of society.

The notion of health promotion is extremely important within the HFA policy framework and within PHC services along Alma Ata lines. This was an area where considerable policy development was needed, outcomes of which are reflected in the 1991 revisions to the European HFA targets (WHO/EURO 1993) and in the latest health policy framework for Europe, Health21 (WHO/EURO 1999); some of this work is considered later in this chapter. The 1999 public health White Paper included a recognition that 'major new Government policies should be assessed for their impact on health' (SoSfH 1999, para 4.45). This use of health impact assessment represents an important step in encouraging all sectors to contribute to health promotion and protection.

Two particularly important elements in PHC delivery are settings-based approaches to health promotion, and the need for intersectoral or multisectoral collaboration with coordinated action of the health sector with other sectors in the economy, and the development of effective partnerships between the many different agencies involved. The use of settings-based approaches can be seen in the Healthy Schools and Healthy Workplaces initiatives, while initiatives such as New Deal, Sure Start, New Opportunities Funding, regeneration (SRB) funding and Neighbourhood Renewal are all designed to support partnership working.

The complexity of different agencies and organisations that need to be brought together provides a major challenge. As Taket and White (2000) conclude in their review of different models for joint working or partnership, there is a 'complexity of factors that affect the outcomes of multiagency work'. While it is possible to identify barriers to, and facilitating factors for, successful outcomes (however defined), generally such facilitating factors are found to be neither necessary nor sufficient, and barriers, while preventing successful outcomes in some contexts, can also be found in other contexts where successful outcomes are obtained. Similar conclusions are supported by Henwood's (1999) review of the Community Care Development Programme. Hiscock and Pearson (1999), based on a study of joint working between health and social services carried out in 1994 and 1995, concluded that joint working can be jeopardised by staff's preoccupations with changes within their own organisations. In the current context of frequent organisational change in the NHS, this is particularly relevant. Examples of successful partnership working are discussed later in this chapter. *Partnership in Action* (DoH 1998) signalled the introduction of new flexibilities, available following the passing of the Health Bill in January 1999, which helped remove the barriers to joint working between health and social services. A summary of the new possibilities is given in Box 3.3. The 1999 Health Act extended the existing duty of partnership between health authorities and local authorities to NHS trusts and primary care trusts, reflecting the need for partnership in service commissioning and delivery, as well as strategic planning (SoSfH 1999, para 10.14).

Primary health care within the NHS

The current organisation of PHC in the NHS was set up in the White Paper published in 1997 (SoSfH 1997). This promised: 'a system we have called "integrated care", based on partnership and driven by performance' (para 1.3), and set in motion a ten year programme to 'renew and improve the NHS'. In the UK, PHC within the NHS is mainly, but not solely, provided outside hospitals to people who are living in the community. Sometimes services are provided to people in their homes, as when a family doctor makes a home call, or a community nurse visits a patient. PHC is often provided through local health centres or clinics, but is increasingly provided in the settings of everyday life – where people work, live, study and socialise (the settings-based approaches to health promotion mentioned above). Some PHC staff, particularly midwives, provide services across hospital and community settings.

PHC is also often the main gateway to care at the secondary and tertiary levels when people are ill. In health service systems like the NHS which include some kind of personal or family doctor (general practitioners in the UK context), people who have a health problem who decide to seek help often approach this doctor first. PHC is especially relevant for promotion of public health and figures importantly in strategies of 'the new public health movement'. PHC is often (though not exclusively) based on relatively simple technologies and frequently requires an understanding of the social and environmental context for health as well as professional skill in techniques and procedures. For example, health promotion professionals working to reduce smoking will aim to encourage individuals to change their own behaviour and will also aim to promote change in public or private organisations, such as restrictions on smoking in public places or workplaces or on tobacco advertising. This work will require communication and facilitation skills as much as medical knowledge.

Box 3.3 Removing the barriers to joint working and supporting partnership

Pooled budgets: health (HA or PCT) and social service (LA) budgets

Lead commissioning: one authority transfers funds and delegates functions to the other so that they can commission both health and social care

Integrated provision: NHS Trust or PCT provides social care services beyond the level possible previously or a social services in-house provider provides a limited range of community health services

Primary health care teams

The PHC team is a term used to describe the group of professionals most closely involved in providing PHC to an individual or family. Giving a precise definition is hard, since in different places the term will be understood in rather different senses reflecting the particular local configurations of services that exist. Figure 3.1 depicts what are usually always included (the 'core' NHS team) and other potential members. Notice that the concept is often limited to health and personal social services related staff, although in line with earlier discussion, it would be more appropriate to include a much wider group: the receptionists and practice manager at a health centre; individuals, families, communities; workers in other sectors. Note also that with contracting and new funding flexibilities, some services provided by the voluntary or private sectors, or by local authorities, may be funded from NHS budgets.

NHS staff working in PHC may be employed by NHS hospital trusts, primary care trusts, integrated trusts, mental health trusts or general practices. Considerable variation exists across the country.

Primary care trusts, discussed below, which were introduced in the 1997 health White Paper, represent the core organising mechanism for the future.

Primary care trusts (PCTs)[1]

The structure of PHC in the NHS in England is now organised around primary care trusts (PCTs), the first wave of which went live on 1 April 2000. PCTs evolved out of the earlier primary care groups. Primary care trusts were established as free-standing bodies accountable to the Strategic Health Authority for commissioning care, with added responsibility for the provision of community health services for their population. These services may include district nursing, health visiting, physiotherapy, chiropody and speech therapy. Such trusts may include community health services transferred from NHS Trusts. Primary care trusts are able to run community hospitals and other community services. All or part of an existing community NHS trust may combine with a PCT in order to better integrate services and management support. Groups of PCTs sometimes also share services and management support.

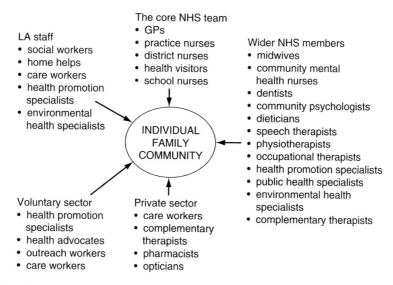

Figure 3.1   The primary care team – the NHS core team and others potentially involved

---

[1] The discussion here is in terms of England, structures are slightly different in other parts of the UK.

According to the DoH (2002a) the main roles of PCTs are:

- Improving the health of the community
- Securing the provision of high quality services
- Integrating health and social care locally

PCTs are required to have clear arrangements for public involvement including open meetings. PCTs are required to use a three year planning cycle and to formulate local delivery plans (LDPs) that focus on the health and social care priorities set out in the DoH's Planning and Priorities Framework guidance (DoH 2004). LDPs are then collated by strategic health authorities into a report for the whole strategic health authority area.

The White Paper argued that the arrangements provided give PCTs

'the responsibility as well as the tools and incentives with which to develop prompt, accessible and responsive services for local people. They will be encouraged to play an active part in community development and improving health in its widest sense. Health visitors and health promotion professionals will have a strong contribution to make in identifying health needs and implementing the programmes that best address them. Other primary care professionals, such as dentists, optometrists and pharmacists, will need to be drawn in to contribute as appropriate to the planning and provision of services.'

Current health policy places great emphasis on partnership and involvement, and the mechanisms of local strategic partnerships are designed to provide a focus for partnership working. A local strategic partnership (LSP) is a single non-statutory, multi-agency body, which matches local authority boundaries, and aims to bring together at a local level the different parts of the public, private, community and voluntary sectors. LSPs are key to tackling deep-seated, multi-faceted problems, requiring a range of responses from different bodies. Local partners working through an LSP will be expected to take many of the major decisions about priorities and funding for their local area.

LSPs are central to the delivery of the New Commitment to Neighbourhood Renewal – National Strategy Action Plan (SEU 2001). A five-year evaluation and action research programme of the LSPs has been commissioned. Recent results from this document the wide variety of different structures, membership and engagement achieved in the different LSPs, as well as the major challenges that LSPs face in terms of achieving transparency and involvement, and in shifting priorities in spending (ODPM 2004).

From the end of April 2004, the responsibilities of PCTs were increased to include being responsible authorities within local crime and disorder reduction partnerships (CDRPs). This places on PCTs the responsibility to work in partnership with other responsible authorities (police, fire and local authorities) to tackle crime, disorder and the misuse of drugs. Each CDRP needs to complete an audit of crime and disorder, anti-social behaviour and drug misuse for their area by the end of September 2004 and formulate a strategy in consultation with local communities to be published by April 2005.

Primary health care in the community – key issues and initiatives

As the previous section has indicated the organisation of PHC provision is changing, at what often seems, for those involved in it, a very rapid pace. This section picks up some of the important issues identified earlier, reviews briefly a number of studies/projects that illustrate current developments and introduces a range of current research. The issues to be addressed are: health promotion; tackling health inequalities; health and regeneration; and, contributing to CDRPs, the example of domestic violence.

Health promotion – everybody's business

As was mentioned earlier, the Alma Ata concept of PHC stresses the importance of promoting and protecting health. A programme in health promotion was established in the WHO

Regional Office for Europe in 1984, taking as its starting point the need to clarify some of the concepts and principles involved in the promotion of health. The definition of health promotion adopted was:

> '... the process of enabling people to increase control over, and to improve, their health. This perspective is derived from a conception of 'health' as the extent to which an individual or group is able, on the one hand, to realise aspirations and satisfy needs; and, on the other hand, to change or cope with the environment. Health is, therefore, seen as a resource for everyday life, not the objective of living; it is a positive concept emphasising social and personal resources, as well as physical capacities.'

(WHO/EURO 1984, p. 653–4)

Along with this comes a recognition that health promotion requires action not only within the health services, but within other sectors as well: 'health promotion ... encompasses actions to protect or enhance health, including legal, fiscal, educational and social measures' (Whitehead 1989, p. 7). Elsewhere this type of model of health promotion has been referred to as the 'empowerment model' (Wallerstein & Bernstein 1988; Whitehead 1989), with the former linking it to Freire's pedagogy. The key features of the empowerment model are that it is positive, dynamic, enabling and participative. It aims to perform a delicate balancing act between recognising the constraints on healthy choices faced by people due to the environments (in the widest sense) in which they live and work, and strengthening people's potential for taking action to improve their health (without slipping into victim-blaming). Health promotion programmes and initiatives therefore involve a wide spectrum of activities including advocacy, mediation, enabling etc. This model of health promotion is the one underlying the various HFA policies, see chronology in Box 3.1. What is more debatable is how well this understanding has been taken up within UK health policy where there are still struggles over this model of

health promotion (see for example: Kickbusch 1997; Naidoo 1986; Ziglio 1997).

Following on from work developing basic principles and concepts of health promotion, further work was initiated to explore mechanisms by which these might be put into practice. The first of these was a project aimed at exploring the concept of the 'healthy city' (Duhl 1986). This commenced in the European Region of the WHO in 1985, involving a small network of European cities (Tsouros 1990). By 1993, the project had grown rapidly, yielding 18 national networks and hundreds of towns and cities actively involved in Europe, North America, and, increasingly, low income countries (Hancock 1993); it had also become known as the Healthy Cities movement, or Healthy Communities in some parts of the world. Besides the European region, WHO has supported healthy city activities in the African region, the eastern Mediterranean region and the western Pacific region (WHO 1994). The work has drawn explicitly on experience outside the health sector. The sources of this experience include community development workers, as well as broad social movements with origins in the community/voluntary sector, such as feminist, black and minority ethnic, civil rights and green organisations and groups. A valuable emphasis of much of the successful healthy cities work has been in stressing the importance of the local context for the selection of priorities for action and of the importance of achieving widespread involvement in, and commitment to, local action. This has particularly involved work around community participation and intersectoral collaboration, two of the themes of HFA. The early work on healthy cities has since led to the development of other approaches based in particular settings, such as health promoting schools, workplaces and hospitals (WHO/ EURO 1993).

Work in another area, 'healthy public policy', built on the earlier experience and responded to the danger of reducing health promotion to a variety of victim-blaming strategies by emphasising the importance of policy in all sectors in creating social, physical and economic environments where 'healthy choices become the easy choices':

> 'Healthy public policy is the policy challenge set by a new vision of public health. It refers to policy decisions in any sector or level of government that are characterised by an explicit concern for health and an accountability for health impact. It is expressed through horizontal strategies such as intersectoral cooperation and public participation.'
>
> (Adelaide Conference on Healthy Public Policy 1988).

The notion of healthy public policy is argued to provide a foundation for promoting physical and social environments that support the adoption of healthy patterns of living (WHO/EURO 1993). Its aim is to ensure equitable access to the prerequisites for health, whether in the form of consumer goods, supportive living environments, or services that contribute to healthy living. It seeks to stimulate action and the development of specific mechanisms so that decision makers at all levels and in all sectors are aware of the consequences for health of their decisions, and are willing to accept their share of responsibility for health in their communities. The commitment to health impact assessment for new policy (SoSfH 1999, para 4.45) reflects the UK government's intention to seek healthy public policy in the future.

Tackling health inequalities

Within the UK, major inequalities in health exist, by income, occupation, ethnicity, geography (the north–south divide). Many are persistent or even widening (Acheson *et al.* 1998). Of particular concern are the health inequalities suffered by groups whose needs are marginalised by mainstream service provision and/or those suffering social exclusion. Tackling health inequalities is one key challenge facing PHC, and requires the creation of effective partnerships, as well as effective intersectoral and multisectoral action.

A growing body of research demonstrates different ways in which the health of disadvantaged groups has been improved. Some studies have demonstrated the key role that voluntary sector organisations can play; one example is presented in Box 3.4 below, and others are reviewed in Taket (1999). Chapter 5 describes the important role that community development approaches can play in tackling health inequalities, also illustrated by the example in Box 3.4.

Box 3.4   Racial harassment as a health issue

Tower Hamlets Health Strategy Group (THHSG) is a voluntary organisation seeking to promote the health of the people of Tower Hamlets, East London. A major part of the role of the group is undertaking action research projects to develop and evaluate appropriate innovatory forms of health-related service provision, which address previously unmet needs for underserved groups within the local communities. Its voluntary sector position has also facilitated the ability to challenge, where appropriate, professional views current in mainstream services. In estate-based health promotion work carried out in the late 1980s (under a community development philosophy – see Chapter 5) with Asian women living in local authority housing, a major issue raised by the women as affecting their lives was racial harassment. The women's strategy of avoidance by minimising time spent outside the home severely curtailed their activities and led to increasing feelings of isolation. The identification of racial harassment as a health issue was something that was initially resisted quite strongly by the health authority (demonstrating clearly the institutional racism affecting statutory services). After continued pressure from the THHSG, this was eventually accepted as a health issue that required a response on the part of the NHS, and was responded to through the provision of training to NHS workers about how to support individuals suffering racial harassment.

The 1999 public health white paper contains acknowledgement that tackling racial harassment still remains an issue – both outside and inside the NHS (SoSfH 1999, para 9.30).

Health Action Zones (HAZ) have been one recent policy initiative aimed at stimulating innovation, and particularly at tackling health inequalities:

'New Health Action Zones will blaze the trail...The accent will be on partnership and innovation, finding new ways to tackle health problems and reshape local services. Health Action Zones will be concentrated in areas of pronounced deprivation and poor health, reflecting the Government's commitment to tackle entrenched inequalities. An early task for each Health Action Zone will be to develop clear targets, agreed with the NHS Executive, for measurable improvements every year.'

(SoSfH 1997, para 10.6)

National and local evaluation of the achievements of HAZs (Barnes *et al.* 2005; Bauld & Judge 2002) have shown mixed success in identifying and implementing ways of reducing health inequalities, with the most successful innovations being integrated into mainstream service provision as the HAZ funding ended.

Health and regeneration

The next topic to be considered in this section is regeneration programmes. These provide an example of multisectoral initiatives that have considerable potential for addressing the health inequalities existing in particular localities. Funding to support regeneration programmes is available through the single regeneration budget (SRB) scheme supported by the Department of Transport, Environment and the Regions.

Traditional regeneration programmes have concentrated on employment, on the physical environment, and on housing redevelopment. Obviously these have impacts, direct and indirect, on health. It is only comparatively recently however, that, during the 1990s, the design and implementation of regeneration programmes began to take health issues explicitly into account. A publication from a 1998 conference (THHSG/HEA 1998) summarised much of the work in the field. More recently this has been taken a step further, through the modification of the objectives allowed in programmes supported by SRB funding to include 'enhancing the quality of life, health and capacity to contribute to regeneration'. This expansion of the remit of SRB funding opened the door to a successful regeneration bid led by a health authority (now a strategic health authority) and focused around the health sector; this example is described in Box 3.5. Other HAs have since followed suit.

Box 3.5 Health and regeneration – the example of Redbridge and Waltham Forest

'The Health Ladder to Social Inclusion' is the first broad health-based single regeneration budget programme (SRB) in the country. It is now led by City and East London Strategic Health Authority and is a seven-year programme, involving many different organisational partners, across public, voluntary and private sectors. The programme commenced in November 1999, and the major spending started in April 2000. Approximately £8 million SRB funding is involved, with at least an equivalent amount in matched funding from the various different partner agencies. The SRB involves projects in the following four main areas:

- Jobs and training
- Capacity building
- Access to PHC services
- Public health

The area covered by the SRB Programme comprises 19 electoral wards, with a total population of approximately 2150000. This population has a higher proportion of black and minority ethnic residents than average for London (30% in Waltham Forest bid area and 34% in Redbridge bid area), poorer health and greater mental health needs than other parts of these two local authority areas.

Box 3.5 (Continued)

The target groups for the SRB programme are:

- People suffering social disadvantage in the SRB area (including homeless and those living in temporary accommodation)
- Black and minority ethnic communities and refugee communities
- Young people
- Older people

The bid was the outcome of an extensive process of consultation and partnership working, involving statutory, voluntary, community and private sectors. It also built on the considerable experience of the community health project in the South of Waltham Forest, which was recognised locally, nationally and internationally for its work with socially excluded communities, including refugees and black and minority ethnic communities. The SRB programme will make use of the new flexibilities introduced in *Partnership in Action*, (see Box 3.3).

Contributing to crime and disorder reduction partnerships (CDRPs), the example of domestic violence

The last topic to be considered in this section is domestic violence as an example of the contribution that the health service can make to CDRPs. Domestic violence is a major crime issue, accounting for almost a quarter (23%) of all reported violent crime (BCS 2000), but it is also a generally unacknowledged public health issue. Intimate partner abuse, often termed domestic violence, is the abuse and control of a person by their current or former intimate partner. Partner abuse occurs in all types of relationships, both same sex and heterosexual, but the highest prevalence is found for abuse against women. A review of population based studies across the world found that between 10% and 69% of women reported being physically assaulted by an intimate male partner at some time in their lives (Heise *et al.* 1999). Thus, for women, domestic violence has a higher lifetime prevalence than breast cancer.

Abuse is associated with both acute and chronic medical problems that are frequently treated in the health care system, with associated resource consequences for the health care system. The cost for the NHS of physical injuries alone from domestic violence is estimated at around £1.2 billion a year (Walby 2004). Domestic violence affects women from all age groups, all ethnic and religious groups, at all income levels. It represents a health problem for those experiencing it, and health impacts are not limited to short-term injuries. Domestic violence can lead to acute and chronic physical injury, miscarriage, loss of hearing and vision, and physical disfigurement. It often leads to depression and alcoholism, and sometimes to suicide. Children are also affected – many women and children develop post-traumatic stress disorder, and experience years of distress. Despite the many opportunities for abused women to disclose in the health care setting, research has shown that approximately 3% to less than 10% of all abused women are identified by health care professionals (Yam 2000). These statistics show the unrealised opportunities for health care professionals to enable abused women to improve their lives.

Recently, there have been a number of projects within the health service exploring how this important public health issue can be tackled, most particularly in primary care settings. There is an increasing body of research (see for example studies reviewed in Taket *et al.* 2003, 2004; Taket 2004) that demonstrates that health professionals can make an important difference to the health and well-being of women and children by providing information about the specialised services that exist, and enabling women to access specialised services.

A number of projects have investigated routine enquiry in health service settings, i.e. aiming to ask all women about experience, if any, of domestic violence, on her own in a private and confidential area, with a female interpreter if necessary. Routine enquiry can be carried out in many different ways: in well women clinics; in general practice by GPs or practice nurses; in the antenatal or maternity services setting to name just a few. The aim of routine enquiry is to facilitate, and not force, disclosure. It must remain the woman's choice as to if, when, and to whom, she discloses. Evaluations of projects have demonstrated that routine enquiry is feasible and sustainable, and acceptable to the vast majority of women (both those who have experienced abuse and those who have not). Many women report that, without being asked directly, they will not disclose their experience. Finding out about locally available specialised support services is important in helping women to consider their options, and receiving the clear message from trusted health professionals that domestic abuse is unacceptable, and *not* their fault, is extremely important. Although many health professionals, prior to training, are apprehensive about raising the topic, once trained and implementing routine enquiry, health professionals report that they find it useful.

Looking to the future

This short closing section offers a brief review of the challenges facing PHC for the future. Perhaps the single largest challenge facing PHC is that of reducing health inequalities, tackling particularly the multiply disadvantaged positions that black and minority ethnic groups often find themselves in.

The importance of tackling inequalities has been fully recognised in health policy, and this chapter has earlier presented examples of some promising avenues of approach. Much work however remains to be done in evaluating the various initiatives underway and then acting on the knowledge gained. This connects to the second challenge to be mentioned here, that of developing the evidence base for PHC practice, a task specifically for research as discussed in chapter 7, which runs alongside the challenge of reshaping the delivery of PHC to utilise this evidence base in practice.

Another major challenge for all of those working within PHC is the pace of organisational change.

Here, a continuation of the tension between drive for seeking 'better' forms of organisation leading to a rapid succession of initiatives requiring changes, and letting one change settle in, before rolling out the next, can be expected. An enormous change agenda has already been set for the future following the move to PCTs, with the full implementation of the new GP contract, as well as initiatives such as the use of salaried GPs, the development of walk in centres and healthy living centres. Major changes can still be expected in the roles of different health professionals (DoH 2002b) and the development of the advanced practitioner in particular will open up new opportunities for nurses and others working in the community. At the time of writing, in August 2004, further structural changes are still under consideration, and a new White Paper on public health is imminent. Exactly what these will imply is not yet clear.

Another area remaining a challenge for the future is ensuring a truly multiprofessional basis for PHC. A continuation of changes in skill mix and role development within all professional groups can be expected. In talking of a 'primary care led NHS', the WHO concept of PHC implies that it is important that this is led multiprofessionally, and not reduced to a GP-led NHS. The dangers of a GP-led NHS are the perpetuation of a restricted understanding of PHC and, in particular, a lack of attention to protection and promotion of health; see Box 3.6.

The WHO concept of PHC introduced in this chapter implies an extensive and important role for the nursing profession in PHC. The WHO Regional Office for Europe, the International Council of Nurses (ICN), and the International Council of Midwives (ICM), issued a joint call in February 2000 for a Europe-wide public health campaign for nurses, health visitors and midwives. This is intended as an initiative to strengthen the impact that nurses, health visitors and midwives have on improving health in the context of WHO's Health21 health for all policy framework. The campaign will emphasise the importance of developing effective teamwork skills and engaging in interdisciplinary teams to promote health, and provide care and treatment.

Box 3.6 Contradictions in policy?

He [Tony Blair] promised that GPs were "central to the delivery of our vision for the health service", driving change and co-ordinating the different "levels of care" from basic community and social services through to the acute hospital sector and rehabilitation. The health secretary later amplified this, saying that GPs would be at the centre of a "single system shaped around the needs of the patient".'

(Health Service Journal 23 March 2000, p. 13, reporting the GP2000 conference)

'General practice is a fundamental part of health care. At its centre is the care provided to people who are ill or believe themselves to be ill, and at its heart a doctor–patient relationship based on mutual trust and personal attention focused on the individual.' John Chisholm, Chairman, General Practitioner Committee, BMA, writing in the foreword to Mihill (2000), which forms a major part of the General Practitioner Committee's policy review process. It contains only four references to health promotion, only one of the many doctors quoted in the report explicitly mentions health promotion as a part of general practice.

Taken together these quotes illustrate the ambiguity surrounding the multiprofessional nature of PHC and the importance of the promotion and protection of health within it. They seem explicitly to draw on a much more restricted notion of PHC than that envisaged within the WHO concept, and which is required to address health inequalities. As a further example of the potential difficulties, note the study of Barclay *et al.* (1999) into priorities for palliative care services, which found considerable differences between GPs and district nurses in terms of views on service adequacy and priorities for future development.

It will also stress the overwhelming significance of developing 'family health nurses' as a force for health improvement throughout the European Region. In the UK, this is reflected in the recommendation that the health visitor develops a family-centred public health role (SoSfH 1999). In the words of Kirsten Stalknecht, President of ICN:

'It is clear that nurses and midwives are at the heart of most effective health care teams, especially the PHC team. Using their varied capacities and expertise, nurses and midwives working in many different capacities will make major contributions to Health21. Nurse policy-makers, managers, educators and clinicians are already leading initiatives that improve the health of the population as a whole, and narrow the gap in health. The Health21 nurse and midwife movement will make all these contributions more visible and should inspire new initiatives.'

References

Acheson, D. *et al.* (1998) *Independent inquiry into inequalities in health*. The Stationery Office, London.

Adelaide Conference on Healthy Public Policy (1988) *Report on Second International Conference on Health Promotion*. Adelaide, South Australia.

Barclay, S., Todd, C., McCabe, J. & Hunt, T. (1999) Primary care group commissioning of services: the differing priorities of general practitioners and district nurses for palliative care services. *British Journal of General Practice*, **49**(440), 181–186.

Barnes, M., Bauld, L., Benzeval, M., McKenzie, M. & Sullivan, H. (eds) (2005) *Health Action Zones: partnerships for health equity*. London, Routledge.

Bauld, L. & Judge, K. (eds) (2002) *Learning from Health Action Zones*. Aeneas Press, Chichester.

BCS (2000) *British Crime Survey, 2000*. Home Office, London.

Bomberg, E. & Peterson, J. (1993) Prevention from above? the role of the European Community. In: *Prevention, Health and British politics* (M. Mills ed), pp. 140–160. Avebury, Aldershot.

DoH (1998) *Partnership in action: new opportunities for joint working between health and social services*. Department of Health, London.

DoH (2002a) *Shifting the balance of power*. Department of Health, London.

DoH (2002b) *HR in the NHS Plan – More Staff Working Differently*. Department of Health, London.

DoH (2004) *National Standards, Local Action: Health and Social Care Standards and Planning Framework*, 2005/05–2007/08. Department of Health, London.

Duhl, L.J. (1986) The healthy city: its function and its future. *Health Promotion*, **1**(1), 55–60.

EC, European Commission (1993) *Commission communication on the framework for action in the field of public health.* COM(93) 559 final, 24 November 1993, Brussels.

Gish, O. (1992) Malaria eradication and the selective approach to health care: some lessons from Ethiopia. *International Journal of Health Services*, **22**(1), 179–192.

Godlee, F. (1995) The World Health Organization: WHO in Europe: does it have a role? *British Medical Journal*, **310**, 389–394.

Hancock, T. (1993) The evolution, impact and significance of the healthy cities/healthy communities movement. *Journal of Public Health Policy*, **14**(1), 5–18.

Heise, L., Ellsberg, M. & Gottemoeller, M. (1999) *Ending Violence Against Women*. Population Reports, Series L, No. **11**. Baltimore: Johns Hopkins University School of Public Health, Population Information Program, December. http://www.jhuccp.org/pr/l11edsum.shtml, accessed 12 Feb 2003.

Henwood, M. (1999) *The community care development programme: building partnerships for success: an evaluation report to the Department of Health.* Department of Health, London.

Hiscock, J. & Pearson, M. (1999) Looking inwards, looking outwards: dismantling the "Berlin Wall" between health and social services? *Social Policy and Administration*, **33**(2), 150–163.

Kickbusch, I. (1997) Think health: what makes the difference? *Health Promotion International*, **12**(4), 265–272.

Kokkonen, P.T. & Kekomäki, M. (1993) Legal and economic issues in European public health. In: *Europe without frontiers: the implications for health.* (C.E.M. Normand & P. Vaughan eds), pp. 35–43. Wiley, London.

Mihill, C. (2000) *Shaping tomorrow: issues facing general practice in the new millennium.* BMA, London.

Milburn, A. (2000) Keynote speech to NHS Confederation Conference, July 2000.

Naidoo, J. (1986) Limits to individualism. In: *The politics of health education.* (S. Rodmell & A. Watt eds), pp. 17–37. Routledge, London.

ODPM (2004) *LSP Evaluation and Action Research Programme, Case-Studies interim report: A baseline of practice*, May 2004. London, Office of the Deputy Prime Minister.

Pannenborg, C.O. (1991) Shifting paradigms of international health. *Asia Pacific Journal of Public Health*, **5**(2), 176–184.

SEU (2001) *A New Commitment to Neighbourhood Renewal – National Strategy Action Plan.* Cabinet Office, London.

SoSfH, Secretary of State for Health (1997) *The New NHS: Modern, Dependable.* Cm 3807, 9 December 1997. The Stationery Office, London.

SoSfH, Secretary of State for Health (1999) *Saving Lives: Our Healthier Nation.* Cm 4386, 5 July 1999. The Stationery Office, London.

Taket, A.R. (1999) *Tackling health inequalities in communities: the role of the voluntary sector.* Paper presented at conference on 'Researching for health: challenges and controversies', Heriot-Watt University, Edinburgh, 20–22 September 1999.

Taket, A.R. (2004) *Tackling domestic violence: the role of health professionals.* Home Office Development and Practice Report 32. London, Home Office. Available at http://www.homeoffice.gov.uk/rds/pdfs04/dpr32.pdf

Taket, A.R., Beringer, A., Irvine, A., & Garfield, S. (2004) *Tackling domestic violence: exploring the health service contribution. Evaluation of the Crime Reduction Programme Violence Against Women Initiative health projects.* Home Office Online Report 52/04. Available at: www.homeoffice.gov.uk/rds/pdfs04/rdsolr5204.pdf

Taket, A., Nurse, J., Smith, K., Watson, J., Shakespeare, J., Lavis, V., Cosgrove, K., Mulley, K. & Feder, G. (2003) Routinely asking women about domestic violence in health settings. *British Medical Journal*, **327**, 673–676.

Taket, A.R. & White, L.A. (2000) *Partnership and participation: decision-making in the multiagency setting.* Wiley, Chichester.

THHSG/HEA (1998) *Putting health on the regeneration agenda.* Proceedings of a conference held at London Guildhall University on 2nd April 1998. HEA, London.

Tsouros, A.D. (1990) *World Health Organization Healthy Cities Project: a project becomes a movement – review of progress 1987–1990.* Milan, SOGESS.

Walby, S. (2004) *The cost of domestic violence.* University of Leeds, Leeds.

Wallerstein, N. & Bernstein, E. (1988) Empowerment education: Freire's ideas adapted to health education. *Health Education Quarterly*, **15**(4), 379–94.

Whitehead, M. (1989) *Swimming upstream: trends and prospects for education in health.* King's Fund, London.

WHO (1994) *The Work of WHO 1992–1993 – Biennial Report of the Director General.* World Health Organization, Geneva.

WHO/EURO (1984) Summary report of the working group on concepts and principles of health promotion. In: *Measurement in health promotion and protection*. (1987) (T. Abelin *et al*.), pp. 653–658. World Health Organization, Regional office for Europe, Copenhagen.

WHO/EURO (1985) *Targets for health for all*. WHO Regional Office for Europe, Copenhagen.

WHO/EURO (1993) *Health for all targets: the health policy for Europe*. Updated edition, September 1991. WHO Regional Office for Europe, Copenhagen.

WHO/EURO (1999) *Health 21 – the health for all policy framework for the WHO European Region*. WHO Regional Office for Europe, Copenhagen.

WHO/UNICEF (1978) *Primary health care: report of the International conference on Primary Health Care, Alma-Ata*. World Health Organization, Geneva.

Yam M. (2000) Seen but not heard: battered women's perceptions of the ED experience. *Journal of Emergency Nursing*, **26**, 464–470.

Ziglio, E. (1997) How to move towards evidence-based health promotion interventions. *Promotion and Education*, **4**(2), 29–33.

Further reading

For a discussion of the challenges that PCTs face and their possible future, see:

Lewis, R., Dixon, J. & Gillam, G. (2003) *Future directions for primary care trusts*. London, King's Fund.

Roche, D. (2004) *PCTs: an unfinished agenda*. IPPR, London.

For research into the changing structure of primary health care and evaluation of its effects:

Audit Commission (2004) *Transforming primary health care: the role of primary care trusts in shaping and supporting general practice*. Audit Commission, London.

Commission for Health Improvement (2004) *What CHI has found in primary care trusts*. CHI, London.

Glendinning, C. (1999) GPs and contracts: bringing general practice into primary care. *Social Policy and Administration*, **33**(2), 115–131.

Malbon, G., Mays, N., Killoran, A., Wykes, S. & Goodwin, N. (1999) *What were the achievements of total purchasing pilots in their second year (97/98) and how can they be explained?* King's Fund, London.

Regan, E., Smith, J., Goodwin, N., McLeod, H. & Shapiro, J. (2001) *Passing the Baton: final report of a national evaluation of primary care groups and trusts*. HSMC, Birmingham.

Wilkin, D., Coleman, A., Dowling, B. & Smith, K. (eds) (2002) *The National Tracker Survey of Primary Care Groups and Trusts 2001/2: Taking responsibility?* NPCRDC, Manchester.

For the publications connected to the evaluation of partnership working in the context of LSPs:

http://www.neighbourhood.gov.uk/lsp_evaluation.asp

For a more detailed treatment of the work of the WHO up to the mid 1990s:

Curtis, S.E. & Taket, A.R. (1996) The widening international perspective on health. In: *Health and Societies: changing perspectives*. Arnold, London.

Chapter 4 **Communication, Skill and Health Care Delivery**

David Dickson and Patrick J. McCartan

NORTHBROOK COLLEGE LIBRARY

Introduction

Communication has always been regarded as a fundamental part of nursing (Castledine 2004; Thorsteinsson 2002). Its importance is clearly articulated within the Nursing and Midwifery Council's Code of Professional Conduct (NMC 2002), which highlights that registered nurses are responsible for ensuring that they safeguard the interests of their patients and develop and maintain appropriate relationships. The centrality of communication is also emphasised by the Royal College of Nursing who consider communication skills to be embodied in several of the defining characteristics of nursing (RCN 2003). In particular, the RCN highlight that nursing interventions are concerned with information, education, advice, advocacy, empowerment and commitment to partnership. Over the past decade NHS reforms, along with developments in technology, education and research have forced nurses to re-examine the way they deliver care (Albarran & Whittle 1999). In particular, it has been necessary for nurses to re-appraise the way in which they communicate within their practice, not only with patients, but also with other caregivers and at a broader national level.

Patients are no longer passive recipients of care, but, as highlighted within clinical governance (DoH 1997), patients are actively encouraged to become involved and enter into partnerships with caregivers. This move from a task-centred orientation to care to patient-centred communication is a challenge for nurses. Rather than making assumptions about what nursing care a patient needs or wants, nurses are now required to employ communication skills that encourage patients to participate and negotiate in decision making regarding their own care (McCabe 2004). The growing health literacy of patients has consequently increased their independence, making it more likely for patients to question and challenge nurses about the care delivered. The importance of communication has been widely examined, including studies that have demonstrated the effects on patient satisfaction (McCulloch 2004), the impact on the quality of care (Goode 2004), and the influence on litigation for malpractice (Fentiman 2003).

An additional communication challenge to nurses working within the community setting is the need to collaborate with the growing number of different professionals and agencies involved in the delivery of care. This requires nurses communicating, and working in partnership, with professionals employed by organisations outside the NHS. To avoid duplication and lapses in care, and to promote a seamless service, Moore (2003, p. 180) suggested that 'nurses will need to learn advanced communication skills that will enable them to speak the language of other providers, commissioners and service users'.

There are also communication challenges for nurses at a wider national level. Arising from the DoH (1998) consultative publication *A First Class Service: quality in the new NHS*, it was agreed that standards would be set through national service frameworks (NSFs) and the National Institute for Clinical Excellence (NICE). These national standards have been, and will continue to be, developed via consultation with the relevant reference groups. As nurses have a major role in the delivery of care in the community setting, and are currently taking on new roles in the form of nurse consultants and specialist practitioners, it is important that they can collaborate effectively with others at a policy-making level (Stichler 2002). This will require nurses to have the necessary interpersonal skills and confidence to contribute meaningfully in such situations.

This chapter will explore the concept of interpersonal communication, tease out its key features and discuss their relevance to nursing practice. A skill-based model of the communicative process will be outlined and applied to nurse–patient interaction, drawing upon empirical and analytical sources from the nursing literature.

Interpersonal communication

Attempts to define the term 'communication' proliferate within the nursing literature. This has resulted in some confusion and blurring of definitions, reflecting the complexity of the concept. Summarised by Rosengren (2000, p. 37), communication is '…both complex and brittle, composed of several series of sometimes very subtle actions and behaviours, which as a rule are felicitous but quite often less than completely successful'. Morrison and Burnard (1997) presented it as a complex phenomenon, concluding that one can only truly understand the concept by breaking it down into manageable components. Traced back to its Latin roots the verb 'to communicate' means 'to impart', 'to share', 'to make common' – meanings reflected in many of the definitions available in the current literature. From the more detailed publications available, Hewes and Planalp (1987) distilled two central themes: *intersubjectivity*, which has to do with striving to understand others and being understood in turn; and *impact* which represents the extent to which a message brings about changes in thoughts, feelings, or behaviour.

Interpersonal communication is viewed as a sub-type of the general term 'communication' and defined, in a generic sense, 'as the skills we employ when interacting with other people' (Hargie & Dickson 2004, p. 4). Described by Hartley (1999), interpersonal communication focuses upon communication which is essentially non-mediated (or face-to-face), takes place in a dyadic (one-to-one) or small group setting, and in form and content is shaped by, and conveys something of, the personal qualities of the interactors as well as their social roles and relationships. Several features of interpersonal communication have particular relevance for nurse–patient interaction.

Interpersonal communication is a transactional process

The notion that interpersonal communication is a linear process has been replaced by a more transactional conceptualisation emphasising the ongoing, dynamic quality of the activity. For Riley (2004), the process is reciprocal. The nurse, for example, when speaking is also receiving messages from the patient. Similarly, when receiving messages the nurse is simultaneously sending messages. While this is pertinent to all interactions, it is particularly salutary in sensitive situations like breaking bad news. The nurse must be mindful of how the altering of any one of the elements of the transactional process may bring about corresponding changes at other stages which may affect the system as a whole. As the nurse and patient act and react to each other in a system of reciprocal influence (which involves feedback and validation), ongoing adjustments are made to the communication that unfolds (Arnold & Boggs 2003).

Describing the communication process as transactional implies mutuality, sharing and the conjoint creation of meaning. A corollary gaining recognition in the nurse–patient interaction literature, is that the ultimate effectiveness of the outcome is not the sole responsibility of the nurse (Morse *et al.* 1997). With the growing emphasis on patient empowerment (Tran *et al.* 2004) and shared decision making (McCabe 2004), the notion of mutuality will increasingly influence and alter the nurse–patient relationship.

Interpersonal communication is purposeful

Another commonly cited feature of interpersonal communication is its purposefulness (Wood 2004). When interacting interpersonally an individual employs purposeful or goal-directed behaviours to achieve a desired outcome (although often with little conscious awareness), as opposed to chance or unintentional behaviours. It is this purposefulness which both provides impetus and gives direction to the transaction (Hargie & Dickson 2004). Purposefulness is a central tenet of the nurse–patient therapeutic relationship which is viewed as 'a goal-directed, focused dialogue between nurse and client that is specifically tailored to the needs of the client' (Duxbury, 2000, p. 22). Recognising that nurse communication has attracted consistent criticism for being often routine, instrumental and shallow (Fletcher 1997; McCabe 2004), describing communication as purposeful does not imply task-centred instrumentality in relationships with patients. Goals can be varied reflecting the multidimensionality of communication itself.

Interpersonal communication is multidimensional

The notion that communication is multidimensional has significant relevance for the community nurse–patient relationship. The term implies that messages exchanged are seldom unitary or discrete. Hargie *et al.* (2004) asserted that communication takes place at different levels simultaneously. While one level is concerned with substantive content, another focuses on relationship aspects that help determine how participants define their association with others. For the practitioner within the community setting, relational issues involving the extent of dominance and affiliation (or liking) are important. Sutcliffe *et al.* (2004) stressed the significance of this distinction in understanding the caregiver–patient interaction.

Negotiating the relationship

Content is probably the more immediately recognisable dimension of interpersonal communication, dealing as it does with the subject matter of talk (e.g. discussing problems the patient has encountered since the previous visit; explaining how to self-medicate). When interacting at a 'content level', relational communication simultaneously defines the type and extent of the association between the interactors, reflecting, for example, the degree of dominance and liking. Dominance is determined by equality or inequality in interaction, resulting in either a symmetrical or complementary relationship. Because of their status or power, community nurses often work within a complementary relationship wherein they are considered 'superior' to the patient. This can affect any communication between

them (Ellis *et al.* 2003). These issues are central in the discussions focusing on the intrinsic nature of the nurse–patient encounter and the need to move towards a more (symmetrical) patient-centred, patient empowered approach (Lawson 2002). While there are some reservations concerning patient empowerment (Hewitt-Taylor 2004; Salmon & Hall 2004) there is a growing acceptance that patients must be more involved in treatment decisions (Bulsara *et al.* 2004; Lloyd & Bor 2004).

The extent and importance of affiliation in nurse–patient interactions is also considered an important relational issue, particularly at a time when there is a growing reliance on technology within nursing (Barnard & Sandelowski 2001; Kyle 2001). While many theorists consider the interpersonal domain to be pivotal in caring (e.g. Arnold & Boggs 2003; Riley 2004) there is conflicting evidence regarding its prominence in actual nursing practice (McCabe 2004; Reynolds & Scott 2000). Furthermore, patients do not always want or expect close emotional contact with their carers, rather they perceive practitioner expertise and the delivery of physical care to be more important (Burkitt Wright *et al.* 2004).

Projecting identity

In addition to dominance and affiliation issues, relational communication also enables one to project one's own identity. By using particular verbal and nonverbal skills people send out messages concerning 'who and what they are, and how they wish to be received and reacted to by others' (Hargie *et al.* 2004, p. 20). For instance, the type of nurse–patient conversation and the wearing of a uniform can impact both positively and negatively on the patient's perception of the nurse. The nurse using formal-type language with little social discourse can convey an image of being 'busy' with little time to spend with the patient (Burnard 2004). Similarly, while a nurse in a uniform might be making a statement about status and power (Lefebvre 2003), this attire is sometimes construed as adding to the nurse's subservience and anonymity (Pearson *et al.* 2001).

Confirming identity

Through relational communication the nurse can also either confirm or invalidate the sense of identity being presented by the patient. In confirming, the nurse acknowledges the existence of the patient as being of value. Invalidation or disconfirmation, however, fails to do either (Arnold & Boggs 2003). This can have major consequences for the therapeutic nature of the nurse–patient relationship (Northouse & Northouse 1998; Slevin 1999).

Interpersonal communication is inevitable

This thinking is represented in the often-quoted maxim that under circumstances where people are aware of the presence of others, 'one cannot not communicate' (Watzlawick *et al.* 1967, p. 49). Such a stance asserts that all behaviour conveys a message. (This proposition is contentious though.) As a consequence, in addition to the generally acknowledged forms of communication such as using words or gesticulations, not saying or doing anything may in itself be viewed as sending out a message. Some theorists take an opposing position in this debate, suggesting that not all behaviour is communication and arguing that being overly-inclusive in this respect renders the term 'communication' largely redundant (Trenholm & Jenson 2000). Rosengren (2000) contended that intentionality bestows special communicative status upon interaction. Accordingly, while some behaviours such as blushing, sweating or spontaneous yawning, might be expressive of bodily or psychological states and thereby informative, they would not be deemed to be properly communicative. This conceptual distinction makes informing, but not necessarily communicating, inevitable. The implications are significant for concepts such as that of skill.

Communication is irreversible

You occasionally hear the saying 'I wish I hadn't said that'. Unfortunately, once a verbal or a nonverbal message has been sent it cannot be retracted (Ellis *et al.* 2003). A nurse may disclose to the patient how a cancer is reacting to treatment, unaware of the fact the patient has not been informed that a treated 'mole' was malignant!

While the personal and relational consequences of the nurse's actions can sometimes be retrieved through using communicative devices such as apologies, justifications and accounts (Reardon 1987), the nurse cannot change the fact that the patient has heard it. As pointed out by Hargie *et al.* (2004, p. 19) 'initial care with words and actions prevents lasting hurt and dented relationships'.

Having reviewed some of the central features of interpersonal communication and where they fit into quality nursing practice, the chapter will continue by exploring what makes communication skilled.

Communication and skill

The centrality of service provider/user communication in the quest to deliver quality nursing care is axiomatic. Reference in this regard to communication as a skill has also become commonplace (e.g. Duman & Clark 2003; Saunders 2003). (The terms 'social skills', 'helping skills', 'human skills', 'interviewing skills' and even 'problem-solving skills' are often used as synonyms.) Pithily put by Farley and Hendry (2004, p. 410), 'Nurses need good communication skills'. The challenge has been taken up by nurse educators to put training programmes in place to uplift competencies in this domain (e.g. Bowles *et al.* 2001; Cooke *et al.* 2003; Quinn 2000), in keeping with policy directives (DoH 2000a). Given such prominence, it is perhaps surprising that this particular application of the concept of skill in the nursing literature has a decidedly 'given' quality. While exceptions can be found (e.g. Chant *et al.* 2002), little effort has been expended on addressing the issue of what precisely it means to construe interpersonal transactions involving end users (or for that matter other care professionals) as skilful.

Musings on the nature of skill are much more conspicuous in current theorising in the literature on communication, per se. While alternatives can be found, Metts and Grohskopf (2003, p. 365) capture consistencies in thinking when they defined communication skills as '...acquired abilities to use interpretative and communication resources, which are manifested in observable behaviour with some degree of regularity, to achieve desirable outcomes'. For Hargie (1997, p. 12) the key features are that it is a '...process whereby the individual implements a set of goal-directed, interrelated, situationally appropriate social behaviours which are learned and controlled'. Elaborating on this line of thought, the following have been teased out as core qualities of interpersonal skill (Dickson 2001):

Utility

Communication that proves successful in bringing about a desired end state is held, other things being equal, to be more skilful than that which fails (Miczo *et al.* 2001), although Berger (2003) stipulated that it must additionally be shown to do so on a reasonably consistent basis. He goes on to note that there is also a requirement for efficiency of action in attributing judgements about skill. The least effort-intensive or the most direct way of completing the task is usually regarded, other things being equal, as the most skilful in a social situation of options.

Behavioural facility

Behaving skilfully implies that the performance is smooth and effortless. Switching attention to the underpinning cognitive processes, Greene (2003) revealed how well-honed skills seldom strain the individual's limited capacity to process information, permit additional tasks to be carried out at the same time, and are often accomplished with only minimal conscious awareness.

Contextual propriety

This criterion has to do with, as put by Spitzberg (2003, p. 581), '...the extent to which behaviour meets the standards of legitimacy or acceptability in a context'. What counts as a skilful way of conducting oneself in one situation may be entirely inappropriate in another: the approach taken with one patient may not be the most appropriate with another. While flexibility and adaptability are central to skilful action (Hargie & Dickson 2004) there is evidence that nurses may not always be sufficiently adept in this regard, failing to tailor their interactions to the needs and characteristics of the individual patient (Caris-Verhallen *et al.* 1999). Of course, this requirement is a core principle of *The NHS Plan* (DoH 2000a), as pointed out by Sarah Mullally, the Chief Nursing Officer for England (Mullally 2003).

Normativity

This extends the previous point by introducing considerations of standards of acceptability of conduct, warrantability of goals, and recognised codes of professional conduct. The fundamental point is made by Wiemann (2003, p. ix) that 'There is also an ethical aspect to communication skills in that they can be used for good or ill...'. The nurse as skilled communicator is expected to be: sensitive to the psycho-emotional as well as physical needs of the patient and equipped to deal with these in offering support through active listening and empathy (Reynolds & Scott 2000); equipped to enter into a relationship that is not prescribed by narrow and traditional task-based roles (Slevin 1999); capable of working collaboratively in a partnership arrangement where power and control are shared with service users (Martin 1998); able to adopt a patient-centred approach to care delivery (Chambers-Evans *et al.* 1999); and adept at providing information as required in an open and comprehensible way (Duman & Clark 2003).

Accusations of poor levels of communication skill persistently levelled at the nursing profession (e.g. McCabe 2004; Wilkinson *et al.* 2003) can invariably be traced to violations of one or more of these expectations. More deep-seated, ideological tensions between nursing as the provision of clinically efficient physical care versus relational-focused personal care, which directly impact role prescriptions, are also implicated (Meerabeau 2004).

In addition to these four cardinal qualities, Spitzberg and Cupach (2002) identified a further two that are commonly associated with people skills: fidelity and satisfaction. Although neither is conceptually unproblematic, skilled communication is accordingly deemed to carry meaning clearly and to produce a greater sense of gratification for those involved.

Communication skill: a conceptual framework

A model of the concepts and processes involved in skilled interaction, deriving largely from a social-cognitive perspective, will now be briefly outlined (see Figure 4.1). It draws upon Argyle's model of social skill (Argyle 1983), as elaborated by Dickson *et al.* (1997) and Hargie and Dickson (2004). This perspective has been applied to health communication (Skipper 1992), including nursing in hospital (McCann & McKenna 1993) and community settings (Crute 1986; Dickson 1999) as well as to conflict mediation (McGrane 2003). Briefly put, this model of skill depicts interactive partners as essentially purposeful planners and decision makers; influenced by their personal histories, attributes and characteristics including emotional states and predispos-

itions; sensitive and responsive to each other, their social environment and the effects of their actions; and operating within a layering of embedded communicative contexts. In addition to the immediate personal–situational framework that shapes interaction, broader organisational and cultural factors can be posited as influential. The significance of this way of thinking should not be overlooked. Notions of interpersonal skill as alternatively method- or content-based can be traced back to Trower (1984). As content, skills are specific sets of behaviour such as questioning, listening, acting assertively, and the like. There is an implicit assumption in much of the nursing literature that communication skills are of this ilk. A consequence, rightly pointed out by Doane (2002) in criticism of this (as she calls it) 'behavioral

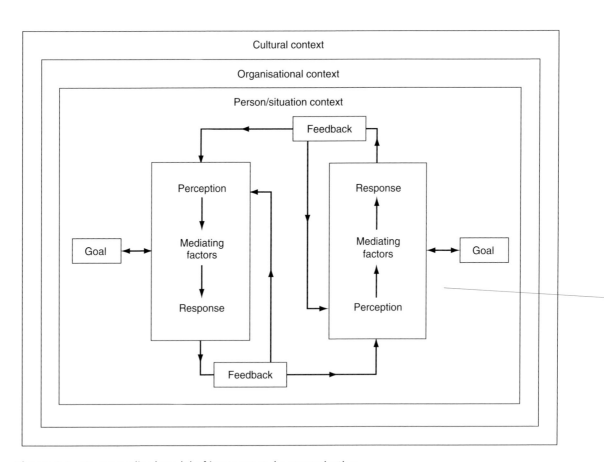

Figure 4.1 Contextualised model of interpersonal communication

skills' approach, may be to breed fixed, inflexible ways of relating on the part of the nurse. A different position is taken here favouring skill being specified, not in terms of behaviour per se, but rather the ongoing processes of monitoring, reflective adaptation and adjustment, within the parameters outline above, as participants work at achieving, modifying or abandoning their interactive goals. (When we talk of skills as 'things' in this chapter these process qualities should be assumed to be features of the behaviour.) It seems to us that there is no inherent quality in activities like questioning, listening, or any of the other commonly cited 'skills', by dint of which they can be unswervingly categorised as such.

Goals

Communication is held to be essentially purposive and goal-directed (Berger 2003; Wilson 2002). As put by Wilson and Sabee (2003, p. 18), 'Many contemporary theories assume that speakers produce messages to accomplish goals and thus develop and enact plans for pursuing goals...' Projected outcomes give direction to, and also mobilise effort in, interacting (Dillard 1990). Likewise, the goal-oriented nature of nursing has been highlighted by, for example, Arnold and Boggs (2003, p. 124) who explained that 'developing professional goals helps the nurse select concrete, specific nursing actions that are purposeful and aligned with individualized client needs'.

Concentrating specifically on community nursing, communication for Spradley and Allender (1996) serves to:

- Offer information for decision making at all levels
- Motivate by clarifying detail so that there is agreement about what to do
- Facilitate affective expression and effect a closer working relationship
- Control behaviour by establishing expectations and setting boundaries

Additionally, communication sometimes has a role-related or ritualistic function.

The goals of the nurse may be complementary or at odds with those of the service user or other health care professional. Patients may even be unsure as to what their goals should be because of unfamiliarity with the situation and circumstances of illness. Premised upon an ideology of participation and partnership, an initial goal of the nurse (a meta-goal) may be to work towards developing agreed personal goals (Arnold & Boggs 2003). The importance, in community health care nursing, of all parties moving together to achieve conjointly agreed health outcomes is heavily stressed (Orr 1992).

For the most part, interactors pursue a multiplicity of goals during interaction, mirroring the different dimensions of interpersonal communication already mentioned. Traditionally, nurses have accentuated those serving instrumental purposes (Chant *et al*. 2002; Kruijver *et al*. 2001; McCabe 2004). Correspondingly, they seem much more confident in their physical care than in their levels of communicative competence (Corner & Wilson-Barnett 1992). Nurses have also rated higher their communicative abilities to deal with clinical or community situations requiring essentially authoritative approaches such as informing, confronting or prescribing, compared with those requiring facilitative alternatives including supportive, catalytic or cathartic involvement (Morrison & Burnard 1989). In a more recent extension of this work, Ashmore and Banks (2004) investigated student nurses' actual use of these types of skills in clinical role-play scenarios, rather than merely their perceptions of their abilities. While the results were open to different interpretations, evidence emerged of limited or flawed supportive communication. Paradoxically, it is just those authoritative approaches to care with which the nurse feels more comfortable that are regarded as often misapplied, according to much contemporary thinking on community nursing practice. Accordingly, Lee and Garvin (2003) advocated replacing the term information transfer (which connotes a one-way, one-sided monologue) with information exchange (based upon a more egalitarian two-way sharing of expertise) when referring to health information provision for patients.

Perception

Our perceptions of the other, our circumstances and indeed ourselves, are fundamental to skilful interaction. While the ability to demonstrate acceptable levels of observation is a requirement of the nurse (Scott 2003), the fundamental nature of the process means that acuity and accuracy are never guaranteed. This is particularly so when it comes to making judgements of others. How we read them typically owes as much, if not more, to ourselves in perceiving as it does to the person being perceived: 'There is no "immutable reality" of the other person awaiting our discovery' (Wilmot 1995, p. 150). A range of perceptual barriers to successful communication in community nursing is accordingly explored by Dickson (1999) and Newman (2003).

Social perceiving is essentially selective, inferential and heavily dependent upon the knowledge structures, expectations and attributional processes of the perceiver. Lack of perceptual sensitivity also means that important interactive detail is neglected. Nurses regarded as excellent were able, amongst other qualities, to spot unexpressed patient needs through their sensitivity to nonverbal behaviour (Redfern & Norman 1999). But it seems that in many cases inaccuracies persist when tuning in to patients' worry, anxiety and stress (Biley 1989; Lauri *et al.* 1997) such that nurses have been accused of frequently failing to notice or misconstrue emotional cues (Faulkner & Maguire 1984). Referring specifically to mental health nurses, Proctor and Welbourn (2002) stressed that they need to display greater 'emotional intelligence'. These tutors go on to lament the under-representation of this area in training.

Self-awareness on the part of the nurse is a further requirement if quality interpersonal engagement with service users is to be enjoyed. As put by Betts: (2003, p. 74) 'Effective communication requires people to maximise self-awareness, both in terms of how behaviour is perceived by others and also in understanding one's own motivations and blind spots.'

Mediating factors

These refer to a complex of cognitive and affective processes by means of which strategies for action emerge in keeping with perceptions of unfolding events, as goals are pursued. However, these processes seldom occupy much conscious attention, as a rule, when operating under familiar sets of circumstances (Bull 2002).

Intrapersonal components of interpersonal communication operating at this stage are discussed in terms of the organising, processing and evaluation of information, decision making and the selection of action plans (Berger 2003; Canary 2003; and Hargie & Dickson 2004; Kreps 1988). For Wyer and Gruenfeld (1995) the sub-processes leading to a strategic interpersonal response include:

- *Semantic encoding* – the interpretation of messages in keeping with available semantic concepts and structures
- *Organisation* – the arranging of information into mental representations of the person, thing, or event
- *Storage and retrieval* – the storage of these representations in memory and their subsequent selective access as and when required
- *Inference processes* – decisions to respond are shaped by inferences about the implications and consequences of that action
- *Response generation* – of over-riding importance here are the strategies selected to bring about targeted goals and objectives

Response

In accordance with goals pursued, particular action strategies are decided upon and operationalised in verbal and non-verbal (including vocal) responses. It is widely recognised, and for some time, that those who are ill may reveal themselves nonverbally in important ways, as well as being particularly sensitive to cues of this type picked up from carers (Friedman 1982). Non-verbal vocal responses (as distinct from *body language*) are often collectively referred to as *paralanguage* (i.e. *how* what is said, including such speech features as the nurse's intonation, tone and quality of voice). It is frequently through paralanguage that the attitudes and emotional states of the speaker are revealed (Knapp & Hall 1997). Carers' paralinguistic cues have also been associated with patients' ability to recall various kinds of verbally transmitted health information (Northouse & Northouse 1998).

Non-verbal and verbal communication intermesh in sophisticated ways (Jones & LeBaron 2002), although the former is held to convey primarily affective information about emotions, attitudes, identities and such like, while language carries cognitive detail of events, ideas, happenings and so forth. When it comes to health communication, though, language often fails owing not only to the actual words used, but also to the underlying concepts and systems of understanding brought to bear. Meanings are very much in people, not in words! Patients' need to have understanding of their condition and treatment (Fleitas 2003; Schmidt 2003) often goes unmet because of the use of jargon and inappropriate verbal codes (Chapman *et al.* 2003). Apart from blatant jargon and esoteric medical terms, more mundane expressions like 'risk factor' may not always succeed in conveying the intended message to, for example, patients with myocardial infarction and their families (Turton 1998). Nurses, though, are identified as being uniquely positioned to act as 'information brokers' between health care users and physicians (Fleitas 2003: Griffie *et al.* 2004) placing a special premium upon their ability to explain effectively in language that can be readily grasped by the recipient (Duman & Clark 2003).

Feedback

Through feedback, judgements can be made as to the extent to which messages have been successfully received and with what impact. Monitoring patient reactions enables subsequent nurse communication to be adapted and regulated appropriately. As such, communicative success is only possible when information about the outcome of a message is made available to the sender for subsequent action (Lumsden & Lumsden 2003).

Adequate self-monitoring of performance is a further important component of feedback. The importance of the nurse's self-awareness has already been emphasised in promoting effective interpersonal interaction.

Person/situation context

Communication is heavily context bound. Interaction takes place, most directly, within a person–situation context that shapes what unfolds (Hargie & Dickson 2004). Likewise, in reviewing variables that impact upon nurse–patient communication, Caris-Verhallen *et al.* (1997) categorised them as pertaining to the nurse, the patient and the situation. Not only is what ensues a feature of personal characteristics and predispositions of both nurse and service user (and including knowledge, values, attitudes, age, gender, personality and socio-economic background) but is co-determined by situational factors such as the roles demanded and rules which pertain. Physical features of the setting, including opportunities for privacy, are also relevant.

Situational factors, of course, have a particular bearing on work in the community. Home visits for the elderly have been found to have direct benefits when measured in terms of mortality and admission to long-term institutional care (Elkan *et al.* 2001). But nursing in the home brings with it an additional role not encountered in the institutional setting – that of 'guest' (Baly *et al.* 1987) – with possibilities of role conflict and confusion. Being a guest is held by Trojan and Yonge (1993) to contribute to the initial phase of establishing a caring relationship when nursing older people. Furthermore, the use of phatic communication (i.e. communication used to mark relationship ties rather than carry content) by the community nurse, to this end, is illuminated by Burnard (2004).

The home as environmental setting can also constitute a source of distraction and disturbance, of course, getting in the way of meaningful engagement. Intrusive noise is mentioned by Taylor and Campbell (1999) in the form of television, radio and other people. Lack of privacy can be an additional factor curtailing facilitative communication with service users. Certainly, Lomas (2004) cited the careful selection of an appropriate location in best practice guidelines to be taken into account by nurses in the challenging task of breaking bad news.

Organisational context

The organisation represents a further framework of communication channels and structures, norms, expectations, opportunities (and barriers), impinging upon what happens between nurse and service user. Lammers *et al.* (2003) identified size, complexity, formalisation, climate and history as organisational features with a particular relevance for communication and service quality. Unfortunately, institutional structures of health care delivery often run counter to the deployment of good interpersonal skills (Chant *et al.* 2002). Specific causes include staff shortages and care management practices resulting in lack of time with patients; definitions of 'good' nursing that foreground physical care to the detriment of psychosocial needs; norms of the ward and attitude of the ward sister; lack of emotional support for staff; and even the wearing of uniforms (Hagerty & Patusky 2003; McCabe 2004; Scott 2003; Wondrack 1998). Indeed, Menzies-Lyth (1988) went as far as to suggest that such systems are subconsciously put in place as a form of emotional defence for staff.

Limited time available to talk with, and listen to, patients would appear to be a persistent consequence of work allocation and budgetary strategy. In a study of health visitors working with older people, Rogers (2003, p. 384) reported that, 'all the respondents, both generic and specialist, felt hampered by lack of time'. This was exacerbated by management attitudes and consequent resource allocation that seemed to devalue this particular user group. That said, Grainger (1995) found, from her work on nursing older people in residential care, that while nurses complained about not having enough time to talk to the residents, when they did have spare time on their hands, they spent it chatting with other nurses. Additionally, Thompson (1994) reviewed some evidence to suggest that there is little correlation between time spent with the patient, per se, and quality of communication entered into.

Managerial styles and influences are additional factors that can impinge upon quality of communication with patients. Staff who are disempowered through exposure to controlling, non-participative management practices and sharp hierarchies of authority are poorly equipped to engage with patients in empowering ways (Cuff 1997; Yam & Rossiter 2000). There is certainly good evidence that the particular ward on which they worked had a profound effect upon nurses' communication with cancer patients (Wilkinson 1991). In addition to management expectation, emotional support provided is another factor. In reviewing some of the findings, Chant *et al.* (2002, p. 19) identified '...the role of inadequate social support and support structures to deal with emotional distress as a barrier to effective communication'.

Cultural context

More broadly still, cultural and sub-cultural variables have a bearing on the different features of the communicative process between nurse and patient. Culture, in short, can be regarded as '...a set of attitudes, behaviors and symbols shared by a large group of people and usually communicated from one generation to the next' (Shiraev & Levy 2004, p. 4). The view is stridently expressed by Arnold (2003, p. 267) that, 'Culturally sensitive communication is essential when providing holistic nursing care for clients from different cultural backgrounds'. In reaction to advancing pluralism and the multi-ethnic nature of UK society, health policies are being put in place to safeguard equality in health care provision (e.g. *The Vital Connection*, DoH 2000b). Service users from minority groups are expected to have their cultural differences accommodated.

Inter-cultural differences run much deeper than possible differences in language, although these are not to be dismissed (Dunckley *et al.* 2003), encompassing not only much of the nonverbal channel of communication but beyond to the underlying social order itself and the meanings and values that give it form. When a nurse and patient from radically different cultures come together, it is not only that they may have different language codes to represent a shared world,

Their social worlds may overlap only marginally. Such cultural diversity can impact at the level of what health and illness means to each, understandings of how one becomes unwell, how one should express one's illness and pain, and how cure can be effected (Street 2003). 'Depression', for example, does not appear in the Chinese lexicon. There it is more acceptable for patients to present with multiple somatic symptoms (Arnold 2003). The interpersonal process of caring, with attendant patterns of accustomed interaction, is also highly contextualised in this way. Griffie *et al.* (2004) revealed, for instance, that amongst some peoples, including Greeks and Ethiopians, openness and truthfulness in explaining an unfavourable diagnosis or prognosis can be regarded as unnecessarily cruel to the extent of even harming the patient.

Returning to the model presented in Figure 4.1, while these are held to be the most significant contexts impacting upon the interpersonal process, there is no assumption that these are the only ones. Indeed, in developing a similar conceptual framework around the medical consultation, Street (2003) specified additional political–legal and media contexts.

Conclusion

Communication lies at the heart of quality nursing care. The picture emerging from the literature on nurse–patient interaction is one that portrays nurses recognising the value of these skills (Bugge *et al.* 1999), feeling less confident in their abilities in this regard (especially in adopting more facilitative approaches) than those to do with providing physical care (Corner & Wilson-Barnett 1992), expressing a need in some cases for further training (Jarrett & Payne 1995), and being frequently criticised for engaging in low-grade communication at odds with patient-centred care (Chant *et al.* 2002; McCabe 2004). But does it matter?

From an evidence-based practice perspective, there is defensible research suggesting that patients who enjoy good quality communication tend to be more satisfied with the care received, exercise greater adherence to agreed/recommended treatment regimens and courses of action, and make more rapid recoveries with fewer complications. (See reviews by Brown *et al.* 2003; Dickson *et al.* 1997; Stewart 1995). Most of this work has concentrated upon the effects of providing information for patients/carers, being sensitive to their psycho-emotional needs, and adopting a patient-centred approach. The majority of the studies have also been conducted in medical settings, evoking a call for more research of this type specifically in nursing (Caris-Verhallen *et al.* 1997). Still, empirical investigations that are available in nursing again point to a substantial role for communication (see reviews by Brown 1999; Thompson 1994; Wilkinson *et al.* 2003).

Truly skilful interaction, as elaborated in this chapter, requires adaptive flexibility in reaching joint goals within a complex of contextualisations, including personal, situational, organisational and cultural factors. The challenge for the next generation of nurse–patient communication research is to begin to disentangle those nurse, patient, and contextual variables under which communication of a particular type leads to positive and acceptable service user outcomes.

References

Albarran, J. & Whittle, C. (1999) Specialist and advanced nursing practice: the debate. In: *Current Issues in Community Nursing: Specialist Practice in Primary Health Care* (J. Littlewood ed), Churchill Livingstone, Edinburgh.

Argyle, M. (1983) *The Psychology of Interpersonal Behaviour*. Penguin, Harmondsworth.

Arnold, E. (2003) Intercultural communication. In: *Interpersonal Relationships: Professional Communication Skills for Nurses*, 4th ed. (E. Arnold, & K. Boggs eds). Saunders, St Louis, Missouri.

Arnold, E. & Boggs, K. (2003) *Interpersonal Relationships: Professional Communication Skills for Nurses*, 4th ed., Saunders, St Louis, Missouri.

Ashmore, R. & Banks, D. (2004) Student nurses' use of their interpersonal skills within clinical role-plays, *Nurse Education Today*, **24**, 20–29.

Baly, M., Robottom, B. & Clark, J. (1987) *District Nursing*. Heinemann Nursing, London.

Barnard, A. & Sandelowski, M. (2001) Technology and humane nursing care: (ir)reconcilable or invented difference? *Journal of Advanced Nursing*, **34**, 367–75.

Berger, C. (2003) Message production skill in social interaction. In: *Handbook of Communication and Social Interaction Skills* (J.O. Greene & B.R. Burleson eds). Lawrence Erlbaum Associates, Mahwah, New Jersey.

Betts, A. (2003) Improving communication. In: *Interpersonal Communication in Nursing; Theory and Practice*, (R. Ellis, B. Gates & N. Kenworthy eds). Churchill Livingstone, Edinburgh.

Biley, F. (1989) Nurses' perception of stress in pre-operative surgical patients. *Journal of Advanced Nursing*, **14**, 575–81.

Bowles, N., Mackintosh, C. & Torn, A. (2001) Nurses' communication skills: an evaluation of the impact of solution-focused communication training. *Journal of Advanced Nursing*, **36**, 347–354.

Brown, J.B., Stewart, M. & Ryan, B L. (2003) Outcome of Patient-Provider Interaction. In: *Handbook of Health Communication* (T. Thompson, A.M. Dorsey, K.I. Miller & R. Parrott eds). Lawrence Erlbaum Associates, Mahwah, New Jersey.

Brown, S. (1999) Patient-centred communication. *Annual Review of Nursing Research*, **17**, 85–104.

Bugge, C., Smith, L. & Shanley, E. (1999) A descriptive survey to identify the perceived skills and community skill requirements of mental health staff. *Journal of Advanced Nursing*, **29**, 218–228.

Bull, P. (2002) *Communication Under the Microscope: The Theory and Practice of Microanalysis*, Routledge, Hove and New York.

Bulsara, C., Ward, A. & Joske, D. (2004) Haematological cancer patients: achieving a sense of empowerment of strategies to control illness. *Journal of Clinical Nursing*, **13**, 251–258.

Burkitt Wright, E., Holcombe, P. & Salmon, P. (2004) Doctors' communication of trust, care, and respect in breast cancer: qualitative study. *British Medical Journal*, **328**, 864–867.

Burnard, P. (2004) Phatic communication and community nursing, *Journal of Community Nursing*, **18**, 8–10.

Canary, D.J. (2003) Managing interpersonal conflict: a model of events related to strategic choice. In: *Handbook of Communication and Social Interaction Skills* (J.O. Greene & B.R. Burleson eds). Lawrence Erlbaum Associates, Mahwah, New Jersey.

Caris-Verhallen, W., Kerkstra, A. & Bensing, J. (1997) The role of communication in nursing care for elderly people: a review of the literature. *Journal of Advanced Nursing*, **25**, 915–933.

Caris-Verhallen, W., Kerkstra, A. & Bensing, J. (1999) Non-verbal communication in nurse-elderly patient communication. *Journal of Advanced Nursing*, **29**, 808–818.

Castledine, G. (2004) The importance of the nurse–patient relationship. *British Journal of Nursing*, **13**, (4), 231.

Chambers-Evans, J., Stelling, J. & Godin, M. (1999) Learning to listen: serendipitous of a research training experience. *Journal of Advanced Nursing*, **29**, 1421–1426.

Chant, S., Jenkinson, T., Randle, J. & Russell, G. (2002) Communication skills: some problems in nursing. *Journal of Clinical Nursing*, **11**, 12–21.

Chapman, K., Abraham, C., Jenkins, V. & Fallowfield, L. (2003) Lay understanding of terms used in cancer consultations. *Psycho-Oncology*, **12**, 557–566.

Cooke, S., Wakefield, A., Chew-Graham, C. & Boggis, C. (2003) Collaborative training in breaking bad news to patients. *Journal of Interpersonal Care*, **17**, 307–309.

Corner, J. & Wilson-Barnett, J. (1992) The newly registered nurse and the cancer patient: an educational evaluation. *International Journal of Nursing Studies*, **29**, 177–190.

Crute, V. (1986) *Microtraining in Health Visitor Education: An Intensive Examination of Training Outcomes, Feedback Processes and Individual Differences*. Unpublished PhD Thesis, University of Ulster.

Cuff, D. (1997) Sharing in Partnership. In: *Contemporary Community Nursing* (S. Burley, E. Mitchell, K. Melling, S. Chilton & C. Crumplin eds). Arnold, London.

Department of Health (1997) *The New NHS: Modern, dependable*. DoH, London.

Department of Health (1998) *A First Class Service – Quality in the new NHS*. DoH, London.

Department of Health (2000a) *The NHS Plan*. DoH, London.

Department of Health (2000b) *The Vital Connection: An Equalities Framework for the NHS*. DoH, London.

Dickson, D. (1999) Barriers to communication. In: *Interaction for Practice in Community Nursing* (A. Long ed). MacMillan, Houndmills, Basingstoke.

Dickson, D. (2001) Communication skills and health care delivery. In: *Community Health Care Nursing*, 2nd edn. (D. Sines, F. Appleby & E. Raymond eds). Blackwell Science, Oxford.

Dickson, D., Hargie, O. & Morrow, N. (1997) *Communication Skills Training for Health Professionals*. Chapman and Hall, London.

Dillard, J. (1990) The nature and substance of goals in tactical communication. In: *The Psychology of Tactical*

Communication (M. Cody & M. McLaughlin eds). Multilingual Matters, Cleveland, England.

Doane, G.A.H. (2002) Beyond behavioral skills to human-involved processes: relational nursing practice and interpretive pedagogy, *Journal of Nursing Education*, **41**, 400–404.

Duman, M. & Clark, A. (2003) Patient information: Part 1. Why provide information? *Professional Nurse*, **19**, 58–59.

Dunckley, M., Hughes, R., Addington-Hall, J.M. & Higginson, I.J. (2003) Translating clinical tools in nursing practice, *Journal of Advanced Nursing*, **44**, 420–426.

Duxbury, J. (2000) *Difficult Patients*. Butterworth-Heinemann, Oxford.

Elkan, R., Kendrick, D., Dewey, M., Hewitt, M., *et al.* (2001) Effectiveness of home based support for older people: systematic review and meta-analysis, *British Medical Journal*, **323**, 719–725.

Ellis, R.B., Gates, B. & Kenworthy, N. (2003) *Interpersonal Communication in Nursing*. Churchill Livingstone, Edinburgh.

Farley, A. & Hendry, C. (2004) Be prepared: how to take the fear out of giving a presentation, *Professional Nurse*, **19**, 410–412.

Faulkner, A. & Maguire, P. (1984) Teaching Assessment Skills. In: *Recent Advances in Nursing, 7, Communication.* (A. Faulkner ed). Churchill Livingstone, Edinburgh.

Fentiman, I. (2003) Litigation and doctor–patient communication. *Clinical Risk.* **9**, 180–181.

Fleitas, J. (2003) The power of words: examining the linguistic landscape of pediatric nursing, *MCN*, **28**, 384–388.

Fletcher, J. (1997) Do nurses really care? Some unwelcome findings from recent research and inquiry. *Journal of Nursing Management*, **5**, 43–50.

Friedman, H. (1982) Nonverbal communication in medical interaction. In: *Interpersonal Issues in Health Care* (H. Friedman & M. DiMatteo eds). Academic Press, New York.

Grainger, K. (1995) Communication and the institutionalised elderly. In: *Handbook of Communication and Ageing Research* (J. Nussbaum & J. Coupland eds). Lawrence Erlbaum Associates, Mahwah, New Jersey.

Goode, M.L. (2004) Communication barriers when managing a patient with a wound. *British Journal of Nursing*, **13**, (1), 49–52.

Greene, J.O. (2003) Models of adult communication skill acquisition: practice and the course of performance improvement. In: *Handbook of Communication and Social Interaction Skills* (J.O. Greene & B.R. Burleson eds). Lawrence Erlbaum Associates, Mahwah, New Jersey.

Griffie, J., Nelson-Marten, P. & Muchka, S. (2004) Acknowledging the 'Elephant': communication in palliative care, *American Journal of Nursing*, **104**, 48–57.

Hagerty, B.M. & Patusky, K.L. (2003) Reconceptualizing the nurse–patient relationship, *Journal of Nursing Scholarship*, **35**, 145–150.

Hargie, O. (1997) Communication as skilled performance. In: *The Handbook of Communication Skills* (O. Hargie ed). Routledge, London.

Hargie, O. & Dickson, D. (2004) *Skilled Interpersonal Communication: Research, Theory and Practice*. Routledge, Hove and New York.

Hargie, O., Dickson, D. & Tourish, D. (2004) *Communication Skills for Effective Management*. Palgrave Macmillan, Basingstoke.

Hartley, P. (1999) *Interpersonal Communication*. Routledge, London.

Hewes, D. & Planalp, S. (1987) The individual's place in communication science. In: *Handbook of Communication Science.* (C. Berger & S. Chaffee eds). Sage, Beverly Hills, California.

Hewitt-Taylor, J. (2004) Challenging the balance of power: patient empowerment. *Nursing Standard*, **18**, 33–37.

Jarrett, N. & Payne, S. (1995) A selective review of the literature on nurse–patient communication: has the patient's contribution been neglected. *Journal of Advanced Nursing*, **22**, 72–78.

Jones, S.E. & LeBaron, C.D. (2002) Research on the relationship between verbal and nonverbal communication: emerging integrations. *Journal of Communication*, **52**, 499–521.

Knapp, M. & Hall, J. (1997) *Nonverbal Communication in Human Interaction*, 4th edn., Fort Worth. Harcourt Brace College Publishers.

Kreps, G. (1988) The pervasive role of information in health and health care: implications for health care policy. In: *Communication Yearbook 11.* (J. Anderson ed). Sage, Beverly Hills, California.

Kruijver, I.P.M., Kerkstra, A., Bensing, J.M., & van de Wiel, H. (2001) Communication skills of nurses during interactions with cancer patients, *Journal of Advanced Nursing*, **34**, 772–779.

Kyle, W.L. (2001) The influence of technology in nursing practice with elder care facilities. *Vision*, **7**, 20–23.

Lammers, J.C., Barbour, J.B. & Duggan, A.P. (2003) Organizational forms of the provision of health care: an institutional perspective. In: *Handbook of*

Health Communication (T. Thompson, A.M. Dorsey, K.I. Miller & R. Parrott eds). Lawrence Erlbaum Associates, Mahwah, New Jersey.

Lauri, S., Lepisto, M. & Kappeli, S. (1997) Patients' needs in hospital: nurses' and patients' views. *Journal of Advanced Nursing*, **25**, 339–346.

Lawson, M.L. (2002) Nurse practitioner and physician communication styles. *Applied Nursing Research*. **15**, 60–62.

Lee, R.G. & Garvin, T. (2003) Moving from information transfer to information exchange in health and health care. *Social Science and Medicine*, **56**, 449–464.

Lefebvre, M. (2003) Nursing uniforms:dead or alive? *Nursing News*. **23**, 23.

Lloyd, M. & Bor, R. (2004) *Communication Skills for Medicine*. Churchill Livingstone, Edinburgh.

Lomas, D. (2004) The development of best practice in breaking bad news to patients, *Nursing Times*, **100**, 28–30.

Lumsden, G. & Lumsden, D. (2003) *Communicating with Credibility and Confidence*, Wadsworth, Belmont, California.

Martin, G. (1998) Communication breakdown or ideal speech situation: the problem of nurse advocacy. *Nursing Ethics*, **5**, 147–157.

McCabe, C. (2004) Nurse–patient communication: an exploration of patients' experiences. *Journal of Clinical Nursing*, **13**, 41–49.

McCann, K. & McKenna, H. (1993) An examination of touch between nurses and elderly patients in a continuing care setting in Northern Ireland. *Journal of Advanced Nursing*, **18**, 838–946.

McCulloch, P. (2004) The patient experience of receiving bad news from health professionals. *Professional Nurse*, **19**, 276–280.

McGrane, F.M. (2003) *One-to-one Dispute Resolution in the Workplace: A Skills Perspective*. Unpublished PhD Thesis, University of Ulster, Jordanstown.

Meerabeau, E. (2004) Be good, sweet maid, and let who can be clever: a counter reformation in English nursing education? *International Journal of Nursing Studies*, **41**, 285–292.

Menzies-Lyth, I. (1988) *Defence Systems as Control Against Anxiety*. Tavistock, London.

Metts, S. & Grohskopf, E. (2003) Impression management. Goals, strategies, and skills. In: *Handbook of Communication and Social Interaction Skills* (J.O. Greene & B.R. Burleson eds). Lawrence Erlbaum Associates, Mahwah, New Jersey.

Miczo, N., Segrin, C. & Allspach, L. (2001) Relationship between nonverbal sensitivity, encoding, and relational satisfaction, *Communication Reports*, **14**, 39–48.

Moore, D. (2003) Communicating with the wider world. In: *Interpersonal Communication in Nursing* (R.B. Ellis, B. Gates & N. Kenworthy eds). Churchill Livingstone, Edinburgh.

Morrison, P. & Burnard, P. (1997) *Caring and Communicating*. MacMillan Press, Basingstoke.

Morrison, P. & Burnard, P. (1989) Students' and trained nurses' perceptions of their own interpersonal skills: a report and comparison. *Journal of Advanced Nursing*, **14**, 321–329.

Morse, J., Havens, G. & Wilson, S. (1997) The comforting interaction: developing a model of nurse–patient relationship. *Scholarly Inquiry for Nursing Practice: An International Journal*, **11**, 321–343.

Mullally, S. (2003) The importance of top-quality patient information. *Professional Nurse*, **19**, 65.

Newman, A.M. (2003) Self-concept in the nurse–patient relationship. In: *Interpersonal Relationships: Professional Communication Skills for Nurses*, 4th ed. (E. Arnold & K. Boggs eds). Saunders, St Louis, Missouri.

Northouse, L. & Northouse, P. (1998) *Health Communication*. Appleton & Lange, Stamford, Connecticut.

Nursing & Midwifery Council (2002) *Code of Professional Conduct*. NMC, London.

Orr, J. (1992) The community dimension. In: *Health Visiting: Towards Community Health Nursing* (K. Luker & J. Orr eds). Blackwell Scientific, Oxford.

Pearson, A., Baker, H., Walsh, K. & Fitzgerald, M. (2001) Contemporary nurses' uniforms – history and traditions. *Journal of Nursing Management*, **9**, 147–152.

Proctor, K. & Welbourn, T. (2002) Meeting the needs of the modern mental health nurse: a review of a higher education diploma in nursing communication module. *Nurse Education in Practice*, **2**, 237–243.

Quinn, F.M. (2000) *Principles and Practice of Nurse Education*, 4th edn. Stanley Thornes, Cheltenham.

Reardon, K. (1987) *Where Minds Meet*. Wadsworth, Belmont.

Redfern, S. & Norman, I. (1999) Quality of nursing care perceived by patients and their nurses: an application of the critical incident technique. Part 2. *Journal of Clinical Nursing*, **8**, 407–421.

Reynolds, R. & Scott, B. (2000) Do nurses and other professional helpers normally display much empathy? *Journal of Advanced Nursing*, **31**, 226–234.

Riley, J. (2004) *Communication in Nursing*, 5th edn. Mosby, St Louis.

Rogers, E. (2003) Health visitors and older people: 'thinking out of the box', *Community Practitioner*, **76**, 381–385.

Rosengren, K. (2000) *Communication: An Introduction.* Sage, London.

Royal College of Nursing (2003) *Defining Nursing.* RCN, London.

Salmon, P. & Hall, G.M. (2004) Patient empowerment or the emperor's new clothes. *Journal of the Royal Society of Medicine.* **97**, 53–56.

Saunders, S. (2003) Why communication skills are good for theatre nurses. *Nursing Times,* **100**, 42–44.

Schmidt, L.A. (2003) Patients' perceptions of nursing care in the hospital setting, *Journal of Advanced Nursing,* **44**, 393–399.

Scott, G. (2003) Has nursing lost its heart? *Nursing Standard,* **18**, 12–13.

Shiraev, E. & Levy, D. (2004) *Cross-cultural Psychology: Critical Thinking and Contemporary Applications,* Pearson, Boston.

Skipper, M. (1992) *Communication Processes and their Effectiveness in the Management and Treatment of Dysphagia.* Unpublished DPhil Thesis, University of Ulster.

Slevin, O. (1999) The nurse–patient relationship. In: *Interaction for Practice in Community Nursing* (ed. A. Long). MacMillan, Houndmills, Basingstoke.

Spitzberg, B.H. (2003) Methods of interpersonal skill assessment. In: *Handbook of Communication and Social Interaction Skills* (J.O. Greene & B.R. Burleson eds). Lawrence Erlbaum Associates, Mahwah, New Jersey.

Spitzberg, B.H. & Cupach, W. (2002) Interpersonal Skills. In: *Handbook of Interpersonal Communication* (M.L. Knapp & J.A. Daly eds). Sage Publications, Thousand Oaks.

Spradley, B. & Allender, J. (1996) *Community Health Care Nursing: Concepts and Practice.* Lippincott, Philadelphia.

Stewart, M. (1995) Effective physician–patient communication and health outcomes: a review. *Canadian Medical Association,* **152**, 1423–1433.

Stichler, J.F. (2002) The nurse as consultant. *Nursing Administration Quarterly,* **26**, 52–68.

Street, R.L. (2003) Communication in medical encounters: an ecological perspective. In: *Handbook of Health Communication* (T. Thompson, A.M. Dorsey, K.I. Miller & R. Parrott eds). Lawrence Erlbaum Associates, Mahwah, New Jersey.

Sutcliffe, K.M., Lewton, E. & Rosenthal, M.M. (2004) Communication failures: an insidious contributor to medical mishap. *Academic Medicine,* **79**, 186–194.

Taylor, M. & Campbell, C. (1999) Communication skills in the operating department, *British Journal of Theatre Nursing,* **9**, 217–220.

Thompson, T. (1994) Interpersonal communication and health care. In: *Handbook of Interpersonal Communication* (M. Knapp & G. Miller eds). Sage, Thousand Oaks, California.

Thorsteinsson, L.S.C.H. (2002) The quality of nursing care as perceived by individuals with chronic illnesses: the magical touch of nursing. *Journal of Clinical Nursing,* **11**, 32–44.

Tran, A.N., Haidet, P., Street, R.L., O'Malley, K.J, Martin, F. & Ashton, C.M. (2004) Empowering communication: a community-based intervention for patients. *Patient Education & Counselling,* **52**, 113–121.

Trenholm, S. & Jenson, A. (2000) *Interpersonal communication,* 4th edn. Wadsworth, Belmont.

Trojan, L. & Yonge, O. (1993) Developing trusting, caring relationship: home acre nurses and elderly clients. *Journal of Advanced Nursing,* **18**, 1903–1910.

Trower, P. (1984) A radical critique and reformulation: From organism to agent. In: *Radical Approaches to Social Skills Training* (P. Trower ed). Croom Helm, London.

Turton, J. (1998) Importance of information following myocardial infarction: a study of the self-perceived needs of patients and their spouse/partner compared with the perceptions of nursing staff. *Journal of Advanced Nursing,* **27**, 770–778.

Watzlawick, P., Beavin, J. & Jackson, D. (1967) *Pragmatics of Human Communication.* W.W. Norton, New York.

Wiemann, J.M. (2003) Foreword. In: *Handbook of Communication and Social Interaction Skills* (J.O. Greene & B.R. Burleson eds). Lawrence Erlbaum Associates, Mahwah, New Jersey.

Wilkinson, S. (1991) Factors which influence how nurses communicate with cancer patients, *Journal of Advanced Nursing,* **16**, 677–688.

Wilkinson, S.M., Leliopoulou, C., Gamble, M. & Roberts, A. (2003) Can intensive three-day programmes improve nurses' communication skills in cancer care? *Psycho-Oncology,* **12**, 747–759.

Wilmot, W. (1995) The transactional nature of person perception. In: *Bridges not Walls: A Book About Interpersonal Communication* (J. Stewart ed). McGraw-Hill, New York.

Wilson, S.R. (2002) *Seeking and Resisting Compliance: Why People Say What They Do When Trying to Influence Others.* Sage, Thousand Oaks, California.

Wilson, S.R. & Sabee, C.M. (2003) Explicating communicative competence as a theoretical term. In: *Handbook of Communication and Social Interaction*

Skills (J.O. Greene & B.R. Burleson eds). Lawrence Erlbaum Associates, Mahwah, New Jersey.

Wood, J. (2004) *Interpersonal Communication: Everyday Encounters*, 4th edn., Wadsworth Belmont.

Wondrack, R. (1998) *Interpersonal Skills for Nurses and Health Care Professionals*. Blackwell Science, Oxford.

Wyer, R. & Gruenfeld, D. (1995) Information processing in interpersonal communication. In: *The Cognitive Basis of Interpersonal Communication* (D. Hewes ed). Lawrence Erlbaum Associates, Hillsdale, New Jersey.

Yam, B. & Rossiter, J. (2000) Caring in nursing: perceptions of Hong Kong nurses, *Journal of Clinical Nursing*, **9**, 293–302.

Chapter 5 Community Development in Public Health and Primary Care

Jane Wills

Introduction

Primary care organisations have been placed at the centre of health services development in the major changes that have taken place in the organisation of health services in recent years. In addition to their role in the treatment of ill health and the commissioning of secondary care services, they are also expected to take the lead in improving the health of their local populations. Public partnership and involvement is enshrined in recent health policy initiatives and the focus on a needs-led service has revived interest in community development approaches.

The NHS Plan (DoH 2000) sets out the vision of a service where care is shaped around the convenience and concerns of patients, their carers and the public – where all will have more say over their own treatment and more influence over the way in which the organisation works. The rationale behind this draws on a growing understanding that:

- Patients' experience of care is intimately tied to the effectiveness of that care – patients' views can help to improve the impact of health care services
- The way care is provided affects more than satisfaction with care, but also patients' physiological, functional and psychological outcomes
- Health care services need to adapt to the changing needs and aspirations of better-informed and more assertive patients/public (Crawford *et al.* 2002; Florin & Dixon 2004)

Participatory approaches to involvement can cover a broad spectrum of attitude and purpose. Taylor (2003) describes these as the consumerist approach in which people are asked for their views on specific issues or services, the representative approach where members of the public sit on advisory groups and committees to community development which involves active engagement with a defined group of people over an extended period of time in order to identify and tackle some of the issues that determine their health and quality of life.

These moves to greater public involvement pose the twin challenges for the NHS of transferring power and ensuring that decisions are representative of a public view. Many of the barriers to involvement are linked to the culture of health care professionals that fosters a belief in professional expertise and does not value lay understandings and priorities. Developing appropriate methods to effectively involve the public and their ability to recognise, evaluate and address health problems are further challenges.

This chapter commences with a short outline of the policy context for community development and approaches to health improvement and then explores the term 'community development' and the related concepts of social capital, capacity building and social inclusion.

The second half of the chapter moves on to discuss some of the challenges and opportunities commonly associated with community development approaches including appropriate and compatible methods of evaluation. These will be illustrated by a brief case study of an innovative community health project.

The current context for community development practice

This section outlines the underlying themes of national policies and strategies and how they relate to communities and community development.

The 'Third Way' political philosophy of New Labour embodies values of individual rights, duties and responsibilities as well as social justice and fairness. Public sector services are to be strengthened by firm performance management coupled with a simultaneous move to devolved services, a shift from the market competition of the late twentieth century. These values have given rise to specific strategies and policy initiatives including:

- Devolved services allowing local flexibility and freedom, with additional 'earned autonomy' for best performing services
- Quality assurance through clear standards and performance criteria
- Partnership working to erode professional barriers and enable the delivery of seamless services
- A positive focus on disadvantaged or excluded groups
- A community focus to build capacity and encourage communities to be active providers as well as users of services (Naidoo & Wills 2005)

Government policy has emphasised the importance of participation by users and the public in the modernisation agenda for health and social care. The NHS Executive (1998) published a document on developing strategies for public participation in the NHS, which recommended using community development as a key part of health needs assessment and as a means of engaging communities in solving local health problems in partnership with statutory agencies. A significant lever was added through the Health and Social Care Act 2001 section 11 Strengthening Accountability. A range of new bodies has been set up with the aim of ensuring that, 'the voices of patients, their carers and the public generally are heard and listened to through every level of the service, acting as a lever for change and improvement' (DoH 2001a, para. 2.1). A patient advice and liaison service (PALS) offering a one stop advisory service has been established in each hospital and primary care trust. This acts alongside an independent complaints advocacy service (ICAS). Every NHS trust and PCT has, in addition, a patient forum (PPIF) that represents community views on the quality and design of local health services to the strategic health authority boards. The commitment and recognition of the need for involvement as a key function of the modernisation agenda is summarised by the New Economics Foundation: 'Our institutions are starting to appreciate that a lack of accountability breeds a lack of legitimacy and trust. We are starting to understand that society is now so complex that no decision will stick unless it has involved everybody with a stake in it' (Lewis & Walker 1998, p. 1).

Local government has also undergone a modernisation programme including a more responsive and community oriented approach. A new duty has been imposed on local authorities under the Local Government Act 2000 to take the lead role in drawing up a community strategy alongside local neighbourhood strategies, to enhance local well-being through creating employment opportunities, reducing crime, improving housing and reducing the gap between the better off and disadvantaged areas. This process is overseen by a Local Strategic Partnership that can enable 'local communities to articulate their needs and priorities' (DETR 2000, p. 38).

Alongside this focus on involvement and participation there has been a renewed focus on 'the community' as the site where needs are both defined and met. A recognition that the issues facing local communities – such as social exclusion, regeneration and neighbourhood renewal – are complex and demand multi-agency working means that 'joined-up thinking' and 'joined-up working' have become the catch phrases for making connections across public services and between these services and the public themselves.

There has been a raft of initiatives intended to transform the country's most deprived and excluded areas. Health inequalities are now clearly linked with the concept of social exclusion, the latter being defined as:

'...What happens when individuals or areas suffer from a combination of linked problems such as unemployment, low incomes, poor housing, a high crime environment, poor health and family breakdown.'

(www.socialexclusion.gov.uk)

This concept of social inclusion in which everyone, whatever their circumstances, is encouraged to make use of opportunities to participate in society, permeates policy announcements variously titled as for example: Health Action Zones, Education Action Zones, New Start, Sure Start, New Deal for Communities, Fresh Start – New Deal for Lone Parents, New Deal for Disabilities and New Deal for Employment, alongside support from the New Opportunities Fund (the Lottery) to develop Healthy Living Centres.

A Social Exclusion Unit was introduced by the Labour Government of 1997/2001 and was charged with exploring the scale of the problems in Britain's poorest areas and advising on how they might be tackled. It set up eighteen policy action teams (PATs) to fast track policy thinking on some of the most intractable problems, sometimes referred to as the 'wicked issues', for example, anti-social behaviour, drugs and substance misuse and youth disaffection. Following what has been described as '…one of the most exhaustive studies into social deprivation and regenerative strategy' (Wintour *et al.* 2000), the PAT recommendations were published in April 2000 as the government's draft *National Strategy for Neighbourhood Renewal* (Social Exclusion Unit 2000). The role of local communities in neighbourhood based regeneration programmes is central and means that community development has now ceased to be seen as experimental and radical but much more mainstream in policy and service delivery.

Defining community development

This section discusses:

- Definitions of community development and how it differs from community-based health promotion
- Historical perspectives on community development
- The related concepts of social capital and capacity building

There is no one widely accepted definition of community development. The Standing Conference on Community Development published a definition of community development that clarifies it as a process:

'Community development is a way of working that encourages individual and collective action around the common needs and concerns identified by the community itself…It is about changing power structures to remove the barriers that prevent people from participating in the issues that affect their lives.'

(Standing Conference on Community
Development www.sccd.org.uk)

Some of the key principles underpinning 'community development' are summarised in Box 5.1

The rise in popularity of community development approaches in the UK is relatively recent but it is a not a new concept. It can be traced back to late nineteenth-century America where its roots lie in colonialism and strategies for social control. At that time black self-help groups

---

Box 5.1   Some key principles of community development

- A collective endeavour to identify and act on issues of concern to individuals and communities
- Involves local leaders and local people to tackle the problems identified
- Is emancipatory – empowering communities, building their confidence and capacity
- Emphasises community participation in the promotion of more equitable and accessible services
- Recognises the importance of social networks and social support
- Provides support to challenge and influence the development and implementation of public policies
- Requires organisations to respond to the identified needs of communities
- Promotes social inclusion and emphasises tackling discrimination
- Aims to reduce inequalities
- Values 'joined up', inter-sectoral working

were organised by the Republican Party to improve agricultural productivity. This approach was extended to teach Native Americans better management of land, health and education with little emphasis upon empowerment or autonomy (CPHVA 1999).

In the UK the rise of community development approaches can be traced to the Community Development Project launched by the Home Office in 1969. Twelve projects were funded to determine new ways of responding to the needs of those living in neighbourhoods with high social deprivation (Jones 1990). The underlying philosophy and principles were essentially radical, progressive and concerned with social equity, based on an analysis of the socioeconomic and political structures responsible for poverty. However, conflicts with government policy ensued and project workers began to question the government's intentions – control of the poor, defusion of the threat of racial and urban unrest. Rather inauspiciously, funding for the projects was withdrawn (Tones & Tilford 2001). In the 1970s and early 1980s numerous community development health projects were set up, mostly funded and located outside the NHS. Inner city decline prompted projects to tackle neighbourhood renewal, sexual health, and youth and leisure provision. Key features of these projects reveal their radical dimensions:

- They are located outside the health professions
- They are concerned with inequalities in health and health care provision
- They promote a collective awareness of the social causes of ill health
- They challenge the professional monopoly of information about health and ill health
- Activities centre on work with small groups of local people (Rosenthal 1983)

An understanding of power and control in relation to, for example, the use and ownership of information, the role and agenda of professionals or the active discrimination against certain groups inform the theoretical basis of community development. Community development approaches have long been associated with the work of Paulo Freire, a Brazilian educationalist. Freire worked on literacy programmes with poor peasants in Peru and Brazil and saw education as the political and social means of changing power relationships (Freire 1972).

Community development as an approach needs to be distinguished from community-based health promotion. The latter has meant programmes or services reaching out to or located in communities as a means of breaking down the boundaries between organisations and users. These projects may be designed and delivered according to the needs of communities but tend to be set within government or health professionals' agendas (Gilchrist 2003). Community development prioritises issues identified by the community themselves and seeks improvements in quality of life – material, environmental or social – that may indirectly lead to better health. They also help to address the problems that are collectively identified as being barriers to the concept of ownership of well-being. In order to achieve this collective approach the key processes involved are individual and community empowerment (Lindsey *et al.* 1999).

'Empowerment' is a notoriously slippery concept that is widely used but differently understood. It can be defined at individual, organisational and community levels. In a broad sense it means 'people gain control in their own lives in the context of participation with each other to change their social and political realities' (Wallerstein 1993, p. 219). If individuals are to become empowered, they need first of all to recognise their own powerlessness. Freire (1972) described this as 'conscientisation', a process of change in awareness and knowledge concerning a person's own position in the world in relation to others. The rise in consciousness of their situation enables individuals to identify their own needs, rather than having them prescribed by others. Community empowerment 'involves individuals acting collectively to gain greater influence and control over the determinants of health and the quality of life in their community, and is an important goal in community action for health' (Nutbeam 1998, p. 354). A central purpose of community development is to strengthen the range and quality of organisation in communities both at the level of networks and local activities but also increasing participation and influence so that communities can begin to identify needs and lobby for change. At the organisational level the central tenets of empowerment are described as the exercise of power, information sharing and involvement in decision making. This will, on the one hand, assist in empowering the individual within the organisation itself, and on the other enable the organisation to influence policies within the wider community (Israel *et al.* 1994).

On a critical note, the true nature of community development is beginning to be more widely contested. Is it driven by the democratic vision it espouses or is it a means of social engineering to promote 'competent and quiescent communities'? Labonte (1990) suggests that community empowerment has become romanticised. He warns that communities may not always be healthy and empowering in their interactions. One of the dangers of this may be that when sustainable change does not occur, 'we may cease victimising powerless individuals only to victimise powerless communities' (Labonte 1990). Further, it has been argued that the decentralised decision making that is such a feature of community development diverts attention away from the lack of control communities have over economic resources (Petersen 1994) and it becomes a means of 'gilding the ghetto' – having little impact on major health inequalities and merely focusing on the felt needs in one area or group.

The government's commitment to consultation and involvement is clear but this needs to be distinguished from empowerment where the objective is to strengthen communities. The ways in which communities are involved in decision making and the design and delivery of programmes and services has been the subject of much debate. Several writers have developed typologies of participation (Arnstein 1969; Brager & Specht 1973; Wilcox 1994) that describe levels or stages of participation. These models make a hierarchical distinction between approaches to involvement according to the amount of power sharing involved and the degree of influence over decisions, attempting to distinguish between consultation, participation

and empowerment. People can be involved in the services that affect or may affect them at a variety of levels and in a number of ways, ranging from very little to complex relationships:

- *Information* – ensuring that relevant information about service planning reaches the public e.g. surveys, leaflets and focus groups
- *Consultation* – asking people's views and advice about plans, policies and services e.g. public meetings and consultation documents
- *Participation* – identifying a problem and asking the public to make a series of decisions within defined limits e.g. the site of a health care facility
- *Partnership* – working together to set objectives, make plans and decide funding priorities, e.g. patients and carers in service planning groups
- *Delegated control* – giving authority and money to a community to plan services, choose providers and run the services.

The meaning of the word 'community' has also long been contested in sociological and policy terms. Jewkes and Murcott (1996) claim there are at least 55 different definitions in use. It is often conflated with neighbourhood yet many different kinds of communities exist. Geographically defined communities are convenient for agencies that want to work within boundaries, but living in the same place does not necessarily guarantee a common view. More recently, the emphasis has been on communities of interest with shared needs such as 'teenage mothers' or 'people with learning disabilities'. Marginalised communities are those whose contributions are invisible. They may experience discrimination and may not make use of traditional or mainstream services. Examples of such groups are asylum seekers, travellers and homeless people. Other communities are those defined by service use; shared interests or occupation; or by characteristics such as culture, religion and sexual orientation (Smithies & Webster 1998).

The question of who to involve in a 'community' is similarly complicated. Early attempts to increase participation focused on a strategy of involving those who were most accessible, who tended to be local leaders. For example, attempts to reach ethnic minority groups frequently employ strategies of contacting faith leaders or using existing groups that meet at religious buildings. Identifying 'activists' and those used to participating in groups – those in tenant groups or parents' associations – may also be seen as ways of increasing involvement and getting a 'lay voice'. Where there is no clear constituency these representatives tend to be drawn from voluntary sector agencies. 'These constraints result in the community representatives being drawn from one small part of the voluntary sector, the larger funded organisations' (Jewkes & Murcott 1998, p. 855).

Personal networks both sustain communities and contribute to the effectiveness of community activity. It is not surprising then that there has been so much interest in the concept of social capital, the term used to describe networks and shared norms that facilitate co-ordination and co-operation for mutual benefit and create civic engagement. It is a relatively new concept that has aroused considerable debate about how it should be defined and measured. It originated with the work of Robert Putnam in Italy and the USA (Putnam 2000; Putnam *et al.* 1993). Putnam found that the very poor living in urban areas in the USA who have a few relatively intense family or neighbourhood ties are trapped in their poverty whereas those with a wider network of weaker contacts do better.

There is a body of evidence that suggests that low social capital and social exclusion arising from poverty or discrimination is linked to poor health. Wilkinson (1996, 2000) has powerfully demonstrated the links between relative income inequality and health status, arguing that poor people who witness the wealth of richer neighbours but feel they can do little to close the gap are likely to experience stress and discontent. It has also been demonstrated that where the levels of social capital are high, associated health benefits are evident. For example, reductions in infant mortality and increases in life expectancy (Putnam *et al.* 1993), lower levels of deaths from stroke, accidents and suicide and improved survival from heart disease (Kawachi & Kennedy 1997) have all been linked to social capital. It is

a concept that is growing in popularity as it relates to the renewed interest in the broader determinants of health, and in particular the importance of the influence of social indicators for health and well-being. For communities to be empowered and strengthened, there has to be a level of mutual trust and co-operation. In this way the concept is helpful as it provides a framework to examine the processes through which formal and informal social connections and networks can protect people against the worst effects of deprivation (Morgan 2000).

The related concept of 'community capacity' refers to 'the set of assets or strengths that residents individually or collectively bring to the cause of improving local quality of life' (Easterling 1998). Capacity building is a systematic approach to build the confidence and ability of individuals, community and voluntary groups/organisations to more fully participate in the regeneration of their neighbourhoods. So it may be used in a functional way to equip people for particular jobs through skills training or NVQ accreditation or it may involve personal or organisational development. The term 'releasing capacity' is therefore often preferred to reflect the view that local people are not 'empty vessels' and do have valuable experience, knowledge and skills.

Making it work – key issues in successful community development

This section discusses:

- The core elements of a community development approach
- Some of the challenges for practitioners and organisations from a community development approach
- A case study of a community development project

Working within a community development framework can provide community practitioners with a number of opportunities and challenges. Some of these opportunities are about building healthy alliances and more responsive services. Some of the challenges relate to issues of professional autonomy, bureaucratic accountability, and fear of loss of professional power. Figure 5.1 provides a useful framework illustrating the process of community development work. It identifies some of the tasks and skills involved in this process.

Forging alliances or partnerships with local people, other community workers, and voluntary and lay groups is fundamental to effective community development work. Practitioners need to build on their existing store of community knowledge to form partnerships and networks in order to identify health needs. In deprived communities, however, the motivation of local people to be involved or take any action may be low. This may be due to a perception that they cannot change anything, or that the agenda reflects primary care trust (PCT) concerns, that they might be asked to step up 'the ladder of

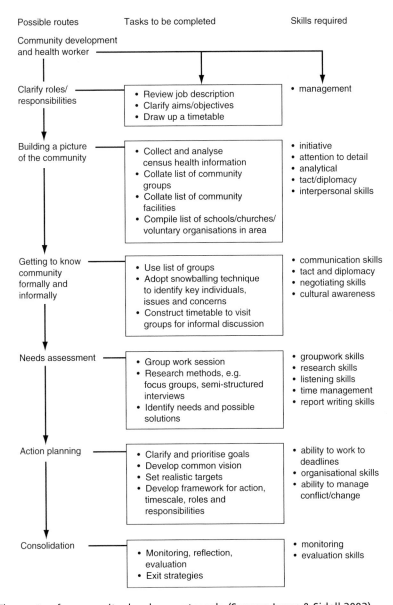

Figure 5.1   The route of community development work. (Source: Jones & Sidell 2002)

involvement' and do more than they want to or that they are outsiders to small cliques that are leading change in their community.

Successful community development also depends on an acknowledgement of the need to start with the priorities identified by the local community (see Chapter 6). Historically, a medical model of health that encourages a focus on pathology has dominated health and social care. This is at odds with a community development approach. A clear identification of community needs as a prerequisite is essential and must include issues wider than patterns of disease and illness and encompass a more social definition of health. The actual needs identified by a community may be radically different from the policy priorities and agendas of local authorities and primary care trusts.

For example, a community development project in east London (www.poplarharca.com) set out to strengthen the 'community' of residents on several local housing estates by working with tenant boards. The project worked at four levels:

- With individual residents, helping them to become more active
- With local groups or organisations to help them be more effective
- With a network of groups and organisations to help them co-operate
- With agencies and other sectors to help them understand the dynamics of community life and help them deliver their services in ways which better meet the needs of the community

The philosophy of community development holds that people should have a say and be involved in a meaningful way, and that their ideas and solutions to the problems facing them are listened to and action taken. For example, a needs assessment undertaken by the Leyton Community Health Project in East London identified that young people wanted:

- Direct access to information
- Support and guidance to promote mental health and physical well-being
- Young people having a say in service design and delivery

- Adults and professionals working alongside them to achieve these aims

As a result, a young peoples' pilot outreach project was set up and run by a nurse, a drugs outreach worker, a sexual health worker and a counsellor with a drop in session at a local school. The pilot project highlighted that action was needed on a number of fronts:

- Development of a less fragmented, more holistic approach to identifying and responding to young peoples' health needs
- Provision of health support in primary schools
- Independent access for young people (i.e. with no requirement for an adult to access the service on their behalf)
- Advocacy and brokerage into a range of other services
- Liaison with the Child and Adolescent Mental Health Service to bring their workers out into non-traditional settings in the community

Whilst young people had been involved in the setting up and advertising of the outreach project, a community health project manager drove it forward and developed it into a young peoples' independent access service named Face 2 Face. It now has one central access point for young people in the community and six school based outreach 'drop in' clinics operating on a hub and spoke approach. This example raises questions about the role of the practitioner in community development and the extent to which they move beyond being a catalyst and facilitator.

The Leyton Community Health Project was nationally acclaimed as a best practice example and formed the basis of a further bid for regeneration funding. However it raises key questions about the sustainability of initiatives and their continued funding. Where new services have been developed as a result of community consultation their potential for exerting a powerful influence on mainstream service provision should be actively pursued as shown here in the development of the young people's service. However, once projects do become mainstream there is always the potential for them to become subject to organisational pressures and lose their drive and innovation.

Box 5.2   Key outcomes of the Poplar Harca project using the LEAP evaluation framework

The key outcomes are:

(1) Healthy people who have

- Awareness and knowledge
- Confidence, choice and control
- Independence and self-reliance
- Connections to community

In the Poplar Harca project many residents felt able to move from volunteering to paid work.

(2) Strong communities characterised by

- Community skills
- Equalities
- Community organisation
- Community involvement

In the Poplar Harca project, the community health development worker has helped to set up and sustain activities such as a food co-op, a play-scheme, a community newspaper and a second-hand shop. In addition, residents and stakeholders report improved general outcomes for health such as greater trust and confidence in public sector agencies, a breaking down of isolation and a 'shut in culture' and increasing contacts and communication.

(3) Quality of life – likely to be context specific but include indicators in the following

- Community economy
- Community services
- Community health and safety
- Community culture
- Local democracy

Measuring the effects of community development initiatives on health is a complex undertaking. This is partly due to the broad range of social, economic and environmental factors encompassed within community development approaches. More traditional research methodologies may not be able to adequately reflect the need for outcome measures that are sympathetic to the differing agendas of the various interest groups involved. The extent to which evaluations of community development initiatives in the past have been well designed has been questioned as

they do not necessarily address the community members' questions of 'am I healthier?' or 'is our community better than before?' (Dixon & Sindall 1994). Equally, evaluations that focus on outputs rather than process outcomes will fail to adequately reflect the successes and failures of community development work. There are frameworks for evaluating community development approaches to improving health and well being. For example, the Achieving Better Community Development (ABCD) framework (Barr & Hashagen 2000) and the Learning Evaluation and Planning Model (LEAP) (Hashagen 2003) both provide a structure within which community development work to promote health may be measured and evaluated. LEAP for Health suggests three levels of impact that can be seen in the outcomes of the Poplar Harca project described above (see Box 5.2).

The role of community health professionals

This section discusses:

- Why community nurses should be engaging in community development work
- How it relates to their scope of practice
- What are the competencies and aptitudes required to carry out this kind of work

The last decade has seen an increase in community participation and collective action together with an expansion of community based health projects. Initiatives arising from government strategies such as New Deal for Communities and Sure Start are attempting to address health inequalities and to assist in empowering local communities to establish elements of power and control over their own life circumstance.

The Department of Health health visitor and school nurse practice development initiative (DoH 2001b) identified community development as an effective way to tackle the issues restricting people's health choices. It identified community health professionals, with their considerable knowledge and unique roles within the local communities they serve, as being in an ideal position to be at the forefront of these initiatives. They possess an abundance of knowledge about the health and social needs of their communities and about how those needs can be met. Their everyday experience of home visiting and their long-term knowledge of individuals, families and networks built up over time are valuable resources. As a result they are well placed to identify community leaders and build alliances with local groups. Community health practitioners also have a role to play in the recruitment and support of lay health workers from the local community who are key players in community health development programmes.

A fundamental shift is required, however, to enable practitioners to change their focus of practice in order to address not only the individual and the family but also the wider community. Community development necessitates a change in 'mind set' from a task- to a community-orientated form of practice recognising the individual as part of a collective group with specific needs. This may also pose an additional threat or challenge to practitioners who may find it difficult to relinquish their supposed superior knowledge and power (Jones & Wiggle 1987).

Practitioners wishing to be more proactive in their communities require skills, training and support to do so. In order for this to occur community development must become an integral part of the fundamental role of the community practitioner. One of the ten key areas in the National Occupational Standards for the Practice of Public Health is 'Working with and for Communities to Improve Health and Well-Being' (see www.skillsforhealth.org.uk). Some of the skills that have been identified as necessary to undertake this role are summarised in Box 5.3 below.

Other core skills identified in the literature on effective community development work but which are not necessarily developed in professional training are summarised in Box 5.4.

Employing authorities may also view community development with some degree of scepticism (Naidoo & Wills 2000). This may contribute to the difficulty of obtaining an overall acceptability for community development within the remit of professional practice. Corporate agendas are not always compatible with the philosophy and aims of community development.

> **Box 5.3 Skills necessary to work with and for communities to improve health**
>
> Facilitating the development of people and learning in communities
>
> Creating opportunities for learning from practice and experience
>
> Supporting communities to plan and take collective action
>
> Facilitating the development of community groups and networks
>
> Enabling people to address issues related to health and well-being
>
> Enabling people to improve others' health and well-being
>
> Working with individuals and others to minimise the effects of specific health conditions

---

Long-term involvement with communities is essential for strategies to develop and to be effective. However, this conflicts with the dominant political philosophy with its emphasis upon competition, league tables and the desire for immediate results. Crucially, this approach and the issues identified by communities may conflict with operational caseload demands or the traditional remit of the service. Much of community development work is resourced by short-term funded projects that do not recognise the time required to work successfully in this way. The funding for initiatives such as Sure Start and New Deal for Communities is longer term but there is vagueness about the sustainability of programmes once central funding is withdrawn. Historically, the shift in approach to community development has proved problematic with a reluctance to alter intervention styles and to work with a broader agenda that tackles the underlying factors affecting health and well-being (Chalmers & Bramadat 1996).

Conclusion

Primary care organisations clearly recognise the importance of public involvement but historically have focused on individuals as patients and understand involvement from this perspective of consulting with patients as users of services. As well as being an unfamiliar field,

---

Box 5.4 Skills required for community development

Building relationships with key partners	Multi-agency, community and inter-professional joint planning and consultation.
Appropriate organisational and leadership styles	Facilitative approach; conflict management; group work experience.
Communication with people at different levels	Speaking the language of diverse groups and organisations.
Humility	Accepting other people's ideas and knowledge; egalitarianism.
Maintaining confidentiality	Awareness of potential dilemmas and conflicts of interest within and between groups.
Flexibility	Working across boundaries; managing change.
Negotiating skills	Dealing with resistance; setting realistic time scales; not promising things you cannot deliver; securing organisational backing.
Awareness of equal opportunities	Anti-discriminatory practice; sensitivity to issues of gender and race.
Accountability	Clarity of roles and responsibilities.
Advocacy/lobbying	Empowerment in everyday decision making; providing choices about, and influence over, service provision.
Evaluation skills	What have the benefits been to the community, short/long term?
Research awareness	In-built, dynamic research approach; utilising evidence-based practice.
Team working	Working and learning together.
Interpersonal skills	Strengthening social relationships.
Health promoter	Skilled in health needs assessment and building healthy public policies.

---

public involvement may also be viewed as a threat to professional expertise and autonomy. The shift required to move to a position where members of the public are valued as equal experts is significant. Although primary care organisations are increasingly working in partnerships relating to community development and regeneration activities (Gillam & Smith 2002), in many instances public involvement is regarded as a 'time consuming indulgence' – desirable and helpful but not necessary. Although there are detailed guidelines for involvement, for example *Strengthening Accountability* (DoH 2003), understanding how to engage local people is very dependent on individual practitioners. Yet reliance solely on the medical model of health and professional expertise ignores many fundamental socio-economic determinants of health and fosters an unhealthy dependency

and passivity amongst patients. An understanding of the benefits of public involvement and skills in supporting public involvement and community development are vital aspects of the role of the community health practitioner today.

References

Arnstein, S. (1969) A ladder of citizen participation, *Journal of American Institute of Planners*, **35**(4), 216–224.

Barr, A. & Hashagen, S. (2000) *Achieving Better Community Development*, Community Development Foundation, London.

Brager, G. & Specht, H. (1973) *Community Organizing*. Columbia University Press, New York.

Chalmers, K. & Bramadat, I. (1996) Community development: theoretical and practical issues for community health nursing in Canada. *Journal of Advanced Nursing*, **24**, 719–726.

Community Practitioners and Health Visitors Association (CPHVA) (1999) *Joined up Working: Community Development in Primary Care.* CPHVA, London.

Crawford, M.J., Manley, C., Weaver, T., Bhui, K., Fulop, N. & Tyrer, P. (2002) Systematic review of involving patients in the planning and development of health care. *British Medical Journal,* **325**, 1263–1265.

Department of the Environment, Transport and the Regions (DETR) (2000) *Preparing Community Strategies: Guidance to Local Authorities.* DETR, London.

Department of Health (2000) *The NHS Plan: a plan for investment, a plan for reform.* DoH, London.

Department of Health (2001a) *Involving Patients and Public in Health Care.* DoH, London.

Department of Health (2001b) *Health Visitor Practice Development Resource Pack.* Department of Health, London.

Department of Health (2003) *Strengthening Accountability: involving patients and the public practice guidance.* DoH, London.

Dixon, J. & Sindall, C. (1994) Applying the logics of change to the evaluation of community development in health promotion. *Health Promotion International* **9**(4), 297–309.

Easterling, D. (1998) *Promoting Health by Building Community Capacity: Evidence and Implications for Grant Makers.* The Colorado Trust, Denver.

Florin, D. & Dixon, J. (2004) Public involvement in health care. *British Medical Journal,* **328**, 159–161.

Freire, P. (1972) *Pedagogy of the Oppressed.* Penguin, Harmondsworth.

Gilchrist, A. (2003) Community development and networking for health. In: *Public Health for the 21st Century: new perspectives on policy, participation and practice,* J. Orme, J. Powell, P. Taylor, T. Harrison & M. Grey (eds) The Open University, Buckingham.

Gillam, S. & Smith, K. (2002) In: *The National Tracker Survey of PCGs and PCTs 2001/2. Taking responsibility,* (D. Wilkin *et al.*) National Primary Care Research Centre, University of Manchester, Manchester.

Hashagen, S. (2003) Frameworks for measuring community health and well being. In: *Public Health for the 21st Century: new perspectives on policy, participation and practice,* J. Orme, J. Powell, P. Taylor, T. Harrison & M. Grey (eds) The Open University, Buckingham.

Israel, B., Checkoway, B., Schulz, A. & Zimmerman, M. (1994) Health education and community empowerment: conceptualising and measuring perceptions of individual, organisational, and community control. *Health Education Quarterly,* **21**(2), 149–170.

Jewkes, R. & Murcott, A. (1996) Meanings of Community, *Social Science and Medicine,* **43**(4), 555–563.

Jewkes, R. & Murcott, A. (1998) Community representatives: representing the 'community', *Social Science and Medicine,* **46**(7), 843–858.

Jones, J. (1990) Community development and health education: concepts and philosophy. In: *Roots and branches,* Papers from the OU/HEA winter school on community development and health. The Open University/Health Education Authority, Milton Keynes.

Jones, L. & Sidell, M. (2002) *The challenge of promoting health exploration and action,* 2nd edn. Macmillan and Open University, Basingstoke.

Jones, J. & Wiggle, I. (1987) The concept of politics of 'integrated community development', *Community Development Journal,* **22**(2), 107–119.

Kawachi, I. & Kennedy, B. (1997) Socio-economic determinants of health: Health and Social Cohesion: why care about income inequality? *British Medical Journal,* **314**, 1037.

Labonte, R. (1990) Empowerment: notes on professional and community dimensions. *Canadian Review of Social Policy,* **26**, 64–75.

Lewis, J. & Walker, P. (1998) *Participation works. 21 techniques of community participation for the 21st century.* New Economics Foundation, London.

Lindsey, E., Shields, L. & Stadjhar, K. (1999) Creating effective nursing partnerships: relating community development to participatory action research. *Journal of Advanced Nursing,* **29**(5), 1238–1245.

Morgan, A. (2000) Community Development: Building Social Capital. In: *London's Health Newsletter.* Issue 5 January 2000, p. 2. NHS Executive, London.

Naidoo, J. & Wills, J. (2000) *Health Promotion Foundations for Practice,* 2nd edn. Ballière Tindall, London.

Naidoo, J. & Wills, J. (2005) *Public Health and Health Promotion: developing practice.* 2nd edn. Ballière Tindall, London.

NHS Executive (1998) *In the Public Interest: Developing a Strategy for Public Participation in the NHS.* DoH, Wetherby.

Nutbeam, D. (1998) Health Promotion Glossary. *Health Promotion International,* **13**(4), 349–364.

Petersen, A. (1994) Community development in health promotion: empowerment or regulation? *Journal of Public Health,* **18**, 213–217.

Putnam, R., Leonardi, R. & Nanetti, R.N. (1993) *Making Democracy Work: Civic Traditions in Modern Italy.* Princeton University Press, Princeton, New Jersey.

Putnam, R. (2000) *Bowling Alone: the collapse and revival of American community.* Simon Schuster, New York.

Rosenthal, H. (1983) Neighbourhood health projects: some new approaches to health and community work in parts of the UK, *Community Development Journal*, **13**, 122–131.

Social Exclusion Unit (2000) *National Strategy for Neighbourhood Renewal*. SEU, London.

Smithies, J. & Webster, W. (1998) *Community involvement in health: from passive recipients to active participants*. Ashgate, Aldershot.

Taylor, P. (2003) The lay contribution to public health. In: *Public Health for the 21st Century: new perspectives on policy, participation and practice*, J. Orme, J. Powell, P. Taylor, T. Harrison & M. Grey (eds). The Open University, Buckingham.

Tones, K. & Tilford, S. (2001) *Health promotion: effectiveness, efficiency and equity*, 3rd edn. Chapman & Hall, London.

Wallerstein, N. (1993) Empowerment and health: the theory and practice of community change, *Community Development Journal*, **28**(3), 218–227.

Wilcox, D. (1994) *A Guide to Effective Participation*. Pavilion, Brighton.

Wilkinson, R. (1996) *Unhealthy Societies*. Routledge, London.

Wilkinson, R. (2000) *Mind the Gap: hierarchies, health and human evolution*. Weidenfeld, London.

Wintour, P., Ward, L. & Hetherington, P. (2000) Bridging Britain's social divide. *The Guardian*. April 1, p. 9.

Chapter 6 Health Needs Assessment, Risk Assessment and Public Health

Elizabeth A. Raymond

Introduction and overview of chapter

This chapter explores the role of health need, health risk and health impact assessments in identifying, agreeing and responding to the health status and health concerns of the individuals, groups and communities who comprise the UK population. In particular, it seeks to draw attention to the contribution which community nurses are in a position to make to such assessments.

Successive UK government documents in recent years (DoH 1989a, b, 2004; Standing Nursing and Midwifery Advisory Committee 1995) have emphasised the notion that health care should be needs-led, and that formal assessment of the health needs of local populations should form an integral part of the purchasing and provision of services. This may seem like a seductive proposition to potential users of the National Health Service (NHS), implying that need alone is to be the basis for access to health care. The reality is more complex, and the notion of policy led by needs assessment can be a front for a range of disparate intentions, priorities and values. *Health, needs, risk* and *assessment* are four terms which together encompass most of the current and enduring issues and dilemmas confronting policy makers and providers of health care. *Health* and *need* have been referred to by a number of writers as contested concepts (Cowley *et al.* 2000; Milner 1999) and the terms *risk* and *assessment* in the context of health care are no less so.

Practising community nurses find themselves at the interface between many of the differing constructions of these concepts, which creates both opportunities and tensions for them in their daily work. As NHS employees they constitute agents of social control, required to implement national and local policies and in so doing to reflect the prevailing official constructions of health and need. As members of a profession regulated by a Code of Professional Conduct (NMC 2002) which specifically identifies their responsibility as advocates for patients and clients, they may also need to act as agents of social change. As such, they may need to challenge official policy and perceptions, when these appear to be inadequate, in response to users' health experiences and perceptions.

The following discussion takes as a starting point the acknowledgement that public health is the health of individuals within their social setting, and consequently that efforts to gain an understanding of the range and diversity of health experience within any population must be an integral part of any assessments aimed at reducing health inequalities. Populations are abstract entities which do not exist apart from their constituent individuals, who together create the social contexts and the health and social policies impacting on the health of those individuals. Percy-Smith and Sanderson (1992) are clear that any welfare system is concerned with the collective provision of services and facilities to meet individual needs. However, significant differences in perspective on health needs assessment characterise those charged with delivering care to individuals compared with those charged with strategic planning for populations as a whole, and these differences in turn reflect different understandings of the term *health*.

Health – a contested concept or a chimera?

In order to identify health deficits and threats to health there is a need for clarity concerning the nature of health itself, yet literature abounds with alternative definitions and descriptions. A *chimera* is defined figuratively as 'any incongruous conception of the fancy' (Hayward & Sparkes 1984), and it is tempting to suggest that health is such an entity. Robinson (1985 p. 67) describes health as an 'abstract notion . . . a concept fraught with ambiguity, which defies objective definition and quantification' and asserts that 'the abstract ideal of "health as a value" . . . is . . . a fragile and insubstantial notion [which] provides a very vulnerable basis for legitimated professional activity'. Although she is here referring to the problematic commitment of health visiting to health as an ideal and a value, arguably her analysis is as relevant in relation to a national health care system which is perceived as more than a 'sickness service'.

Broadly speaking, health has been conceptualised from:

- A biomedical point of view, which emphasises medical interventions to prevent and treat disease, and is mainly concerned with functional capacity
- A behavioural point of view, which emphasises individual responsibility for health influencing behaviour
- A social point of view, which focuses on social and political determinants of health and emphasises social justice
- A postmodernist point of view, which according to Naidoo and Wills (1998) challenges the adequacy of the preceding perspectives and suggests that no single theory sufficiently explains health experience

According to postmodernism the reality of health is more complex and less predictable than can be accounted for by the previous explanations. This resonates with the experience of community nurses which leads them to be wary of the generalisations implicit in the other perspectives. In relation to their contribution to health needs assessment, however, community nurses need to adopt an eclectic approach, considering the relative significance of each perspective. Community nurses are at the interface between service users and the health care system, where it becomes important to recognise that implicit

in many of the alternative definitions of health lie assumptions concerning the purpose and justification for its promotion. A range of terms is used to describe tools and strategies which relate to the identification and management of need, including:

- Health needs assessment
- Health impact assessment
- Environmental impact assessment
- Health inequality impact assessment
- Integrated impact assessment
- Poverty profiling
- Sickness impact profiling
- Global health status analysis
- Rapid appraisal
- Community and population profiling
- Caseload and work load analysis and profiling
- GP practice profiling

These terms reflect the range of differing perspectives which exist regarding the nature of needs and their assessment and management.

Perspectives on health needs assessment

Cowley *et al.* (2000 p. 133) describe needs assessment as 'messy, variable and multifaceted'. The range of different perspectives on the subject can be summarised as:

- Citizens' perspectives
- Biomedical perspectives
- Social perspectives
- Economic perspectives
- Political perspectives

Citizens' perspectives

Diversity and competing needs
The major difficulty for policy makers is that the citizens of any society are not a homogeneous group either in distinguishing characteristics, relative need, or in attitudes to health. This frequently contributes to a mismatch between local health care provision and need. Wright *et al.* (1998) draw attention to large variation in availability and use of health care by geographical area and point of provision, and a tendency towards an

inverse relationship between the needs of a local population and the availability of care to that population.

Much literature discusses how and why *users* or *consumers* of health care and their *informal carers* should be consulted, but far less attention is paid to the recognition that citizens who are not currently in contact with health care services still have health care needs and views on how those needs should be met. Also, virtually all such members of the public are either *past users* or *prospective users* of health services. Very few infants and mothers experience the processes of pregnancy and delivery without any intervention whatever from health care professionals, and few will survive into extreme old age without experiencing some degree of long-term limiting illness or disability.

Within any geographically-based population group individuals and sub-groups will have competing needs, so that, for example, older people and people in pain and awaiting hip replacements may feel that increased resources for them are more important than improved fertility treatment for would-be parents. Additionally, subjective experiences of health and health deficits will vary between individuals who appear to the observer to share a similar health status.

How individual meanings of health are constructed

Arguably, health as individuals experience it is a means to an end, not a goal in itself, whereas for many service providers improved health is the goal. Lay views of all citizens will be influenced by their expectations of their own health, their awareness and experience of need, their concepts of health, and their beliefs about their own and others' ability to maintain or improve their health. These in turn will be variously influenced by an individual's particular personal aspirations and goals in life, socio-economic status, ethnic and religious affiliations, and even personality.

Identifying diverse needs and perceptions

Given the heterogeneity within society, constructing a form of health needs assessment which can effectively identify and give insight into the range of needs from citizens' perspectives presents a challenge. Billings (2000) identifies two principles which need to underpin effective consultation of the public:

- Enabling those who are usually less able to have a voice to be adequately represented
- Avoidance of tokenism, or a form of consultation without real intention of using the resultant data to inform decision making.

Large scale surveys and statistics cannot be sufficiently sensitive to variations within and between areas and tend to obscure the concerns of groups which are locally in a minority. More time-consuming and labour intensive qualitative methods of data collection have to be used if members of a local population are to be genuinely consulted, and careful thought needs to given to how adequate representativeness can be achieved. Such methods commonly include public meetings, health forums, interviews and focus groups, and rapid appraisal (Appleton & Cowley 2000).

Rapid appraisal

Pickin and St Leger (1993) describe rapid appraisal as a research strategy of particular value in involving local people in the purchasing process, and as having been developed primarily in order to understand the needs of deprived urban communities. It can be undertaken in about ten working days, hence the description *rapid*, and it reflects the World Health Organization primary care philosophy underpinning Health for All targets (WHO 1985), emphasising equity, participation, and multi-agency collaboration. Murray (1999) describes three successful adaptations of rapid appraisal by health care staff in Edinburgh:

- An assessment by an expanded primary care team (health visitor, general practitioner, two social workers and a community education worker) of the health needs of a housing estate with 1200 residents
- An assessment of the specific mental health needs of the same population by a team comprising a community psychiatric nurse, a general practitioner and a psychiatrist

- Assessments by each of three newly employed community psychiatric nurses of local perceptions about mental health and illness within the neighbourhoods to which they had been appointed to work. Part of the purpose of the appraisals was to contribute to the staff's orientation to their new surroundings. Findings from the three neighbourhoods, each of about 40 000 residents, were also combined into a locality mental health profile

Some of the key values of rapid appraisal which Murray identifies include:

(1) *Community orientation* – rapid appraisal is based on the assumptions that individuals need to be understood within their social context, and that contact with individual members of a local population gives greater depth of insight into the wider community
(2) *Necessity of public involvement* – rapid appraisal involves lay members of the local community in assessing and planning
(3) *Multisectoral approach and promotion of networking* – rapid appraisal acknowledges the need for wider perspectives than simply those of health services, and the involvement of local workers outside the health service as key informants is seen as important
(4) *Promotion of equality* – rapid appraisal offers an adaptable means of focusing on the needs of deprived areas

Murray (1999) also draws attention to several limitations of the strategy, including risk of bias in the choice of informants, limitations to the data related to the limited time frame and resources involved, the need for training in the technique, and that co-ordination of the activity can be logistically difficult.

Reviewing the attempted use of rapid appraisal with a larger population, Murray also makes clear that the technique works best with homogeneous communities and is therefore not suitable for use with large populations. Pickin and St Leger (1993) suggest an upper population limit of 12 000.

Ong and Humphris (1994), describing some of the earliest uses of rapid appraisal in the UK health field, identify several stages in conducting it:

- Selecting team members, representing a range of relevant perspectives
- Initial workshop for team members to determine target area, key informants to be interviewed, and key questions to be asked
- Fieldwork – interviews with key informants selected from three broad groups;
  — professionals working within the community, e.g. community nurses, teachers, police
  — recognised community leaders, e.g. religious leaders, local councillors, leaders of self-help groups, playgroup leaders
  — people with insight into local informal networks, e.g. bookie, lollipop person, owner of corner shop, supermarket checkout staff
- Data analysis
- Preliminary identification of needs list
- Comparison of team's ranking of priorities for action with the ranking by the informants
- Open meeting between team, informants, and public to formulate action plans
- Further meeting of team members, informants and public to develop plans and evaluate action taken

Ong and Humphris (1994) draw attention to lessons learned from the early use of rapid appraisal in the UK. Comparison of priorities for action revealed disparity between the team's priorities, the community's priorities, and the team's expectation of the community's priorities. Use of rapid appraisal of itself does not necessarily resolve the tension between differing perceptions, and the involvement of communities in planning and decision making raises issues of power and control, with the challenge to professionals and planners to accept a shift to a shared ownership of the processes involved.

The degree of skill in identifying key informants is also important. The aim is to build up a multifaceted picture from individuals who represent a range of viewpoints, but the extent to which any individual is able to represent the experiences or viewpoints of others remains debatable and likely to be limited.

Finally, health planners continue to rely on the kind of quantitative data associated with biomedical explanations of health and illness, and thus have difficulty in being persuaded of the validity of the kind of qualitative data generated by methodologies such as rapid appraisal.

Biomedical perspectives

Biomedical explanations – a major and enduring facet of public health

The so-called *medical model* of health focuses on threats to health in terms of disease processes, or what might be described as malfunctioning of the mind or body. From this perspective health needs assessment seeks the causes of ill-health largely within the individual and the physical environment. Explanations for mental ill-health are more likely to be seen as either genetic in origin or residing in an individual's ability to adapt to her/his environment than in structural and social inequities.

This understanding of the significance of the environment has been an enduring facet of public health and primary health care in the UK since the middle and late nineteenth century. The impact of the Industrial Revolution, the increasingly crowded and insanitary urban environments which it spawned, and the enhanced mortality and morbidity due to infectious diseases such as the cholera epidemics which swept the country, have left their mark on a century of public health activity. Martin and McQueen (1989) suggest that the legacy has been a concern with the social context of health, which was, however, historically dominated by medical and biological perspectives and largely continues to be so.

Communicable disease epidemics also serve as a continuing reminder that the health relationship between the individual and society is two-way. Individual health choices may imperil others. For example, parents of a healthy, well-nourished child in optimum living conditions may consider that vaccine-associated risk outweighs the risk of measles, mumps or rubella

to their child. Nevertheless, in a metropolis where the healthy and affluent live in close proximity to the poor, homeless families and asylum seekers, failure to achieve a herd immunity places the children of the latter in greater jeopardy. Naidoo and Wills (1994) cite immunisation as an example of a situation where individual freedom may be imposed upon in order to protect the health of the wider community.

Communicable diseases continue to threaten the health of populations world-wide and the complex relationship of the former with the environment and patterns of human behaviour is a significant part of the focus of epidemiological investigations.

The role of epidemiological data

Although medical and biological explanations do not tell the whole story, epidemiological and statistical data collected on this basis make a major contribution to health care policy and practice. Mortality and morbidity statistics not only help to identify new or increasing threats from communicable and other diseases but also offer evidence of the effectiveness or otherwise of health interventions both through preventive action and treatment. Population data such as age structure, ethnicity and socio-economic profiles help to identify patterns of ill-health related to social groups in society. Tools such as sickness impact assessments and global health status analyses help to give some insight into the differing health experience of individuals and groups that cannot be revealed by morbidity statistics alone.

However, the choice of categories of data to collect is not a value-free activity. For example, if specific social groups such as travelling families are not separately identified and compared with more mainstream groups, their differing needs profile may be completely overlooked. Making comparisons between groups in this way can challenge assumptions. Data on travelling families which has been collected consistently suggests they experience poorer health than that of the majority of settled families. However, a proposition to target resources to ex-travelling families now settled in one locality, on the assumption that such health differentials would be perpetuated, was challenged by local health visitors. When data was collected in order to settle this question it was found that the ex-travelling families did not differ significantly from their neighbours, although the local population as a whole was comparatively needy. Targeted resources would have created an invidious and unjust situation.

No strategy is without limitations, but epidemiology, with its tried and tested methods of investigating disease patterns and tracing causes, will always play a significant part in assessing health need and health risk. It is a public health discipline which, despite its biomedical origins, spans both medical and social perspectives. Epidemiogical data identify associations and relationships between health problems and social groups, but epidemiologists seek to explore such relationships further in terms of understanding cause and effect. For example, a 'medical' cause for a typhoid outbreak might be found through identification of a carrier of the disease, but equally poverty and homelessness or poor housing can be seen to be direct contributors to respiratory disease. For the majority of diseases, the correlation between social inequality and inequality of health experience is a strong and enduring one (Benzeval *et al.* 1995).

Social perspectives

A social justice view – inequality, not need
Social perspectives on health incorporate more than an acknowledgement of the impact of social factors on health. A considerable body of literature focuses heavily on issues of social (in)justice, oppression and inequality. From a social justice perspective, the whole notion of health needs assessment can be suspect. Bradshaw, who originated the oft-quoted taxonomy of need (Bradshaw 1972), subsequently challenged the appropriateness of needs assessment as a basis for policy formation (Bradshaw 1994). He argued not only that the concept of need is too imprecise, too complex, and too contentious, but that at the time he was writing the word need had become a smoke-screen to hide the true intention of policy

which, in seeking to reduce public expenditure and cut taxes, was having the effect of increasing inequalities. Writing from a social policy and social justice perspective, he argued that inequality is a more appropriate target for health and social policy than need. His analysis puts the finger on the essential tension between a principle of equity and the principles of efficiency and cost effectiveness which continue to imbue current health policy.

Amongst the synonyms offered by *Roget's Thesaurus* for need are the terms poverty, penury, and destitution. These reflect a social justice concept of need which identifies poverty as a key element related to ill-health. Whilst there is not a simple relationship between poverty and ill-health, the mass of evidence linking the two can also be constructed as evidence of the consequences of social policy (Acheson 1998; Black *et al.* 1980). As UK governments have reduced their contribution in terms of social security and welfare benefits over the last twenty-five years, the gap in income and living standards between the richest and poorest in society has widened (Acheson 1998; Benzeval *et al.* 1995; Black *et al.* 1999; DoH 2002). Black *et al.* (1999) argue strongly that if health inequalities are to be reduced and the nation's health is to be improved, then material deprivation needs to be addressed urgently by institution of a programme to improve benefits to a level that has been determined as minimally sufficient to maintain health.

Poverty profiling
Bond (1999) documents an example in Nottingham of severe deprivation associated with high levels of poor health. The project Bond describes incorporated a poverty profile that revealed three of Nottingham's most deprived electoral wards to exhibit some of the city's worst levels of ischaemic heart disease, stroke and respiratory disease and well above average rates of low birth weight babies, dental disease and hospital admissions following accidents.

Blackburn (1992) views poverty profiling as one element of health needs assessment. She argues that it generates objective and comparable information which sets health information and health need into a social context that aids understanding of how people's experience of poverty shapes their health, and she suggests that a poverty profile should be a component of health profiles compiled by community nurses. Blackburn (1991) and Wilkinson (1996) construe the impact of poverty on health as more than the consequence of material disadvantage. Both authors point to the psychological impact described by Wilkinson as high levels of stress deriving from feelings of fear, vulnerability, helplessness, hopelessness and related negative emotions.

Social justice – disability as a product of social processes

The Disability Movement has particular reason to focus on social justice in relation to health, and Craddock (1996a) draws attention to the movement's contention that disability is the product of social processes and does not result from an individual's impairment but rather from society's failure to meet the individual's needs. Craddock discusses the role of occupational therapists from opposing medical and social perspectives in a way which has a wider application to all health care providers. She focuses on occupational therapy as a profession allied to medicine with an accompanying claim to the right of diagnostic assessment and prescription of treatment even 'when working with medically stable disabled people' (1996a, p. 20). Later (Craddock 1996b) she argues that the continuing definition of occupational therapy interventions as 'treatment' reinforces the dependent role of the disabled person, and that a more appropriate response to disabled clients in the community would be to work in an equal partnership with them. As consultants rather than therapists, social services occupational therapists in particular need to acknowledge client perceptions of their needs and 'focus on the removal of disabling barriers and the supply of necessary equipment to facilitate the activities and lifestyle of the client's choice' (1996b, p. 76).

Several years ago in one health authority, when sufferers from multiple sclerosis were consulted concerning their perceived needs, health care professionals were somewhat startled to learn that an overwhelming concern was with the lack of accessible public toilets – a clear example supporting the importance of a social model of disability.

Day (2000) reports on a survey of nations by the World Health Organization which reflects issues of social justice on an international scale. The survey used a new measure of disability adjusted life expectancy (DALE), where years of serious illness are subtracted from the average age at which a person in a given country dies. This measure revealed that in the year 2000, years lost to serious disability were much higher in poor countries, with the ten countries at the bottom of the league all being in sub-Saharan Africa. Unexpectedly, the United States ranked 24th amongst developed nations, but the high rates of heart disease, violent death, tobacco-related cancers and AIDS cited as explanations for this low position support the same theme of social processes influencing the prevalence of disability.

Both within and between nations, tensions can also arise between social justice perspectives and economic perspectives on needs definition.

Economic perspectives

Need, supply and demand

From an economic perspective in health care the concept of need translates to a *dynamic relationship between demand and supply* of services. The more limited the resources are, the less all that is demanded is likely to be acknowledged as *legitimate need*, and vice versa. Furthermore, a distinction is made between *health need* and *health care need*, so that health needs that cannot be addressed by health care services are excluded. *Health need* itself has been defined from this perspective as *the capacity to benefit* from health care interventions, and *health needs assessment* becomes part of the process of reconciling supply and demand. From Wright and colleagues' point of view (1998) the latter is 'an objective and valid method . . . an evidence-based approach to commissioning and planning health services' (p. 1310). It includes activities that contribute to quantifying demand and indicating value for money, such as methods of measuring ill-health, and assessing the effectiveness of health care interventions in relation to explicitly identified benefits. Whilst they also suggest that health needs assessment involves consideration of questions of priority setting, others have suggested that it can simply be a distraction from the difficult decisions of rationing health care in the context of demand outstripping resources.

Needs assessment and escalating costs

The NHS was originally established with the expectation that costs to the public purse would diminish as the population became fitter (Beveridge 1942). This view of health failed to consider the influence of changed consumer expectations shown by a rise in consumerism with greater concerns about service quality including access, equity, appropriateness and effectiveness (Wright *et al.* 1998), and the impact of continuing technological advancement. Rising health care costs have contributed to current emphases on measurable outcomes of interventions in terms of health gain, where such gain has been defined in terms of measurable 'years added to life' and 'life added to years' or quality adjusted life years (QALYs). These measures examine increased survival rates as a result of interventions, but also consider the quality of such added life. However, as Robinson and Elkan (1996) point out, such measures necessarily involve value judgements about what constitutes quality of life, drawing attention to some of the problems inherent in the notion of measurable health gain.

Demand and the symptom iceberg

The notion of demand from an economic perspective bears some relationship to Bradshaw's description of *expressed need*. Whilst it may be construed as a pressure on the public purse, an alternative view is that demand represents the tip of the iceberg of *felt need*. Hannay (1979) referred to the 'symptom iceberg' in his study of referral patterns, and drew attention to the huge variation in interpretation of symptoms, beginning with patients themselves and going on to the responses of their GPs. Indeed, at every level there are instances where significant health

deficits fail to receive further attention. Wright *et al.* (1998) assert that many patients with angina or multiple sclerosis are not known to either their local GP or a hospital specialist, whilst homeless people and those suffering chronic mental illness may need health care but not demand it.

An economic perspective – a rational approach or a means of avoidance?

In the face of the range of competing views and definitions in relation to health need and health care provision, the language of economics appears to offer a welcome measure of clarity, suggesting that the use of quantitative measures of need, a sound evidence base for choice of effective and efficient intervention, and objective criteria for prioritising action will provide a rational foundation for an equitable health care system. However, the limitation of this approach is that it is in danger of dealing with the messy, diverse reality of human need by simply neglecting to engage with the possible consequences in suffering and distress for those whose needs are not legitimated.

Political perspectives

It is possible to discern a continuing paradox in UK health and social policy. On the one hand, the emphasis in policy in relation to the NHS contains a persistent economic theme of cost-containment and cost-effectiveness which continues to place significant emphasis on the responsibilities of individuals and communities. (DoH 1989a, DoH 1997). On the other hand, social and environmental policy outside the NHS increasingly seems to acknowledge the health impact of many factors in society not historically seen as health-related. However, the foreword to *Tackling Health Inequalities: a Programme for Action* (DoH 2003) reflects the changing emphasis in government thinking from what Tony Blair refers to as a 'one-size-fits-all' approach to services via a needs-led approach, with the emphasis on service provision in response to identified need and all the ambiguities inherent in that concept, to a currently explicit concern with tackling health inequalities at every level.

One expression of this change was the establishment in 2000 of the Health Development Agency (HDA) with its specific remit to function as the national authority on how to improve health and reduce health inequalities. This agency works across the board with all organisations whose remit involves health improvement, including the NHS and local government bodies as well as the voluntary, academic and private sectors. It describes three principles underpinning health needs assessment (Hooper & Longworth 2002):

- Improvement of health and inequalities of populations. This principle is applied by:
  - identifying the most significant factors affecting health
  - making changes that tackle those factors
  - targeting population groups with the most to gain
  - targeting those services which will make the greatest difference
- Integration of identified health improvement strategies into the planning processes used by the targeted services
- Involvement of those who know what the health issues are in a community, those who are concerned about those issues and those who have the ability to make changes happen

In deciding priorities for action the HDA specifies four criteria to be used:

- *Impact* – what factors have the most significant impact on health, in terms of severity and magnitude
- *Changeability* – which significant factors can be effectively changed
- *Acceptability* – what changes can be made which are both the most acceptable and will produce the greatest positive impact
- *Resource feasibility* – what the resource implications of the proposed changes are and whether it is feasible to meet them

The contribution of health care to health

It would be only too easy for members of health care professions to view themselves as the experts on health. However, there is much to support an alternative view that sickness rather than health is the province of most health care professionals, and that their positive contribution to health is more limited than other agencies. Wright *et al.* (1998) make a distinction between *health needs* and *health care* needs, arguing that the former include needs which are not amenable to medical interventions, but require social or environmental interventions, whilst the latter are those that can benefit from health care services. Such a distinction creates helpful boundaries for those charged with rationing limited health care resources, but it also displays a reductionist and comparatively simplistic view of health which fails to address the complex interrelationships between factors impacting on health. It also risks reinforcing unidisciplinary approaches to interventions despite a continuing climate of emphasis on healthy alliances between service providers. Birley (1999; p. 11) asserts: 'Typically, government spends less than 10% of its budget on the health sector, but it is the expenditure in the other 90% that arguably has the most impact on human health.' Robinson and Elkan (1996) point out that epidemiology itself has shown repeatedly that medical interventions have only had a limited impact on the health of populations. Taken together, these assertions suggest that, alone, health care provision overall can only make a comparatively small contribution to health improvement.

Impact assessments and the health impact of public policy

Needs assessment has little meaning or relevance unless needs identified are then effectively addressed and, in recent years, the importance of critically examining both health and non-health policies for their unintended as well as intended health impacts has been recognised.

Milner (1999, p. 40), discussing the health impact of non-health public policy, makes reference to 'the social model of health which acknowledges that population health is determined by a wide range of factors, *most of which are outside the control of the formal health setting*' (my emphasis). Appleby (1999) acknowledges that policies usually have long-term and indirect unintended consequences that may include positive and negative effects on health, whilst Scott-Samuel (1999), citing evidence that public policy is the most important determinant of the public's health, seems to imply that the role of politicians is more influential than that of health professionals.

The Independent Inquiry into Health Inequalities (Acheson 1998), reinforced by the subsequent Tackling Health Inequalities programme for action (DoH 2003) drew attention to the need for the evaluation of any policy likely to impact on health in terms of that policy's effect on health inequalities.

The recognition of this need for policy evaluation has given rise to the development of a number of impact assessment strategies, to some extent interrelated. These strategies focus on the side effects of non-health policies and health policies alike. The four areas of impact which are increasingly being incorporated into policy development both locally and nationally are:

- Environmental impact assessment
- Health impact assessment
- Health inequality impact assessment (sometimes referred to as equity in health impact assessment)
- Integrated impact assessment (focusing on the impact of a policy on a range of different issues together, with an emphasis on joined-up planning) (Health Development Agency 2004)

An example of local or national policy which may give rise to an impact on all of the above areas would be road transport policy, which could impact on air pollution, respiratory health and road accident rates, and inequalities in terms of mobility and access to health facilities as well as trade and business interests.

Impact assessments can be prospective, informing choices between alternative policy options and enabling modifications to proposed policies to maximise health outcomes. They can also be retrospective, offering a means of evaluation.

The documented discussion of the best means of conducting such assessments reveals the paradoxical concerns with necessary cost containment and social justice. Whilst Appleby (1999 p. 7) contends that cost–benefit analysis should be the evaluative technique of choice, converting health loss or gain into financial equivalents such as the Department of Transport's value of a statistical life (£550 000 at 1990 prices according to Appleby), Scott-Samuel (1999) is clear that key principles of health impact assessment include an explicit focus on social and environmental justice.

Public policy and the community nurse

Since all community nurses work in face to face contact with patients and clients in their homes and community settings, they are in a prime position to observe the differential health impact of public policies on different individuals. Some years ago a newly qualified health visitor expressed serious concern at a road improvement scheme which would place an infant welfare clinic beside a newly designated dual carriageway with no safe means for pedestrians to cross the road near the clinic. Her more experienced colleagues maintained that it was not their business to alert the highway authority. Arguably even then those staff failed to recognise their role as responsible citizens, and had this happened today it could be said that an opportunity was missed to contribute to government accident prevention targets. An example of the impact of national policy on which many community nurses would be in a position to make informed comment would be the effects of asylum and immigration policy, that in turn lead to perceptions of social exclusion.

Community nurses also have a role in distinguishing between those health influencing factors over which clients have control and those over which they do not; e.g. the extent to which individuals have control over their diet varies greatly and whilst some have the means and the knowledge to make healthy choices, others do not. Effective health policies will be those that incorporate the capacity to address such individual variation.

Prevention and health: everybody's business – and an individual's responsibility

During the 1970s the preventive function of public health action, which had historically comprised efforts to address adverse living and environmental conditions, also began to incorporate attention to individual lifestyles and behaviours which constituted risk factors in relation to particular diseases. As disease patterns changed and infectious diseases were replaced as the leading causes of death by heart disease and cancers in particular, prevention of ill-health began to be seen as more of an individual responsibility (Department of Health and Social Security 1976). Health promotion and education aimed at behaviour change has increasingly occupied a significant place in public health strategy. However, the simplistic belief that knowledge invariably confers power, and that therefore health information would automatically result in healthy choices has given way to greater understanding of obstacles to sustained behaviour change. Community nurses are amongst those front-line workers who are in a prime position to analyse the obstacles that confront clients in the locality in which they work.

Despite the more recent caveat that behavioural explanations of health can amount to 'victim blaming' where individuals are constrained by social circumstances and unable to adopt healthy behaviours, individual behaviour clearly does contribute both to the health of that individual and of others. The speeding motorist, the drunk driver and the smoker who lights up in the presence of a baby or a vulnerable asthmatic all fail to meet their personal responsibilities for health.

Identifying the needs of vulnerable groups

The term *vulnerable group* is a convenient label to attach to members of society who share common experiences which render them more than ordinarily open to compromised health. It may conjure up images of urban decay and deprivation, and indeed such areas are home to many vulnerable people. However, the use of tools to rank local areas in terms of relative deprivation risks placing many vulnerable individuals and groups living in more affluent areas at greater risk to their health. Those living in poverty do not all live conveniently in ghettos of substandard housing on run-down inner city estates, and indicators of poverty are not all equally appropriate for use in all localities. For example, the Jarman Index (1983) used to calculate underprivileged area scores, includes indices that relate to lack of car

ownership as an indicator. Evans (1997) points out however that car ownership can become a necessity in rural areas where there is a lack of public transport. The same author adds that cottages of those on low incomes in the country are often found next door to the homes of high-earning city commuters. Evans pleads for rurally sensitive indicators of need in order to achieve equity of service provision in comparison with urban areas.

Rather than relying on existing categories of those perceived to be vulnerable, a socially responsible approach to needs assessment requires a continuing review of changing characteristics, patterns and trends in a population which may sustain or alter the relative vulnerability of certain of its members. Some current examples of these include the rural poor, refugees and those suffering from disability. Consideration of needs in rural areas in particular offers some challenges to some of the stereotypical assumptions about vulnerable groups.

Needs assessment in rural areas

Despite the figures indicating that approximately 20% of the UK population, more than ten million people, live in rural areas (NCVO 1994), much literature about needs assessment makes little or no mention of the special problems of rural populations. Several themes emerge in the literature which does exist:

- The National Council for Voluntary Organisations (1994) echoes Evans' (1997) concerns, identifying an absence of relevant and adequate measures of deprivation in rural areas
- Problems of distance, travel and transport emerge as major problems both for access by users to health facilities and for domiciliary provision of services (Brown 1999; Clark *et al.* 1995; Gerrard & Walsh 1997; NCVO 1994)
- Costs of service provision, information and facilities are increased in rural areas, yet choice and quality can often be reduced (Brown 1999; Clark *et al.* 1995; NCVO 1994)

An example of problems of service provision offered by Brown (1999) is that of poor distribution of nursing and residential homes in particular, despite the higher proportion of frail elderly living in rural areas. The significance to individuals is brought home by an account in the Mull and Iona community newspaper (Am Muileach 1999) of a proposed progressive care centre project. The article points out that there are no residential nursing beds on the Isle of Mull, and a woeful shortage of residential care beds. Inevitably, older people end up on the mainland somewhere far from their own environment, and visitors encounter long journeys to see them. Evening visiting is impossible because of the ferry times.

Alternative views on health needs and public health – differing but complementary?

A consideration of different perspectives on what constitutes health need and public health is not merely a theoretical exercise, but raises questions concerning the basis for decisions and actions. There is a risk of thoughtless polarisation of attitudes. For example, community nurses may dismiss the value of large-scale surveys and quantitative data collection as failing to capture the 'real' felt needs of the public and to identify local realities which determine the effectiveness of service responses. From this viewpoint, statistics may be regarded with cynicism as at best incomplete and inaccurate, and at worst ammunition for distortion of the real issues. Conversely, policy makers and economists may view qualitative, anecdotal, and small-scale data as insufficiently precise, objective and representative to be trustworthy. Polarisation in terms of public health perspectives may arise when notions of individual responsibility conflict with those of victim-blaming.

These potential conflicts draw attention to the context-bound nature of all human viewpoints. The dominance of a medical model of health especially during the latter part of the 19th century and the first half of the 20th century coincided with the battle to contain the impact of communicable diseases, with a hierarchical social structure which was only beginning to be questioned, and with the rise of technology and science. Health as the concern and responsibility of each individual emerged during a period of apparent success in eradicating communicable disease with immunisation and antibiotics, to be replaced by chronic diseases arguably resulting from choice of lifestyle in an era of increased affluence for all. More recently, complacency about technological mastery of infectious disease has been rudely challenged by the emergence of new diseases including the HIV/AIDS pandemic, and the resurgence of old diseases newly resistant to immunisation or antibiotics, such as tuberculosis and methicillin-resistant *Staphylococcus aureus* (MRSA).

Marchant (2000) draws attention to an international shift in public health priorities towards chronic non-communicable diseases, led in part by the World Health Organization itself. This has raised both ideological concerns and worries about the accuracy of judgements being made. Those concerned from a social justice perspective argue that emphasis on chronic non-communicable diseases simply widens the gap between the rich and the poor, because these are the diseases of affluent societies and infectious diseases have a hugely disproportionate effect on people in the developing world. Those concerned about miscalculation point to evidence that when funding drops for the battle against infectious diseases, time and again they return, and that with increasing drug resistance we are losing the weapons we have against them.

Marchant's comments are strangely reminiscent of the 19th century, when the rich in the growing towns and cities could no longer fully insulate themselves from the health concerns of the poor as the cholera and typhoid epidemics attacked rich and poor alike. The evidence of history suggests that the range of views on health need and public health all have a relevant contribution to enable the nurse to acquire a full understanding of all the dimensions needing to be addressed in order to most effectively promote the public's health. Not least of such contributions are those offered by practising community nurses.

Health needs assessment – the contribution of community nurses

Three key factors

The particular contribution community nurses can make to the process of health needs assessment is constrained by:

- Their perception of their position as agents of both social control and social change
- The extent to which their potential contribution is recognised and sought by commissioners of services
- The ability of community nurses to articulate their knowledge in language familiar to such commissioners

Community nurses who perceive themselves primarily as employees may on the one hand be at risk of focusing excessively on failures of compliance on the part of clients as the explanation of health deficits – for example low resistance to infection as a result of failure to follow sound dietary advice. On the other hand, recognition of their advocacy role may help them to be more alert to negative health impacts of policies – for example relating the incidence of asthma and respiratory infection to housing policies which result in disadvantaged families living in damp and inadequately heated homes.

It is important that community nurses do not fail to recognise the special nature of the knowledge of people's health experience that they accumulate as a part of everyday practice. In being privileged to enter the homes and lives of people with whom they might not ordinarily have contact, they have a unique opportunity to develop understanding and insight into local patterns of need, knowledge which is not easily accessed in other ways. As an advocate, it becomes the nurse's responsibility to seek ways of sharing that knowledge with service purchasers and providers and influencing policy development.

Percy-Smith and Sanderson (1992) comment that because community nurses have detailed first-hand knowledge of their clients and the problems that they face, they can make a valuable contribution to understanding the causes of health problems. The authors assert that such front-line workers should be fully involved in the policy process and that, in their view, the latter have been a neglected resource. The inclusion of community nurse representatives on primary care trust boards reflects a changing attitude to the ascribed worth of their knowledge. These boards offer a structure within which community nurses

---

Box 6.1 Community nurses' contribution to health needs assessment

- Insight into a local community's strengths as well as its needs
- Knowledge of local 'natural' boundaries
- First-hand insight into clients' health experience and sickness impact
- First-hand insight into the health impact of official policies
- Insight into the needs of informal carers
- Understanding of problems relating to access and equity
- Day-to-day contact with the range of interested parties
- Ability to identify existing and emerging patterns of need within their caseloads
- Ability to provide 'live', contemporaneous caseload data, both statistical and qualitative
- Ability to identify the range and diversity within caseload populations
- Evidence of effectiveness and cost-effectiveness of local interventions

---

have a far more effective channel of communication with local primary care decision makers than previously. It is an opportunity to be exploited, but in order to do so effectively, community nurses will need to appreciate the perspectives, priorities and language of politicians, economists and purchasers. They will also need to be skilled in presenting their evidence of need as they understand it, and in articulating the basis for the service responses they would propose. Indeed, specialist community nurses of the future need a new corporate image of themselves as partners in assessing, planning and managing health interventions in the community as well as what they have always been – skilled providers of existing services.

Box 6.1 lists the contributions community nurses can offer to needs assessment, which are discussed below.

Insight into a local community's strengths as well as its needs

Robinson and Elkan (1996) point out that community nurses function as participants in the social processes of the communities within which they work. They become privy to factors influencing the experiences and behaviour of local people which are not accessed by more formal needs assessment strategies. The presence of recognised local community leaders, active tenants' and residents' associations and other local community groups suggests a strong sense of local community and identity which may make the difference between hope and apathy for those living in a deprived area. Community nurses not only become aware of existing family and informal social support networks, but also of how these networks operate, who is included in them and who is excluded from them.

Local knowledge of such community characteristics can contribute to meaningful dialogue between local people and the relevant authorities, and a deeper understanding of the necessary elements of local health interventions if they are to be successful. However, it is important for community nurses to value such knowledge. Some years ago, health visitors sought to set up a clinic on a 'no-go' east London council estate, with a signal lack of success. Subsequently a community development project was established and, at the request of local tenants, some complementary therapy services were set up. A health visitor recruited to provide baby massage sessions found herself dealing additionally with precisely the child care and management questions that the clinic had been intended to address. When asked why the project succeeded where the clinic had failed, a project manager commented that the former was felt by residents to be something the authorities wanted, whereas they felt that the community project was responding to what the residents wanted. Even the title of a service may be symbolic of ownership by the authorities or the local people, and what feels acceptable to one population group will not necessarily do so to another.

Knowledge of local 'natural' boundaries

Community nurses also come to recognise the 'hidden' boundaries to neighbourhood territory that determine people's willingness to use facilities. Distance may be less important than whether a facility is perceived to be located in one's own group's neighbourhood or not, and one street can be bisected by such boundaries. 'Natural' routes that people use are also not necessarily the most obviously logical, as witness the instances where parents will dash across busy roads with young children rather than struggle over bridges or through underpasses on longer but safer routes. Usage or otherwise of services may not only be affected by territorial and geographical factors, however. In one locality the fear of personal attack prevented mobile elderly people from walking to the nearby new day centre, and despite the close proximity and easy level walking, transport had to be arranged before the centre was used.

Insights such as these can make a crucial contribution to the success of new policies and initiatives.

First-hand insight into clients' health experience and sickness impact, and into the health impact of official policies

In working with clients, patients and families community nurses become aware of the unique multi-faceted web of factors impacting on the health experience of each individual – for example, in one locality high levels of neighbour noise pollution and consequent lack of sleep exacerbated people's pain experience associated with illness. Again, the impact of physical disability when living on benefit on the tenth floor of a tower block is likely to be very different from the impact of the same disability when living on the ground floor in owner occupied purpose built or adapted accommodation, and being a person of independent means.

Insights such as these place community nurses once again at the interface between lay and official understandings of health issues. Phillimore and Moffatt (1994) refer to discounted knowledge in drawing attention to dismissive official attitudes to public fears and concerns. Taking the example of possible health effects of pollution from local industries they discuss the different ways of knowing about the environment and its impact on health. The residents may describe periods of illness they associate with episodes of pollution (experiential, subjective knowledge), whilst scientific predictions may dispute the existence of a cause-effect relationship (scientific, objective knowledge). This kind of tension is at the heart of debates about needs assessment strategies, a debate which ceases to be academic for the community nurse exposed to both sides of the argument. What should have been the action of the health visitor exposed to the social and psychological consequences for a young family of five and their mother resulting from the death from bladder cancer of a father in his 30s? The father in question was an employee in a major chemical industry, and one of a number of employees who became ill in similar circumstances.

The above examples also indicate opportunities for community nurses to observe the impact on individuals of policies in the realms of housing, disability, benefit, employment and the environment.

Insight into the needs of informal carers

Caring for a dependent relative, particularly where that relative is mentally ill, disabled or terminally ill can mean that the carer becomes socially isolated, may find themselves in reduced financial circumstances, and that their needs may be easily overlooked. Community nurses may sometimes be the only regular visitors who are in a position to recognise where existing services are inadequate to meet their needs and to act as advocates on their behalf.

Understanding of problems relating to access and equity

Some years ago in the west of England a complaint arose that parents from a small new town development outside the city were defaulting on paediatric follow-up appointments with their children. The implication was that there was a need to educate the parents to be more compliant. However, contact with the families enabled health visitors to point out the range of problems encountered by these parents. Most of the families were on low income, without access to a car, and typically had two or three children under five years of age. Social support networks and local child care facilities were lacking, and a journey to the paediatric outpatient department involved

two bus rides with all the children and then a climb on foot up a hill with a gradient of 1 in 4. One of the bus services was infrequent, and then on arrival at the outpatient department waiting times could be long. From the health visitors' point of view, the need was for more locally based paediatric outpatient services.

Day-to-day contact with the range of interested parties

In their everyday work community nurses have to deal with a range of statutory and voluntary agencies, and in so doing will become aware of how role boundaries and resource limitations limit the effectiveness of these agencies in addressing complex health care needs.

Whilst under the NHS and Community Care Act 1990 the concept of health need was a narrow one, arbitrarily separated from the concept of social need, Cowley *et al.*'s (2000) study found that the prevalent nursing concept of need was of a complex and variable phenomenon reflecting a nursing ideal of wholeness, or holism. It is perhaps unsurprising that policy makers tasked with addressing needs of whole populations and with limited resources at their disposal tend to create boundaries which delimit so-called legitimate need. Such a strategy arguably redefines an impossible task into a possible one. It is equally unsurprising that nurses confronted daily by their clients' total situations and expressions of felt need should find it almost self-evident that attempts to separate health and social care misrepresent reality.

Community nurses with such an holistic perspective on need are in a prime position to contribute to collaborative and multi-disciplinary approaches to needs assessment.

Ability to provide 'live', contemporaneous caseload data, both statistical and qualitative and to identify existing and emerging patterns of need within their caseloads

One of the insoluble dilemmas of needs assessment is that populations are dynamic entities, and assessments are arguably out-of-date before they are completed. Mobile populations, an influx of migrants, the impact of a recession, the onset of an epidemic and changing social patterns comprise but a few examples of factors which make a final and comprehensive needs assessment an impossibility. The value of caseload data from community nurses as from others working in direct contact with the public is that such data is both up-to-date and 'live' – that is, it is in touch with the current issues for local people.

Ability to identify the range and diversity within caseload populations

One limitation of statistics drawn from a large population is their tendency to average out differences. An important contribution community nurses can make in identifying need lies in caseload knowledge which enables them to recognise small minority groups who become vulnerable locally because they are few in number and may thus be regarded as low in the scale of priorities where emphasis is on the most cost-effective use of resources. Where populations are polarised, for example, where the majority of people occupy one end or other of the social scale, community nurses may be in a position to identify how a given policy or initiative will differentially affect the two groups.

Evidence of effectiveness and cost-effectiveness of local interventions

In summary, community nurses, by virtue of the special knowledge gained in practice, are in a position to make a significant contribution to the needs of local people and to estimates of effectiveness and cost-effectiveness of interventions offered in response. One particular aspect of such estimates is attention to the assessment of risk, both in terms of threats to health and any risks associated with service response. Immunisation programmes offer examples of situations where it is ethically imperative to assess the balance of risk.

Risk assessment

Public policy and risk assessment

A significant element of health impact assessment of any public policy needs to be risk analysis, involving the identification and quantification of environmental health hazards and the relative risks of various options (Milner 1999). Birley (1999 p. 13) defines a *health hazard* as potential harm, a *health risk* as the probability that a health hazard will harm a particular group of people at a particular time and place, and a *health impact* as a change in health risk reasonably attributable to a policy or project. A policy may have an identifiable and measurable cause–effect relationship with a health risk, for example where acceptable limits are set on the industrial discharge of pollutants. In other instances several different policies may combine to produce cumulative effects such that individually they may represent acceptable levels of risk, but together they create an unacceptable health impact. Birley suggests that in particular those health risks that have more complex and multifactorial determinants are susceptible to such cumulative effects.

Scott-Samuel (1999) suggests that potential risk can be assessed in terms of:

- Estimated size of hazard, such as increased air pollution
- Likelihood of the hazard occurring: whether it is definite, probable, or speculative
- Subjective perceptions of risk, including qualitative data from populations that would potentially be threatened

In considering how a policy has the potential to impact on health, Birley (1999) draws attention to the need to address:

- The characteristics of a community that create vulnerability to health hazards, such as poverty, poor immune status, high unemployment
- Risk factors arising from change in the environment, such as alienation, insecurity and fear that may arise as a consequence of resettling communities
- The contribution of health protection agencies, i.e. the available staff and resources, the knowledge and skills within the agencies and their statutory responsibilities. In addition to health services, health protection agencies include services such as police, transport, local government, local community organisations and emergency services

Risk assessment and the community nurse

The risk assessment function of community nurses is inextricably interwoven with their responsibility to search for health needs and their role in health promotion.

As with their potential contribution to identification of need, community nurses are equipped to offer insights into threats to health by virtue of their daily contact with their clients and client groups, as the following examples demonstrate.

Community nurses contribute to a range of screening procedures, and all screening programmes seek to identify either possible indicators of risk to health or actual disease incidence at a pre-symptomatic stage. Community nurses, however, are also able to identify unintended effects of the screening programmes themselves, such as the intense distress and anxiety occasioned by ambiguous or false positive results from screening for breast cancer. Furthermore, they can contribute to cost-benefit analysis of screening for conditions such as hypertension, where there is debate about the necessity for and appropriateness of intervention in all cases. Where identification does not lead to treatment, the negative outcome of anxiety still remains.

Any community nurse may be in a position to identify how unwanted side effects of any particular drug therapy outweigh its therapeutic benefit for given patients. District nurses in particular are likely to encounter adverse drug reactions arising from physiological changes associated with ageing and the prescription of several drugs to an older patient in the management of multiple chronic diseases.

A district nurse may also experience at first hand the unrelenting demands of patients with advancing Alzheimer's disease which are in danger of driving caring relatives to physical or mental breakdown or violence. Equally the nurse may be able to identify how respite care itself may cause deterioration in the behaviour of the patients and so destroy the delicate balance which has enabled the carers to cope. Such insights can inform policies in relation to the development of sensitive and appropriate services that will contribute to the protection of both patients and their informal carers in the home. The in-depth knowledge of the individual experiences of patients, clients and carers equips community nurses to identify areas of risk to health or safety common to the vulnerable groups to which such individuals belong.

Health visitors are able to use their knowledge of child development as well as their assessment of the stressors impacting on adult carers in the family to identify home safety and accident risks, and any community nurse making a home visit may be able to identify environmental hazards due to building design or use. Homeless families may be especially vulnerable where landlords have failed to maintain properties with adequate facilities and safety precautions, whilst elderly patients are at risk in properties not adapted to take account of increasing frailty and infirmity.

Community nurses can also offer a perspective on how patterns of human behaviour in the wider community relate to health risks. Recently, a group of community nurse students commented on the phenomenon of the school run, itemising the effects of parents taking their children to school by car as being:

- Later development of child pedestrians' ability to use the roads safely
- Contribution to lack of exercise in childhood with its effects on resting heart rates and blood pressure
- Increased congestion and risk of road accidents outside schools

Conclusion

This chapter has sought to present some key perspectives and issues surrounding the assessment of health need and health risk which have particular relevance to community nursing practice. Particular messages for community nurses that emerge are:

- Identifying and responding appropriately to health need involves dialogue and partnership with individuals and agencies whose perspectives, priorities and language may differ markedly from those of community nurses
- Community nurses possess insights and knowledge by virtue of their access to clients'

homes and lives which place them in a unique position to offer informed contributions to formal community health needs and risk assessments

- Community nurses need to recognise and value the special insights their work provides them with
- It is not enough for community nurses to wait to be asked for their contributions. They need to be active in contributing to the work of their local primary care trust, not least by briefing their board nurse representatives as fully as possible

Community nurses are not only in daily touch with the health needs and risks confronting their patients and clients; in a world beset by ever faster change in the environment, technology and society, community nurses are placed in a key position to identify newly emerging needs and threats to health. They have the capacity to act as an early warning system, but only if they remain alert to this aspect of their potential role.

References

Acheson, D. (1998) *Independent Inquiry into Inequalities in Health* (Acheson Report). The Stationery Office, London.

Am Muileach (1999) Caring for the community. *Am Muileach* Issue 211, p. 16, June.

Appleby, J. (1999) Health Impact Assessments: Desirable but Difficult. In: *Report on one day seminar on health impact assessment*. DoH, London.

Appleton, J.V. & Cowley, S. (2000) *The Search for Health Needs: Research for Health Visiting Practice*. Macmillan, Basingstoke.

Benzeval, M., Judge, K. & Whitehead, M. (1995) *Tackling Inequalities in Health: An agenda for action.* King's Fund, London.

Beveridge, W. (1942) *Social Insurance and Allied Services (Beveridge Report)*. HMSO, London.

Billings, J. (2000) Lay Perspectives on Health Needs, Chapter 5 In: *The Search for Health Needs: Research for Health Visiting Practice* (J.V. Appleton & S. Cowley (eds). Ch. 5. Macmillan Press Ltd, Basingstoke.

Birley, M. (1999) Procedures and Methods for Health Impact Assessment. In: *Report on one day seminar on health impact assessment*. DoH, London.

Black, D., Morris, J.N., Smith, C. & Townsend, P. (1980) *Inequalities in Health: report of a research working group (Black Report).* Department of Health and Social Security, London.

Black, D. Morris, J.N., Smith, C. & Townsend, P. (1999) Better benefits for health: plan to implement the central recommendation of the Acheson report, *British Medical Journal*, **318**, 724–727.

Blackburn, C. (1991) *Poverty and Health: Working with Families.* Open University Press, Buckingham.

Blackburn, C. (1992) *Poverty Profiling: a Guide for Community Nurses.* Health Visitors Association, London.

Bond, M. (1999) Placing poverty on the agenda of a primary health care team: an evaluation of an action research project, *Health and Social Care in the Community*, **7**(1), 9–16.

Bradshaw, J.R. (1972) A taxonomy of social need. In: *Problems and Progress in Medical Care*, G. McLachlan (ed). Nuffield Provincial Hospital Trust, Oxford.

Bradshaw, J.R. (1994) The conceptualization and measurement of need: a social policy perspective, In: *Researching the People's Health*, J. Popay & G. Williams (eds). Routledge, London.

Brown, D. (1999) *Care in the Country: inspection of community care in rural communities.* DoH and Social Services Inspectorate, London.

Clark, G., MacLellan, M., McKie, L. & Skerratt, S. (1995) *Food availability and food choice in remote and rural areas: Research Project conducted in the Western Isles of Scotland.* Health Education Board for Scotland, Edinburgh.

Cowley, S., Bergen, A., Young, K. & Kavanagh, A. (2000) A taxonomy of needs assessment, elicited from a multiple case study of community nursing education and practice, *Journal of Advanced Nursing*, **31**(1), 126–134.

Craddock, J. (1996a) Responses of the Occupational Therapy Profession to the Perspective of the Disability Movement, Part 1, *British Journal of Occupational Therapy*, **59**(1) 17–22.

Craddock, J. (1996a) Responses of the Occupational Therapy Profession to the Perspective of the Disability Movement, Part 2, *British Journal of Occupational Therapy*, **59**(2) 73–78.

Day, M. (2000) Blighted lives: a new way of looking at how long we live reveals Africa's plight. *New Scientist*, **166**(2242), 19.

DoH (1989a) *Caring for People: Community Care in the Next Decade and Beyond*. Department of Health, London.

DoH (1989b) *Working for Patients*. Department of Health, London.

DoH (1997) *Our Healthier Nation*. Department of Health, London.

DoH (2003) *Liberating the Public Health Talents of Community Practitioners and Health Visitors*. Department of Health, London.

DoH (2004) *The NHS Improvement Plan*. Department of Health, London.

Department of Health and Social Security (1976) *Prevention and Health: Everybody's Business: a reassessment of public and personal health*. HMSO, London.

Evans, C. (1997) Country Life. *Nursing Times*, **93**(50), 24–25.

Gerrard, C. & Walsh, M. (1997) Down on the Farm. *Nursing Times*, **93**(50), 26–28.

Hannay, D. (1979) *The Symptom Iceberg: a study of community health*. Routledge and Kegan Paul, London.

Hayward, A.L. & Sparkes, J.J. (1984) *The Concise English Dictionary*. Omega Books Limited, Ware, Herts.

Health Development Agency (2004) *HDA Impact Report: 2003/04*. HDA, London.

Hooper, J. & Longworth, P. (2002) *Health Needs Assessment Workbook*. NHS Health Development Agency.

Jarman, B. (1983) Identification of underprivileged areas. *British Medical Journal*, **286**, 1705–1709.

Marchant, J. (2000) WHO's way to health, *New Scientist*, **166**(2232), 16–17.

Martin, C.J. & McQueen, D.V. (1989) Framework for a New Public Health In: *Readings for a New Public Health* C.J. Martin & D.V. McQueen (eds). Edinburgh University Press, Edinburgh.

Milio, N. (1986) *Promoting Health through Public Policy*. Canadian Public Health Association, Ottawa.

Milner, S. (1999) The Health Impact Assessment of Non-Health Public Policy. In: *Report on one day seminar on health impact assessment*. DoH, London.

Murray, S.A. (1999) Experiences with 'rapid appraisal' in primary care: involving the public in assessing health needs, orientating staff, and educating medical students. *British Medical Journal*, **318**, 440–444.

Naidoo, J. & Wills, J. (1994) *Health Promotion: Foundations for Practice*. Baillière Tindall, London.

Naidoo, J. & Wills, J. (1998) *Practising Health Promotion: Dilemmas and Challenges*. Baillière Tindall, London.

NHS and Community Care Act 1990. The Stationery Office, London.

The Nursing and Midwifery Council (2002) *Code of Professional Conduct*. NMC, London.

Ong, B.N. & Humphris, G. (1994) Prioritizing needs within communities: Rapid Appraisal methodologies in Health. In: *Researching the People's Health*, J. Popay and G. Williams (eds) Ch. 4. Routledge, London.

Percy-Smith, J. & Sanderson, I. (1992) *Understanding Local Needs*. Institute for Public Policy Research, London.

Phillimore, P. & Moffat, M. (1994) Discounted knowledge: local experience, environmental pollution and health. In: *Researching the People's Health*, J. Popay and G. Williams (eds). Routledge, London.

Pickin, C. & St Leger, S. (1993) *Assessing Health Need using the Life Cycle Framework*. Open University Press, Buckingham.

Popay, J. & Williams, G. (1994) *Researching the People's Health*. Routledge, London.

Robinson, J. (1985) Health Visiting and Health. In: *Political Issues in Nursing* Vol.1, R. White (ed). John Wiley & Sons, Chichester.

Robinson, J. & Elkan, R. (1996) *Health Needs Assessment: Theory and Practice*. Churchill Livingstone, Edinburgh.

Rural team of the National Council for Voluntary Organisations (1994) *Not just Fine Tuning – a Review of Shire County Community Care Plans for Rural Areas*. National Council for Voluntary Organisations.

Scott-Samuel, A. (1999) Methods for Prospective Health Impact Assessment of Public Sector Policy. In: *Report on one day seminar on health impact assessment*. DoH, London.

School Standards and Framework Act 1998. HMSO, London.

Standing Nursing and Midwifery Advisory Committee (1995) *Making it Happen: Public Health – the Contribution of Nurses, Midwives and Health Visitors*. DoH, London.

TSO (1997) *The New NHS: Modern, Dependable*. Cm 3807 The Stationery Office, London.

TSO (1998) *Our Healthier Nation: a contract for health*. Cm 3852 The Stationery Office, London.

Wilkinson, R.G. (1996) *Unhealthy Societies: the Afflictions of Inequality*. Routledge, London.

World Health Organization (1985) *Targets for Health for All. Targets in Support of the European Regional Strategy for Health for All*. World Health Organization Regional Office for Europe, Copenhagen.

Wright, J., Williams, R. & Wilkinson, J.R. (1998) Development and importance of health needs assessment (Health Needs Assessment, Part 1). *British Medical Journal*, **316**, 1310–1313.

Chapter 7 Research Perspectives Applied to Primary Health Care

Pam Smith, Julie Bliss, Pat Colliety, Vasso Vydelingum and Ben Gray

Introduction

This chapter is designed to assist the reader to make links between research, policy and practice as described elsewhere in this book. The chapter can also be read as a 'stand-alone' text that provides the community health care practitioner with the necessary information to consider research methodologies, methods and findings as they apply in everyday practice.

The chapter considers:

- Priorities for nursing and primary health care research
- The knowledge base for primary health care practitioners
- Reflective practice and research mindedness
- The research process
- Selected research examples that demonstrate the application of the research process and use of research in community nursing practice
- General research issues

Priorities for nursing and health care research

Over the past decade, government policy and strategy in the United Kingdom, has put primary care and public health high on the agenda of health and social care delivery (DoH 1990, 1992, 1999a). This agenda is supported by the emphasis on the utilisation of existing staff in new ways and the evolution of new roles. There are also changes to funding primary care through the general medical services (GMS) which shifts the focus from doctors to take account of practice workloads and patients' needs (DoH 2000a, 2002a, 2002b, 2003a; Hawksley *et al.* 2003; Meyrick *et al.* 2001).

This agenda has been supported by a research and development strategy to set priorities and promote a research culture to move the base of clinical practice from ritual to evidence and improve the quality of care of patients, clients and communities (DoH 1991, 1997a, 2000b).

Well established features of the evidence-based health care landscape are the Cochrane Collaboration originating in Oxford in the 1990s, to undertake systematic reviews of trial findings and disseminate them among clinicians and purchasers, and the NHS Centre for Reviews and Dissemination at the University of York. The aim of the York centre is 'to promote the application of research-based knowledge in health care'. This knowledge not only relates to evidence on the effectiveness of treatments but also service delivery and organisation. The National Institute for Clinical Excellence (NICE) is another key feature of the government's drive to raise the profile of evidence-based health care and to ensure that only those interventions with a proven track record of effectiveness are adopted. Kendall (1997), a professor of community nursing, is not alone in the view that '"evidence-based practice" has become the watch-word of the NHS' indeed a view that is even more strongly reflected in the current NHS.

Smith *et al.* (2004) are cautious of the messianic flavour of the evidence-based health movement and invite other approaches to capture evidence through narratives and participatory action research to both complement and offer alternatives to the 'gold standard' of systematic reviews, meta-analysis and randomised controlled trials. Narrative and participatory action research, as we shall see later have much to offer the community nurse practitioner.

Readers will be familiar with the changing discourse of health promotion and public health.

This discourse dates back at least to the 1976 policy document *Prevention and Health: Everybody's Business* when responsibility for maintaining health and well being was explicitly shifted from a collective responsibility at the level of government and firmly placed on individual shoulders. More recently, the *Health of the Nation* document (DoH 1992) was criticised for its narrow focus on five prescribed areas: coronary heart disease and stroke; cancers; mental illness; HIV/AIDS; and accidents. Research and development programmes were set up for each of these areas in order to document and reduce their incidence and investigate treatment outcomes. The responsibility for these programmes was devolved to the regional health authorities, which, in 1996, were incorporated into the Department of Health.

Harris (1993) believed that changes during the early 1990s within the NHS offered opportunities to redress the balance between hospital dominated research programmes of the past and population based primary care and by inference, public health research of the future. Historically, there has certainly been a dearth of research in the field of community nursing in favour of topics associated with the care of hospitalised adults.

The White Paper *Saving Lives: Our Healthier Nation* recognises that social and economic issues play a major role in the nation's health (DoH 1999a). Public health initiatives have been a key feature under the auspices of the health development agency and the continued interest in the development of strategies and toolkits to move the agenda forward. As Wanless (2004) so clearly highlighted, the emphasis for public health practice has to shift from a focus on individual needs to that of the whole population in order to recognise, understand and tackle inequality.

Consequently, priorities such as social inclusion and interdisciplinary health and social care and key innovations such as Health Action Zones, Health Improvement Programmes, Sure Start Local Programmes for the under-fours and regeneration initiatives which operationalise current policies, are of concern and interest to community nurses. The public health electronic library (PHel www. phel.gov.uk) ensures that information about these and other initiatives is widely disseminated.

Partnerships with communities and individuals working together with health authorities, local authorities and the voluntary sector are seen as key to improving health and promoting equity. Schools, workplaces and neighbourhoods are identified as the key settings for action. Professionals from different agencies are expected to work together to achieve this. The imperative for partnership working has been given further impetus in the wake of such tragedies as Victoria Climbié, whose cruel treatment and subsequent death at the hands of her great-aunt went undetected because of a lack of integrated working between the police, health and social services.

Joint assessments between community nurses and social care staff to ensure that patients' health and social needs are considered and the creation of children's trusts to promote effective communication and co-ordination between all those working with children as highlighted by the Laming report (2003) are examples of how working partnerships can be developed. The emergence of new roles for NHS staff (DoH 2002b) and the new mechanism for funding primary care (DoH 2003a) further enhance the partnership process.

As part of implementing the Government's framework to put patients and frontline staff 'at the heart of the NHS' set out in *Shifting the Balance of Power*, strategic health authorities are required to produce a 'transformation plan' to propose ways of delivering the Government's health care agenda (DoH 2003a, 2004). Primary care trusts (PCTs) are identified as taking a lead role in the changes because of their 'unique position across community, hospital and primary care' and at the interface of the NHS and local authority. Initiatives are required to develop both existing staff and new roles to support innovative services such as Hospital at Home and Hospital at Night while taking account of the reduction in junior doctors' hours. Within the NHS there is a move away from working with traditional roles towards looking at what needs to be done and who is the most appropriate person to do it (DoH 2000a, 2002a, 2004) all of which must be underpinned by a sound evidence base.

Since their election in 1997 and their continued office until the current time the Labour Government has introduced a number of cornerstone documents that continue to confirm the prominence of evidence-based practice, research, quality and audit as components of clinical governance (DoH 1997b, 1998, 1999b).

In 1997 a Department of Health document stated:

'The NHS Research and Development strategy aims to create a knowledge-based health service in which clinical, managerial and policy decisions are underpinned by sound information about research findings and scientific developments.'

(DoH 1997a)

The NHS Research and Development strategy has subsequently shifted its emphasis to support these initiatives (DoH 2000b) in a comprehensive rethink set out in the policy document *Research and Development for a First Class Service*. Active research programmes are encouraged, based on locally defined priorities and alliances in order to develop specialist research which 'reflect consultation with NHS users and staff'. The need for a capacity building strategy to take the proposed research forward is also acknowledged.

Saks (2000), in the introduction to a textbook entitled *Developing Research in Primary Care*, observes that although the imperative of evidence-based practice calls attention to the importance of undertaking primary care research, it still remains 'relatively underdeveloped' (p. 1). The increased prominence of public health policy and associated initiatives call for a renewed emphasis on a broad sweep research agenda to incorporate the associated fields of primary care, health promotion and public health to ensure the rhetoric matches the reality.

The importance of research skills to community nurses and public health practitioners is highlighted by a study undertaken by three of the authors of this chapter (Vydelingum *et al.* 2004). They were commissioned by the local strategic health authority to create a vision for and undertake a skills audit of public health among the local community nursing community. This included school nurses, practice nurses, health visitors and district nurses who all identified a range of research, epidemiological and change management skills as being essential for taking the new public health agenda forward.

Changes to local working arrangements such as meeting targets for First Contact, Public Health and Chronic Disease Management, as outlined in the report *Liberating the Talents* (DoH 2002b), also highlight the need for new skills as part of the development of new community nursing roles.

For example, the impact of the new roles on nursing practice and perception are captured in the following quotation featured in a paper by Franks and Smith (2002). A nurse consultant working in the care of older people describes the scope of her new role that allows her to work collaboratively with other professions thus:

'central to this job is trying to forge links between health and social care. I work with entire ward teams of nurses, domestic staff as well as strategically with the PCT (Primary Care Trust). I have told people about my role – the community team, other professionals, trust boards, voluntary organisations...and I'm still doing it two years later'.

From a reading of government policy therefore, there is clearly a need to identify an appropriate knowledge base and flexible and innovative research methodologies and methods for investigating a range of issues associated with health service reform in general and public health and primary care in particular. The next section examines the knowledge, methodologies and methods required to fulfil the research requirements of the current primary health care and public health agendas.

The knowledge base for public health and primary health care practitioners

Primary health care practitioners draw on knowledge from a range of disciplines including medicine, epidemiology, psychology, sociology and anthropology. The field is complex and as such needs a multidisciplinary approach to its practice, education and research.

Epidemiology, often described as the cornerstone science of public health (Mulhall 1996) is concerned with 'the occurrence, distribution and determinants of states of health and disease in human groups and populations' (Abramson 1990, p. 12).

Scientific knowledge, which predominates in medicine and epidemiology, is associated with facts and theories. On closer scrutiny these are not necessarily set in tablets of stone, as the risk factor literature illustrates.

For example, stress, which prevailed as a risk factor in the development of peptic ulcers for decades, was overturned during the 1990s in favour of a bacterial model of disease causation. Researchers demonstrated that there was a strong association between the organism *Heliocobacter pylori* and the occurrence of the condition (Moore 1995). The discovery of this new information was not welcomed by the drug companies at first and indeed financial reasons may have played a part in delaying the uptake of the bacterial rather than the stress theory of causation.

Practitioners need to 'accept that the information and research we talk about today is based on yesterday's understanding'. It is also necessary 'to understand the limitations of our present knowledge' and acquire 'skills to evaluate new information and research findings and to apply this to tomorrow's situations' (Rees 1992).

As clients and patients become well informed through the media and the internet, primary health care practitioners are no longer the only holders of evidence or information about diseases and treatments. They need to become more familiar therefore with critical appraisal of the literature, research methodologies, methods and findings and evaluate them in the light of practice. Ways of doing this are through reflective practice and increasing research mindedness. The practitioner who combines reflection and research mindedness is in a good position to apply research to practise and undertake research.

Reflective practice and research mindedness

Reflective practice described by Benner (1984) and Schön (1987) assists practitioners to work in a reflective and analytic way to recognise their field knowledge, evaluate research findings and guide future practice. Researchers work in similar ways, moving between the field, the literature and their data to make interpretations to generate findings and guide future research.

Research mindedness is defined by the Royal College of Nursing's research group as 'a critical and questioning approach to one's work, the desire and ability to find out about the latest research in the area and apply it as appropriate' (RCN 1982).

For the primary health care practitioner who shares many similar work experiences to social workers the following elements of research mindedness identified in a textbook for social work practitioners seem particularly relevant (Box 7.1).

Although Everitt and colleagues published their textbook in 1992 their original insights on reflective practice and critical thinking are still as pertinent today. This definition of research mindedness reflects an integrated approach to research-based practice. The emphasis for the authors is clearly not simply on doing research but on using its theoretical perspectives and methods to think analytically about and inform practice.

Box 7.1   The characteristics of the research-minded practitioner (Everitt *et al.* 1992). With permission from Palgrave Macmillan

- Constantly defining and making explicit their objectives and hypotheses
- Treat their explanations of the social world as hypotheses – that is, as tentative and open to be tested against evidence
- Aware of their expertise and knowledge and that of others
- Bring to the fore theories that help make sense of social need, resources and assist in decision making with regard to strategies
- Thoughtful, reflecting on data and theory and contributing to their development and refinement
- Scrutinise and analyse available data and information
- Mindful of the pervasiveness of ideology and values in the way we see and understand the world

Research mindedness also allows practitioners to identify their own knowledge and expertise that would otherwise go unrecognised and undetected. Being research minded therefore encourages reflective practice and critical thinking, challenges the status quo and constructs arguments to defend resources and assist decision making (Smith 1997).

A conversation by one of the authors with a district nurse about the types of devices for dispensing medication for people with asthma demonstrates how the reflective and research minded practitioner is able to gather evidence to improve the quality of patient care. The district nurse reported difficulties in prescribing up to date devices for treating patients with asthma. The general practitioner she worked with disapproved of them because of the lack of medical research to show how they benefited patients. Also, the new devices were twice the cost of the old asthma equipment.

The district nurse observed that patients favoured the more modern devices for a variety of reasons: they looked better, were less bulky and easier to dispense. In other words, patients attached social, personal and consumer values to these more modern devices which in turn improved the dispensing and continued use of the asthma medication. Consequently, because patients favoured the more modern devices, compliance improved, which the nurse suggested also made them more successful in medical terms.

Conversation then turned to a research paper in which the quality of life of patients with asthma had been linked to social, personal and subjective factors. Subjective feelings had been shown in the research to improve the quality of life of the patient. Research showed that the patient's personal views, including views that the patient had of health staff and methods of treatment, would significantly influence quality of life. As this example illustrates, personal, aesthetic and consumer choices play a substantial part in the dispensing of asthmatic medication and the quality of the patient's care (Drummond 2000).

The nurse then brought the research paper to the attention of her medical colleague. The research was evidence that the nurse's hunch had a basis and could be applied to general practice. The nurse had shown that patients' subjective and consumer views influenced quality of life and the continued use of asthma medication. The nurse and the doctor had research evidence that the more modern asthma devices would be better in improving quality of life. By reflecting on her practice, the research minded nurse had influenced health care and improved its quality in the general surgery's running of asthma clinics.

Such evidence-based approaches to primary health care practice has been formalised in the rise in nurse prescribing powers through the introduction of extended nurse and supplementary prescribing to provide patients with quicker and more efficient access to medication (DoH 2003b).

The contribution community nurses make to the monitoring and evaluation of health care has long been recognised as evidenced in a series of papers compiled by the Health Visitors' Association (HVA 1994). Local practitioner knowledge, described as qualitative (p. 47) and anecdotal (p. 49) was identified as being particularly valuable. A later document (HVA 1995) cited by Kendall (1997) aimed to accumulate evidence to demonstrate the effectiveness of health visiting to decision makers. However, the authors of the report were seriously challenged in their endeavours. Kendall attributes this to the difficulty of demonstrating the person- or family-centred activity of health visiting, practice nursing or district nursing which does not fit with the type of evidence associated with the 'gold standard' of systematic reviews. Decision makers are more familiar with this form of evidence and need to be convinced, as Popay and colleagues suggest, of the importance of 'subjective meaning, description of social context, and attention to lay knowledge' which qualitative research can offer (Popay *et al.* 1998).

How then can reflective, research minded practitioners go one step further to systematise and consolidate their local knowledge into research questions, projects and evidence? The research process provides a helpful framework that can be used for this purpose.

The research process

The practitioner can begin the research process by keeping a reflective diary to accumulate qualitative and anecdotal evidence for the purposes of informing decision makers, evaluating and assuring quality of care. Reflection and research mindedness are part of the process by which an evidence-based approach to practice is assured. An evidence-based approach to practice means having information from research that will assist in this process. The district nurse, described above, demonstrates how this can be done.

The following discussion is based on a seminar on research mindedness and the research process, prepared by experienced practitioners, while undertaking a postgraduate diploma in nurse education. One of the practitioners was a community nurse, and one of the authors of this chapter (Czuber-Dochan *et al*. 1997).

They selected Macleod Clark and Hockey's 1989 definition of research described as 'an attempt to increase the body of knowledge i.e. what is currently known about nursing by the discovery of new facts and relationships through a process of systematic scientific enquiry'. For Macleod Clark and Hockey 'the essential characteristic of research is its scientific nature'. Czuber-Dochan and colleagues also chose the Department of Health's (DoH 1993) definition of research as the acquisition of knowledge that includes 'gaining information, clarification and illumination as well as translating it (research) directly into policy or practice'. This last point suggests the important role practitioners play in critically assessing the relevance of research for practice.

Drawing on these and other texts, Czuber-Dochan and colleagues characterise research as:

- A process
- Scientific
- Objective
- Systematic
- Problem solving
- Advancement of knowledge
- Exploration of facts and relationships
- An enquiring attitude

They conclude: 'As the list above indicates, we adopted a broad concept of research because we saw it as being representative of the "real world" of nursing. We believed that conceptualising research in this way would provide opportunities to embrace both the art and the science of nursing knowledge. It would also support the notion that nursing, like research was a diverse activity that takes place in a variety of settings' (Czuber-Dochan *et al*. 1997).

The research process refers to the different stages involved in undertaking a research project. Like any process however, although the project is represented as being divided into distinct stages, which follow on from each other, often they are not mutually exclusive and there may be some overlap between them.

The stages of the research process can be grouped in the following way:

- Identifying the research problem and formulating a research question
- Selecting an appropriate research approach or methodology
- Designing the study
- Developing data collecting methods and techniques
- Collecting data
- Data management, analysis and interpretation
- Writing, research presentation and dissemination

Czuber-Dochan and colleagues identified 'advancement of knowledge' as a key component of research. Major changes have occurred in understanding the ways in which knowledge is produced. In a text written by an interdisciplinary group of authors from education, sociology, science policy and political science, the shift from the conventional, scientific mode of knowledge (referred to as Mode 1) to a new mode of knowledge (referred to as Mode 2) is described (Gibbons *et al*. 1994). Mode 1 refers to the hypothetico-deductive linear approaches to knowledge production that are common in academic research. Hypotheses are devised and tested in order to verify theories, make predictions and discover a body of independent objective knowledge.

The new mode of knowledge production is described as 'non-linear' in that it does not depend on hypothesis and theory testing. Rather, the production of Mode 2 type knowledge requires reflexivity, interdisciplinarity and values difference. It can take place in a variety of settings such as factories, hospitals and health centres and draws on a range of sources and processes (including information technology) to support a research agenda that is committed to exploring and legitimating different knowledge forms.

Similarly, it is important to recognise that the usual convention of describing the stages of research as a linear process is also limited, and needs to be sufficiently flexible to manage the production of Mode 2 knowledge. As Smith (2004, p. 114) notes: 'Multiple stakeholders with their competing values, agendas and expectations are involved in the new production of knowledge' and there is an increasing recognition that research designs and approaches need to be sufficiently flexible and responsive to carry out investigations across organisations, disciplines and professions. In the next section, the stages of the research process and a range of research methodologies and methods associated with different types of knowledge are considered.

Taking the research process forward

The research process is a conventional but convenient framework in which to consider research paradigms, approaches and methods when reading about and/or planning a project. The process involves identifying a topic, specifying underlying theories, formulating questions, selecting a suitable approach, specifying methods and devising a plan to take the study forward. This will depend to some extent on whether a qualitative or quantitative research approach is adopted. Ultimately however, the choice of methodologies and methods depends on the researcher's preference but also on the purpose of the research, the topic under study, the subject discipline, the funding body and the resources available. Careful consideration of time and financial budgeting, secretarial support and obtaining ethical clearance is required when planning the research and will repay itself with interest over the remainder of the study. The following sections present a selection of worked examples to demonstrate the application of different aspects

of the research process to primary health care practice.

Research examples

Identifying the research problem: where do research questions come from?

Holloway and Wheeler (2002) suggest that certain criteria should be considered when identifying a research problem. They argue that the topic must be relevant, be of interest to the researcher and the question must be researchable. Brink and Wood (1994, p. 2) define a researchable question as 'an explicit query about a problem or issue that can be challenged, examined and analysed and that will yield useful new information'. Potential topics for research stem from the thoughts, observations and practice experiences of the community nurse.

For example, while working as a district nurse, one of the present authors experienced concern while attending a joint study day organised by the local health and social services. The purpose of the day was to prepare for the introduction of the 1990 NHS and Community Care Act, which recommended a system of single assessment between health and social workers. A social worker expressed concern at the proposal to involve district nurses in the assessment of patients and clients for long term care. (This system has since been superseded by the introduction of the Single Assessment Process (DoH 2002c).) Only social workers, in her view, were able to undertake the assessment taking into account social, psychological and economic need. Her belief was that district nurses would operate from a medical or nursing perspective and only assess physical needs. The author was about to begin a Masters' dissertation and this situation gave her the opportunity she was waiting for: a practice related topic of study. She therefore decided to explore the role perceptions of district nurses and social workers (Bliss 1998).

This interest in district nurses and social workers working together, although originating in the early 1990s continues to be relevant with the move to care trusts at the beginning of the 21st century. Bliss has continued to develop this interest in the way district nurses and social workers collaborate by considering the findings of the Masters' dissertation which identified palliative and terminal care as one area with potential confusion between the two professional groups. The findings had implications for practice, such as clarifying the key role district nurses have as coordinators of palliative care provision (Bliss 2000) within the complex provision of palliative care in the community (Bliss *et al.* 2000). Research funded by the NHS Executive has since explored the effectiveness of different service configurations to provide palliative care (Cowley *et al.* 2002). One aspect of this which may benefit from further research is consideration of how decisions are made by district nurses and social workers involved in developing palliative and continuing care packages (Bliss & While 2003).

The role of the literature review
In order to refine the area of study in the above district nurse and social worker example, a literature review was undertaken. The following key words and phrases were identified as important: collaboration, role theory, government policy pre- and post-NHS reform and team work. A ten-year cut off date prior to the commencement of the original research was identified (i.e. 1984). It became apparent, however, that important references to teamwork from the 1960s would be missed unless the cut off date was revised (i.e. 1964).

The literature review helped the author to refine the research question. Pointers were also provided from previous studies for identifying research approaches and developing data collection tools and analysis that had proved to be effective. For example, the literature review revealed research by Dingwall and Fox (1986) that examined health visitor and social worker perceptions of child protection using a series of vignettes, based on scenarios taken from professional practice. As a result of the literature review, the author decided to consider using vignettes in her own study (see below).

She could have also decided to follow Dingwall and Fox's example of expressing her research question as a hypothesis or tentative proposition that states the expected relationship between phenomena ('type of training affects attitudes towards child care problems'). The hypothesis is often stated in terms of causality such as 'smoking causes lung cancer' or 'type of training affects attitudes towards child care'. The way in which the research problem is set up influences the subsequent study design (see below).

Since Bliss (1998) undertook her study, the world wide web (www) and revolution in computer technology have influenced the ways in which information is accessed and disseminated. Surfing the net is a quick way of gathering infor- mation on research, nursing, and just about anything else imaginable at the touch of a button. Many comprehensive computerised databases are available, including a number of research journals. Examples of tried and tested databases include: CINAHL, MEDLINE, BIDS or EMBASE. These databases may be available as CD-ROMS and online. Online, search engines allow search terms or keywords to be typed in to produce lists of results. The National Electronic Library for Health (NELH www.nelh.gov.uk until March 2005; www.library.nhs.uk after 15th November 2004) has opened up an exciting gateway not only to research but also policy, practice and education literature. The Public Health Library is part of that electronic gateway. An associated part of the electronic age is the growth of the network culture and the possibility to work with colleagues at a distance through the internet. Further discussion on the world wide web and a range of useful databases are presented at the end of this chapter.

Selecting an appropriate research methodology and approach
Silverman (1993, 2001) defines methodology as a general approach to studying research topics which is concerned with the philosophy and theory that drives the research rather than the nuts and bolts of data collection and analysis, such as the specific techniques like observation, interviewing and audio recording, (i.e. the methods).

Paradigm, a term used by the physicist turned philosopher of science, Kuhn (1970), is defined in two basic ways: first, as the range of beliefs, assumptions, values and techniques shared by a scientific community; and second, as the procedures used to solve specific problems and take theories to their logical conclusion. In short, paradigm pertains to the worldview and practical endeavours that drive research.

Guba and Lincoln (1994) state: 'Paradigm issues are crucial; no inquirer, we maintain, ought to go about the business of inquiry without being clear about just what paradigm informs and guides his or her approach' (p. 116).

For behavioural psychologists, epidemiologists studying the distribution of diseases in populations and clinicians conducting clinical trials, the methodology of choice is likely to involve experimentation, careful observation, measurement and control of the phenomena under study. Because this type of methodology is associated with numbers and counting, it is described as 'quantitative'. It is also associated with scientific enquiry underpinned by positivist philosophy and hypothetico-deductionism.

That this is an over-simplification of the nature of scientific enquiry is made evident in the writings of Medawar, an eminent and influential medical scientist, who encourages researchers to think creatively and take risks. He writes:

'The word "science" itself is used as a general name for, on the one hand, the procedures of science – adventures of thought and stratagems of inquiry that go into the advancement of learning – and on the other hand, the substantive body of knowledge that is the outcome of this complex endeavour'.

(Medawar 1984, p. 3)

Similarly, methodologies used in epidemiological studies may include descriptive and explanatory surveys as well as experiments which serve three main purposes: for community diagnosis; aetiology; evaluation of health care.

The preferred methodologies of social scientists such as anthropologists and sociologists are more likely to be interactive or 'qualitative'. Such methodologies include ethnography, grounded theory and phenomenology, which involve participant observation and in-depth interviewing to describe and explain qualities of phenomena. Critical social theory, feminisms, symbolic interactionism and interpretive hermeneutics underpin these methodologies (For further explanations see for example: Goodman & Strange 1997; Harper & Hartman 1997; Wedderburn Tate 1998.)

Issues about paradigms are not without controversy. Whilst it is argued that positivist (quantitative) and naturalistic (qualitative) paradigms should be mixed, Atkinson (1995) had earlier argued that such simplistic polarisation is unhelpful. Some commentators suggest nursing requires its own methodologies and methods to generate knowledge that is uniquely nursing whilst others suggest this limits the nature and scope of enquiry (Cotter and Smith 1998). Similar issues have been debated within the field of health services research (HSR). Popay and colleagues (1998) argue convincingly for the need for interdisciplinary working in order to embrace a pluralistic approach to the study of health across a range of different approaches and methods. In particular, they note the increasing recognition given to qualitative research and the contribution it can make to the field (Black 1994). Bell (1999) prefers to see the quantitative/qualitative distinction as a continuum in which 'no approach prescribes nor automatically rejects any particular method'.

This is good news for primary care practitioners in general and nurses in particular, who often feel the need to justify qualitative research as a 'quirky' alternative to their more quantitatively inclined medical colleagues.

Haase and Myers (1988) make the case for nurses to value and integrate a range of paradigms and approaches by reconciling rather than choosing between qualitative and quantitative research. Their framework is useful for thinking about the feasibility of developing combined approaches to research in a health service that emphasises both quality and cost effectiveness. This framework ties in well with Popay and colleagues' proposals for incorporating a plurality of perspectives in HSR, referred to above.

Evidence

Before designing a study, it is essential to consider the existing body of knowledge on the topic area for research. It is important to review the literature, as discussed earlier, and critically appraise the evidence, synthesise the results and draw conclusions. Such an exercise would identify gaps in either knowledge on the topic area, methodology or theoretical understanding. If there is no or very little published literature on the topic, then a literature search on areas or topics closely related to the research topic should be conducted. For example, a health visitor wishing to study parents' experiences of using cranial osteopathy on their children may find very little published material on the topic owing the recent introduction of such services. However, she may find that a literature search on parents' experiences of using alternative therapies for their children quite informative. It is worth noting at this stage the hierarchy of evidence (Box 7.2). The hierarchy is usually based on the scientific rigour of the studies and the ability of the results to be generalised to the wider population.

> **Box 7.2 Hierarchy of evidence**
>
> - Randomised controlled trials (RCT) with double blind (clinical trials)
> - Well designed RCTs with pseudo-randomisation
> - Well designed RCTs with no randomisation
> - Cohort studies – prospective and retrospective studies with controls
> - Qualitative studies
> - Case studies
> - Expert opinions
> - Anecdotes

Examples of these different types of evidence are presented by Smith and colleagues (2004) in their book *Shaping the Facts: Evidence-based Nursing and Health Care*. James *et al.* (2004) refer to Archie Cochrane's monograph *Effectiveness and Efficiency*, which so strongly influenced the evidence-based practice movement and after whom the Cochrane collaboration was named. They point out that it is often forgotten that Cochrane wrote about the importance of so called 'softer skills' in ensuring quality health care as the following quotation demonstrates:

In 'cure' outcome plays an important part in determining quality, but it is certainly not the whole story. The really important factors are kindliness and the ability to communicate.

(Cochrane 1972, p. 28)

The hierarchies of evidence described above as qualitative studies, expert opinions and anecdotes can often best capture the 'softer skills' of kindliness and communication identified by Cochrane. Investigating such concepts usually falls outside the remit of randomised controlled trials (RCTs) and cohort studies. But even here Pope *et al.* (2004) show there to be exceptions to the rule. They describe the innovative RCT undertaken by feminist scholar Ann Oakley in which she demonstrated the connection between social relations and the health and well being of women and their babies (Oakley 1992).

Baum (1995) points out that public health as a focus of study is complex and requires the integration of qualitative and quantitative methods not only to describe but also understand communities.

Designing the study

When designing a research study it is important that an appropriate research design is selected to take account of the type of research question being considered and the type of evidence required. Examples of research designs frequently used in primary health care research include: experiments and clinical trials; descriptive and explanatory surveys; case studies; participatory approaches. Many of these designs are concerned with evaluation, which is a key interest of primary care research. As Daly and colleagues (1992) observe:

'We would argue that when a given problem is studied, different approaches to research will ask different data and use different frames of analysis.'

Experiments, randomised controlled trials and quasi-experiments

The experimental approach, referred to as the 'randomised controlled trial' (RCT), has been widely applied to the study of interventions on human subjects. Oakley notes: 'The RCT has been increasingly promoted over the last twenty years as the major evaluative tool within medicine' (p. 27).

In order to decide on the specific design for the trial, researchers need to be clear from the outset of their aims and should have one or two clearly stated objectives (Crichton 1990). Study design incorporates every stage of the study including decisions about sampling, size, the techniques by which the subjects will be allocated to a treatment (or non-treatment group), how the intervention will be introduced, statistical applications required and the methods by which the outcome of the study will be evaluated.

The phenomena under study (smoking and lung cancer; occupational groups and attitudes to child care) are broken down or reduced to smaller components known as 'variables'. Smoking, for example, may be broken down into variables such as type and number of cigarettes smoked and over how many years; lung cancer may be examined in relation to variables such as the victim's age and class status. The variables are chosen because they are assumed to have explanatory value that will contribute to theory testing, prediction and new knowledge. Smoking would be the independent or explanatory variable and cancer the dependent variable.

Subjects recruited to take part in studies need to be representative of the population from which they are drawn and bear sufficient similarity to the type of individuals likely to benefit from the intervention. Clear inclusion criteria therefore should be identified for this purpose. It is important that variables related to class, age, gender and ethnicity are taken into consideration. It has been shown that studies have been undertaken with a bias towards white middle class males with a risk that the needs of women, ethnic minority groups and older people will be overlooked. The famous Framingham heart study undertaken in the USA, for example, provided detailed knowledge of the risk factors associated with cardiovascular disease in white middle class men but did not take sufficient account of the specific risks for women and people of different ethnic backgrounds (www.framingham. com; www.nhlbi.nih.gov/about/framingham/ riskabs.htm)

A study of people with strokes who had not been admitted to hospital used a randomised controlled trial to assess the impact of offering them a package of occupational therapy for up to five months, compared with a control group who received 'routine practice' (Walker *et al.* 1999). The results were very encouraging in that the measures used to assess activities of daily living and 'carer strain' suggested that the intervention produced more favourable results compared with the people in the control group.

A 'placebo' group may be added to the experimental and control groups. The placebo group receive a modified version of the treatment or intervention. The reason to introduce a placebo group into the study design is two-fold. First, it helps to discount bias on the part of researcher or patient in their judgement (whether favourable or otherwise) towards the experimental intervention. Second, it provides a control for the frequency of spontaneous changes that may occur in the patient, independent of the intervention under study.

Oakley (quoted in Watts 1999) argues for RCTs to evaluate health promotion interventions rather than the qualitative approaches that have traditionally been favoured in this field. To prove her point she cites evidence that suggests health promotion can actually be harmful (e.g. health visitors' rigorous attempts to prevent old people falling down and breaking bones actually seemed to increase the fracture rate). Her conclusion therefore is that 'the case for evaluation in health promotion is even stronger than elsewhere in medicine because the people you are dealing with are not ill in the first place' (p. 30). Oakley has since spearheaded web-based databases comprising systematic reviews, which demonstrate the effectiveness of promoting health, and a trials register of interventions (http://eppi.ioe.ac.uk). The databases are regularly updated and submitted to the Cochrane Collaboration for Health Promotion and Public Health.

Health impact assessment (HIA) is an evaluation strategy designed to measure the effects of public policies on individual and community health. It has been described as 'great for addressing inequalities'. HIA is recommended in

Saving Lives: Our Healthier Nation (DoH 1999a) and is of two types: prospective (the impact of a new policy on health is evaluated ahead of its introduction to maximise the potential benefits) and retrospective (the impact of a policy is monitored following its introduction). HIA can also be used to inform better decisions for future policy and practice at a local, national and international level (Taylor & Blair-Stevens 2002).

Because HIA is such an important part of government commitment to implementing an effective public health agenda, primary care practitioners need to be aware of the methodologies currently being developed. These methodologies can be applied to a variety of projects, policies and programmes and are represented diagrammatically in Figure 7.1 and Box 7.3 (DoH 1999c).

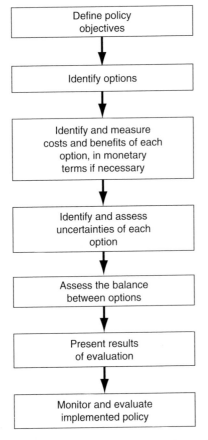

Figure 7.1 Stages involved in appraising policy

> **Box 7.3 Evaluative tools. With permission from the DoH**
>
> The choice of evaluative technique in any appraisal of policy will depend partly on the question to be addressed and partly on availability of data. These approaches to evaluation are summarised here:
>
> - *Cost effectiveness analysis (CEA)*: If alternative (non-health care) policies yield the same type of effect, but at different volumes, then CEA is the appropriate evaluative technique, and the output of the analysis will be expressed in terms of cost effectiveness (CEA) ratios, i.e. 'cost per unit of effect'
> - *Cost utility analysis (CUA)*: This is a special case of cost effectiveness analysis where the effects are measured in some generic way such as quality adjusted life years (QALYS)
> - *Cost benefit analysis (CBA)*: This type of analysis enables an assessment to be made of the worth of implementing a policy or not (rather than implementing policy A vs policy B). CBA converts all costs and benefits to monetary terms: if the value of the costs exceeds the value of the benefits then this suggests that it is not worthwhile to implement the policy

Since the last edition of this text book was published, the Health Development Agency has taken on the leadership of the health impact assessment initiative. There is now an entire website (www.hiagateway.org.uk) dedicated to its dissemination and implementation. The website contains case studies written by practitioners and policy-makers with personal experience of using HIA. The case studies present examples of how using HIA has provided opportunities to increase community participation as well as a mechanism to evaluate the impact of a range of cross-sectoral initiatives including transport, air quality, nutrition and sports facilities (www.hiagateway.org.uk/contacts/personal_experiences). The case studies illustrate the broad remit of public health and the need for the community practitioner to be aware of local initiatives that may impact on, and go beyond, their own role.

Surveys

Most people are familiar with surveys either as investigators or respondents. There are two types: the descriptive survey used to collect biographical, demographic and attitudinal information and the explanatory survey set up to find out 'why?'. The Office for National Statistics regularly conducts a whole range of routine and special surveys. The national census is the prime example of a survey that describes the total population. More usually a representative sample has to be drawn. Controversially, in the 1991 census a whole generation of young men were lost from the census data because they 'disappeared' from the electoral register rather than pay the unpopular and expensive poll tax. Valuable resources were then lost from the inner cities because the level of deprivation was underestimated (Hanlon 1994).

Sapsford and Abbott (1998) describe the Dingwall and Fox study, referred to by Bliss (1998) as a quasi-experiment or type of explanatory survey. This was because the study design manipulated variables to compare health visitor and social worker perceptions of child protection. Twenty participants from each profession were asked to rate what they thought was going on in 20 vignettes. The vignettes, used as proxies for child protection cases, described a set of circumstances or incidents related to child neglect and violence. The findings suggested there were many areas of overlap between the social workers and health visitors and that organisational rather than training differences might account for their reported difficulties in working together (Dingwall & Fox 1986); a finding supported by the Laming Report (2003).

Clinical trials and surveys more often have large samples so they can claim generalisability but Dingwall and Fox make no such claim. Rather they 'hope to establish the value of the approach and to show that the results are sufficiently interesting to justify further investigations'. Gomm *et al.* (2000) suggest that experimental methods are the only ones capable of investigating causality, as it is impossible to decide whether such and such health and social care interventions are effective if it is unclear what causes what effects.

It is important for practitioners to realise that small scale studies, of the sort Bliss was engaged in, are valuable for giving insights on local situations while identifying areas for further enquiry.

Case study

Bliss (1998) decided to use an ethnographic case study to access the differences in role perceptions of health visitors and social workers. Her sample was selected from one community trust involving six district nurses from one clinic and six social workers from the same local authority serving the locality. Selecting the sample from the same area was important since it reduced the variability of the environment in which the participants were working. She then used vignettes during in-depth interviews to complement participant observations and insights. Vignettes removed the need to be present at case conferences. This was important from an ethical point of view since ethical clearance would have been required to attend a case conference. Given the sensitivity of some the cases discussed at conferences, it is possible that clearance would have been withheld.

Case studies are ideal for lone researchers to gain in-depth perspectives on a situation or incident (Bell 1999). A socio-political picture of the organisational context can be constructed and interpersonal relationships described. The case study can be combined with a range of qualitative methodologies. Ethnography for example involves participant observation and interviewing during extended periods of fieldwork.

Different study designs can use similar methods

Even though researchers may employ different study designs they can select similar methods. Bliss (1998) and Dingwall and Fox (1986) used vignettes to study the perceptions of two occupational groups.

Different methodologies and methods give you different answers

Pound *et al.*'s (1995) study describes the use of qualitative in-depth interviews as an alternative to large-scale surveys to explore the components of hospital care valued by people suffering from strokes. The authors explain that previous studies have assumed that patients prefer to stay at home following stroke but, using a different methodology, this study revealed otherwise. Patients were shown to use both technical and psychosocial criteria to evaluate both the process and outcome of their care.

Participatory approaches for community research

A number of research approaches are available to primary health care researchers that involve local participants and contribute to empowering and improving their lives and communities. Community participation is also a key health promotion concept (Smithies & Adams 1993).

Readers will be familiar with action research, a popular methodology with health care researchers (Bate 2000). Action research is usually associated with participatory and collective forms of research although at its most extreme it can be set up as an experiment in which an 'intervention' is tested and its outcomes monitored (Coghlan & Brannick 2001; Sapsford & Abbott 1998). The central tenet of action research is the cyclical process of intervention, evaluation and feedback. Researchers and participants work closely together. Bell (1999) suggests the problem-solving nature of action research makes it particularly appealing to practitioner researchers. Action and other participatory forms of research balance generalisable knowledge and benefit to the community by collaborating as experts and as equals in the research process (Macaulay *et al.* 1999, p. 774).

The public health agenda described above with its emphasis on partnership working and the major NHS reorganisations that are currently underway, particularly within the PCTs, suggests the appropriateness to the community practitioner of understanding the principles of action research to gain insights into the process of developing complex relationships and managing change.

Participatory appraisal

Participatory appraisal, a community research approach, encapsulates the current government commitment to eliminate social exclusion and reduce poverty. It involves multi-agency and partnership working to assess need and involve local communities in order to effect and evaluate change. It also demonstrates the range of methods available to primary health care practitioners.

Chambers (1994) describes participatory appraisal (PA) as: 'a growing family of approaches and methods to enable local "rural or urban" people to express, enhance, share and analyze their knowledge of life and conditions, to plan and to act'.

Investigators involved in participatory methods are concerned with issues of empowerment and the relationship between research and action. The aim of PA is to enable those from marginalised groups to make their needs known while at the same time encourage debate within communities and agencies involved in developmental work with them.

Feurstein's model of participatory evaluation has been adapted by Smithies and Adams (1993) to systematise an approach that is subject to competing agendas and unpredictable outcomes while maintaining a commitment to community development. The model is presented as a cyclical process and emphasises the importance of capacity building to equip local people to develop local initiatives. The model (see Figure 7.2) offers a framework that evaluates and builds on any initiatives forthcoming from the PA.

Data collection methods

Methods are the techniques of doing research: asking questions, observing people and groups, analysing case records, sifting through historical documents and local newspapers (Everitt *et al.* 1992; Silverman 2001). A variety of research methods can be used within a study, irrespective of the underlying paradigm and approach. The use of a multi-method research approach is described as 'triangulation' by which more than one method is used and/or groups of people studied within the same project (Denzin 1989).

The February 2000 issue of the *Journal of Interprofessional Care* was dedicated to the 'new collaboration' in the NHS and explored a range of key issues in a series of research based articles. Topics, approaches and methods included: rapid appraisal of the Health Improvement Programmes

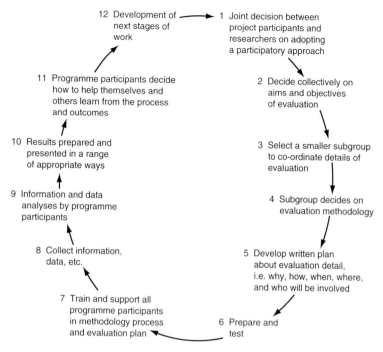

Figure 7.2 The participatory approach to evaluation (Feurstein, as adapted by Smithies & Adams 1993). With permission from Routledge

(HimPs); questionnaire surveys, participatory study, evaluation, in-depth and semi-structured interviews, focus groups and documentary analysis. Also of interest to the community researcher is the use of telephone interviews. One of the authors undertook both face to face and telephone interviews with patients who agreed to participate in a study to evaluate the role of the specialist nurse in the care of people with multiple sclerosis (MS). It was found that both types of interview generated data of comparable quality but the key lay in the technique of the researcher to collect, analyse and elicit rich data (Johnson *et al*. 2001).

Data management, analysis and interpretation

How data are analysed in a study will depend on the research questions being asked and the methodologies and methods being used. Data analysis is often the most time consuming part of the research. For example, if it takes two months to collect data, it is likely to take four months to analyse and interpret them.

In order for researchers to retrieve their data easily and accurately for analysis and interpretation, it is important that, during data collection, they develop systems to ensure this. In quantitative studies, it is likely that the data are collected and recorded on standardised forms, for example self-administered questionnaires and structured interview schedules.

In qualitative studies, the researcher develops ways of recording fieldwork notes during participant observation, such as by keeping index cards to record observations as events take place, for example mealtimes in a day nursery. Interviews are (with the participants' permission) most often tape-recorded and then transcribed to facilitate analysis of the interview contents.

In large-sample surveys, data are likely to be stored in a computer. This will potentially ease and speed up data analysis. If the sample is small, it may be quicker to analyse the data by hand. Data, it should be remembered, are only as good as the operator who enters them into the computer and the logic that inspires decisions about statistical tests. Preparing data for analysis may also be very time-consuming.

Data analysis produces summary statistics (e.g. frequencies and average – mean, median and modes) and appropriate statistical significance tests (Jolley 1991). Statistical analysis can be undertaken using such programs as SPSS (Statistical Package for the Social Sciences) or Minitab; and textual analysis, for example the 'Nudist' and 'Ethnograph' programs which are constantly being revised.

Statistical tests are based on probability theory, and a statistician is usually consulted to advise on the appropriate test given the sample size, type of data and questions being asked. In short, the data are manipulated statistically in order to ensure the results have not occurred by chance. The importance of logic in interpreting results cannot be underestimated. A 'significant' result does not mean that 'cause' and 'effect' are automatically established. First the researcher must ensure that a number of conditions are met if causality between variables is to be demonstrated. Sometimes an accidental link may bind independent and dependent variables together in a 'spurious' relationship, or confounding of results or muddling the picture (Gomm *et al.* 2000).

The hallmark of the qualitative research process is that coding and analysis take place alongside data collection. The researcher then decides what future data should be collected, and from where and whom they should be obtained.

During the process, in-depth descriptions, interpretations and theoretical perspectives are generated. Phenomena are then described through narratives and accounts as a way of understanding, explaining and making inferences.

Melia (1982) in her now classic study used grounded theory (Strauss & Corbyn 1994) and in-depth interviews to study student nurse socialisation. Analysis yielded six conceptual categories, which were then used as a framework for presenting substantive issues raised by the students. The categories were: 'learning and working', 'getting the work done', 'learning the rules', 'nursing in the dark', 'just passing through', 'doing nursing' and 'being professional'. From 'nursing in the dark', for example, she derived further categories, which she labelled 'coping with the dark', 'fobbing off the patient' and 'awareness contexts'.

Latent and content analysis can be used to analyse transcripts and develop themes and categories (Morse & Field 1996). In PA analysis is collaborative and collective and, as described in the example below, permits a variety of needs and concerns to be expressed.

Processed data are referred to as 'findings' or 'results'. Methods of data analysis vary according to the underlying research approach. Qualitative research is presented through words and narratives, quantitative research through numbers and statistical manipulations and also in tables and graphs (Smart 1997) (see Figure 7.3).

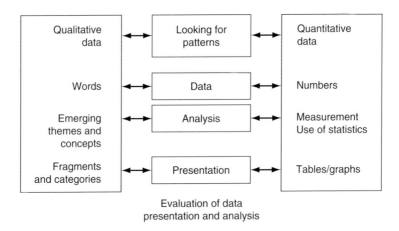

Evaluation of data
presentation and analysis

Figure 7.3 Overview of data analysis. (Source: Smart 1997). With permission from Elsevier Science

A multi-method evaluation of health promotion in clinical placements

A multi-method evaluation was undertaken to describe the health promotion component of clinical placements (Smith *et al*. 1998). Student and qualified nurses, midwives and health visitors took part in the evaluation. The data collection took the form of a questionnaire survey, focus groups in two trusts, a case study of one general practice, telephone and face to face interviews and documentary analysis of educational curricula. The sample was opportunistic and recruitment relied on local contacts. The multi-method approach allowed the researchers to build up a picture of how health promotion was experienced in the clinical setting. Comparisons were made between the findings and the literature.

Of particular interest to the researchers was the fact that different approaches to data collection revealed different stances. In particular a broader notion of health emerged from the focus group discussions. Questionnaire findings tended to restrict respondents to prescriptive views of health promotion. Focus groups are a useful method for community practitioners because they encourage participants to exchange and expand ideas (Kitzinger 1994). Telephone interviews, by saving on travel time, allowed the researchers to widen their sample using the semi-structured schedule that had been employed during face to face interviews.

Example of participatory appraisal

Thirteen people from eight different agencies (e.g. health, social services, education and housing) spent a week learning participatory appraisal skills and using them to review young people's needs and services on an inner city housing estate. The idea was to make young people's experiences of living in a multi-racial area with high unemployment visible. An important outcome of the week was to enable young people and adults to own future developments, such as a health access clinic.

The course participants spent two days in the field where they spoke to 19 adults and 106 young people under 25 years of age, described as a convenience or opportunistic sample.

Methods used included direct observation, semi-structured interviewing, mapping, brain storming, spider diagram, impact ranking, evaluation wheel, informal interview. The use of visual techniques is particularly important to allow people to participate who would normally be excluded because of language or literacy barriers.

The findings produced collaboratively included: the designation of more safe public spaces where people could meet and communicate in socially pleasing surroundings and conduct games, such as soccer. Practical suggestions were made such as the need to provide more litter bins, dog toilets and plant trees and flowers (James 1999).

One of the authors has also used participatory appraisal to evaluate aspects of a Sure Start local programme and to contribute to a health needs assessment of young people in housing need living in an inner city foyer (Smith 2004). The benefit of participatory appraisal is that it is flexible and responsive to local conditions; the disadvantage is that it is time consuming and dependent on a researcher having the skills to facilitate and empower local people. There may also be a tension between the academic need to publish in prestigious journals and the local community's desire to disseminate the findings quickly in newsletters and the popular press.

General research issues

Validity, reliability and generalisability

Regardless of methodological considerations, all researchers must consider issues of validity and reliability. In quantitative research, reliability refers to the extent to which methods and settings are consistent over time, across groups and between researchers. Validity refers to the accuracy and truth of the data being produced in terms of the concepts being investigated, the people and objects being studied and the methods of data collection and analysis being used.

For qualitative researchers the social context in which data are collected is important to consider. During field observations for example, as researchers become increasingly familiar with the research setting, they are able to check the accuracy and recurrence of data in a number of different situations and from a variety of participant perspectives.

Validity and reliability are important concepts in large-scale studies, such as clinical trials and surveys, if the studies are to be generalisable. This is a particular concern in undertaking systematic reviews to ensure the robustness of the findings. Meta-analysis takes account of these issues by reviewing the populations, methodologies and findings of a number of studies on a given topic. Statistical analysis is then applied to assess the significance of the combined results.

In qualitative research, concepts of validity and reliability are not easily transferable. There is a lot of debate and controversy about the best ways to evaluate qualitative research (Koch 1994; Sandelowski 1993). However, Guba and Lincoln (1989) proposed four main methods for establishing rigour in qualitative studies; dependability, credibility, transferability and confirmability:

- Dependability (reliability). Findings of the study need to be consistent and correct to be dependable, so that anyone reading the study will be able to evaluate the sufficiency of the analysis and results from the research process
- Credibility (internal validity). The extent to which readers and participants can recognise the meaning that they give to the situations or contexts or the 'truth value' of the results
- Transferability (generalisability). How the results in one context could be 'transferred' to comparable situations or participants. In some cases, due the small-scale samples utilised, theoretical transferability could be achieved
- Confirmability (objectivity). This method requires an audit or decision trail for readers who can judge the study for the intellectual honesty, researchers' bias and openness to sensitivity to the methods

Presentation and dissemination

Presentation and research dissemination is essential so that findings are made available to be used and applied by others. Researchers may change their style of presentation according to their audience. One of the authors wrote up her research for two journals: the *Journal of Advanced Nursing* (Smith 1987, 1991) and *Nursing Times* (Smith 1989). To the non-researcher, the article in the first journal may appear 'jargonistic', using language that is difficult to understand. In the *Nursing Times* article, the language is more accessible and easier to understand by the field-level practitioner. The issue of whether researchers should write in the first or third person is discussed by Webb (1992). The convention in quantitative research is to maintain objectivity and authority by writing in the third person. Qualitative, and particularly feminist, researchers prefer to write in the first person. In this way, they write themselves into their research accounts and make their methods and findings more transparent to the reader.

The notion of networks is an important part of the modernised health service and have been set up for the purposes of practitioners sharing expertise and knowledge across NHS trusts. The public health networks have been set up primarily to allow public health specialists and practitioners across PCTs 'to share good practice, manage public health knowledge and very importantly act as a source of learning and professional development' (DoH 2004, p. 39). These networks also offer contacts with universities to support research, education and development and joint cross boundary collaborations across PCTs.

The Internet or World Wide Web (www)

The Internet is useful for gathering and sharing information on web pages, by email, in forum discussions and newsgroups. It also influences the way research is conducted and disseminated. Although there has been massive investment in information technology, some practitioners still do not have access to the Internet and inequalities still exist between different parts of the country and different professional groups. This situation is improving as the NHS commits itself to ensuring that its employees have access to e-mail and a vast range of electronically accessible databases. It is essential that access and training are provided to practitioners because of the many uses of information technology and the net. Because information develops at such a fast rate, information published in more traditional media, such as books and journals, are in danger of being out of date before they are published!

Professional, ethical and information sharing issues are associated with research on the net. At present, it is extremely difficult to regulate the Internet or hold individuals or companies responsible for unethical research practices. Copyright on the net is ambiguous, meaning not only is most information free and transcends boundaries, but also individuals and companies are not accountable for bad press of individuals, libellous remarks or improper research and ethical practices. Web service providers say they are unable to regulate what goes on their notice boards or is discussed in forums.

The main message to be taken from this by potential researchers is to be extremely cautious about the information received and transmitted via the Internet. Currently, large amounts of information are available and positive and negative uses of the Internet must be considered.

Research proposals

Monkley-Poole (1997) suggests:

> 'There can be many reasons for writing a proposal apart from "pure" research. For example, similar principles can be applied to writing proposals to obtain resources to introduce change into clinical practice or undertake an audit of services. Proposals can also be submitted to request funding to support study leave or attendance at a conference. In the health service, the move to the market with its emphasis on evidence based health care suggest the need for practitioners to attract monies to fund research and to clearly identify and document research activities being undertaken in the clinical areas.'

A proposal puts forward the argument for why a piece of research is worth doing, how it will add to the body of knowledge and the plans and procedures necessary to successfully complete it. The applicant also includes a short curriculum vitae to demonstrate that she has the necessary experience for the job. When writing any proposal it is important to consider the membership of the panel or committee who will be taking decisions based on its content since each member will have different backgrounds and biases. It is important to be clear and explicit when putting together the proposal especially if the people making decisions about it are likely to be unfamiliar with its approach. Another source of guidance for preparing and submitting a research proposal is provided by Punch (2000).

Funding

Researchers with an interest in particular topics will apply for funding when tenders are advertised. These are found in a variety of places such as nursing journals including the *Nursing Times* or *Nursing Standard*. Newspapers like the *Guardian* or the *Times Higher Education Supplement* are also good sources of information about funding.

In addition, there are a number of websites that assist in identifying funding sources and their purposes such as the *Charities Aid Foundation* (www.cafonline.org) and www.trustfunding.org.uk which replaces *The Directory of Grant Making Trusts. The Association of Medical Research Charities Handbook* (AMRC 2004) has also been replaced electronically. All the information previously contained in the handbook is now available on the organisation's website (www.amrc.org.uk).

Guidelines supplied by funding organisations will contain the relevant information to inform the applicant. These guidelines may also indicate the preferred philosophical and methodological approach to be employed.

Individual funding bodies invite submissions at different times of the year and may offer varying degrees of financial support. It is important, therefore, for the applicant to be realistic when estimating the budget and to request resources that will satisfy anticipated need as 'top-up' funds after the event may not be forthcoming. One source of funding that had been open to nurses especially for the study of education and practice based research was the English National Board for Nursing, Midwifery and Health Visiting now incorporated into the Department of Health funding initiatives and, to a lesser extent, the United Kingdom Central Council for Nursing,

Midwifery and Health Visiting now superseded by the Nursing and Midwifery Council.

An important source of funding is the NHS Service Delivery and Organisation (SDO) research and development programme administered by the London School of Hygiene and Tropical Medicine (LSHTM). Useful advice is provided on their website (www.sdo.lshtm.ac.uk).

The association of the LSHTM with the SDO R&D programme is an example of how funding for research programmes are administered through higher education establishments. Universities may also have research committees that allocate monies to local staff in response to competitive bids. The CHAIN (communication, help, advice, information network), now administered through the NHS University, is an excellent news source on research contacts, bids and specialist practice that it is well worth subscribing to (chain@nhsu.org.uk).

Charities such as the Florence Nightingale Foundation are specifically committed to funding research, travel, training and projects (www. florence-nightingale-foundation.org.uk) while the Foundation of Nursing Studies is committed to supporting practice development, small scale research projects, dissemination and implementation (FoNS 1996, www.fons.org).

Ethical issues

Irrespective of paradigm, approach or method, research proposals should always be scrutinised for their ethical implications and submitted to an ethics committee for approval prior to commencement of the study. Research subjects should also be fully informed of the study's implications before giving their written consent and be able to withdraw without prejudice at any time. Participant observation should not be covert and researchers using this method should be clear about their role.

All research activity must comply with the research governance framework for health and social care (DoH 2001), as in general terms, health authorities and PCTs owe a direct and non-delegable duty of care to NHS patients. The framework clarifies responsibilities and accountabilities that define the setting in which negligence might occur and refers to the responsibility of researchers' employers.

Health authorities are required to set up multi-centre research ethics committees (MREC) and local research ethics committees (LREC) to protect both subjects and researchers. The multi-centre committees cover a cluster of health authorities and the researcher applies to one of these committees when the research is being undertaken in more than one site. When the research is being undertaken in one site only the researcher applies to the appropriate local trust based committee. S/he must also apply to the local research and development committee for permission to commence fieldwork and to request an honorary contract. Ethics committees are also found in universities. Professional bodies, such as the Royal College of Physicians and the Royal College of Nursing, produce guidelines to assist researchers in considering the ethical dimensions of their research proposals (RCN 1993). ARVAC (Association for Research in the Voluntary and Community Sector) has a set of ethical guidelines sensitive to the complex needs of the sector and which focus on the research subjects' rights. Researchers are urged to take account of equal opportunities, in terms of race, gender, disability and sexual orientation and the principles, values, objectives and agendas of the participants. The development of 'mutually beneficial relationships' between researchers and researched, set within the wider 'social, political and economic setting', are seen as key (ARVAC 2000, www.arvac.org.uk).

Unexpected ethical consequences can result from 'neutral', seemingly theoretical science; for example, the application of theoretical physics to the development of the atom bomb did untold harm and formed no part of Einstein's original intentions. Similarly, Darwin's theory of evolution was used by many Victorian biologists to advance pejorative racial stereotypes. This was especially true in Australia during the nineteenth century. Social Darwinism, as it was known, put forward racist stereotypes of aboriginal inferiority that tried to establish European cultural dominance. This approach continues to this day.

Unlike obviously intrusive clinical trials, and research practices such as giving placebos rather than treatment or testing drugs with unknown side-effects, qualitative research is often seen as exempt from the need to be scrutinised by an ethics committee. However, ethical implications of covert research, i.e. research undertaken without the subjects' knowledge, are apparent when findings are reported without subjects ever having known they were being observed.

Consider, too, the ethical implications of interviews about feelings and emotions and the need to consider the participant's view with respect to research on women involving cervical screening (Howson 1999) or young women's experiences of abortion (Harden & Ogden 1999). Such interviews need to be carefully managed so as not to distress the interviewee.

Ethics committees

Ethics committees are set up to regulate good ethical practice in the conduct of health care research. Through the granting of ethical approval, LRECs are ensuring that health care research adheres to the basic principles of the Helsinki Declaration and the EU convention on Human Rights.

The Human Rights Act 1998, active since 2000, contains numerous articles that are relevant to health care research. Protection of right to life (Article 2); prohibition of torture or degrading treatment or punishment (Article 30); right to liberty and security (Article 5); right to respect for private and family life (Article 8) and freedom of thought, conscience and religion (Article 9) should be included for consideration in study proposals to protect the interests and well-being of research participants. Further information on the requirements for ethics committees is available on local PCT websites and the Department of Health website, including COREC (www.corec.org.uk) the Central Office for Research Ethics Committees.

Ethics committees require researchers to prepare written proposals to demonstrate the proposed study's adherence to ethical principles. This may involve the signing of a consent form, following a full explanation of events, before the research commences. This is known as informed consent. Any nurse is within her rights to ask to see the consent form before allowing researchers access to patients.

Research on people with mental health problems, with a learning disability or with children is problematic. This is because these groups are vulnerable to improper research practices. There is the issue of whether children, the learning disabled and mental-health service users may make informed decisions and give their full consent (or whether someone can consent on their behalf). Informed consent is particularly important if one considers the capacities of these groups as they are spelled out in law.

Conclusion

Research is the combination of systematic inquiry and a personal journey. The personal interests and style of each researcher and practitioner influences the questions asked and the approaches taken.

It is hoped the chapter will generate ideas for the reader about the approaches and findings used for the study of community nursing and public health care and their application to practice. In particular, it identifies the knowledge base for primary health care and the topics and methodologies of relevance to the field. Reflective practice and research mindedness are described as part of the primary care practitioner's tool kit for recognising and drawing on experience which in turn contributes to the evidence base which informs research and practice. The World Wide Web plays an important part in making a wide range of materials electronically accessible as part of the policy, practice and research base. Issues such as ethics, proposal writing and funding are also raised to further assist primary care practitioners to apply and use research.

Research in its various guises is no longer an optional extra in the modern health service. Indeed, the current NHS agenda actively supports the development of a critical research culture. This chapter is designed to assist primary care and public health practitioners to shape a role for themselves within that culture in order to meet their own professional and personal needs and those of patients and clients.

Box 7.4   Further reading

Audit Commission Reports – http://www.audit-commission.gov.uk
Cochrane database – http://www.update-software.com/ccweb/cochrane/revastr/ccabout.htm
Department of Health – http://www.dh.gov.uk/dhhome.htm
Eppi-Centre – http://eppi.ioe.ac.uk
Health Impact Assessment – http://www.hiagateway.org.uk
National Institute of Clinical Excellence (NICE) – http://www.nice.org.uk
The National Electronic Library for Health (NeLH) – www.library.nhs.uk
Our Healthier Nation – http://www.ohn.gov.uk
The Public Health Electronic Library (PHel) – http://www.phel.gov.uk
York Centre for Systematic Reviews and Dissemination – http://www.york.ac.uk/inst/crd/

Journals

Links Page – http://www.sciencekomm.at/journals/medicine/nurse.html
Nursing Standard – http://www.nursing-standard.co.uk
The Journal of Advanced Nursing – http://www.blackwell-synergy.com/issuelist.asp?journal=jan
The Nursing Times – http://www.nursingtimes.net/
The Sociology of Health and Illness – http://www.blackwellpublishers.co.uk/journals/SHIL/

Ethics

Central Office for Research Ethics Committees – http://www.corec.org.uk
The Human Rights Act 1998 – http://www.gov.uk/acts/1998/htm

Funding

Foundation of Nursing Studies – http://www.fons.org
Florence Nightingale Foundation – http://www.florence-nightingale-foundation.org.uk
The Association of Medical Research Charities – http://www.amrc.org.uk
Directory of Grant Making Trusts – http://www.trustfunding.org.uk
The NHS Service Delivery and Organisation (SDO) Research and Development programme – http://www.sdo.lshtm.ac.uk

Networks

Communication, help, advice and information network (CHAIN) – http://www.chain.nhsu.org.uk
The Developing Practice Network – www.dpnetwork.org.uk

Statutory Body

Nursing and Midwifery Council – http://www.nmc-uk.org

References

Abramson, J.H. (1990) *Survey methods in community medicine*. Churchill Livingstone, Edinburgh.

AMRC (2004) *The Association of Medical Research Charities* (www.amrc.org.uk).

Association for Research in the Voluntary and Community Sector (ARVAC) (2000) *Code of Good Practice for Researching in the Voluntary Sector*. ARVAC, London, (www.arvac.org.uk)

Atkinson, P. (1995) Some perils of paradigms. *Qualitative Health Research*, **5**(11), 117–124.

Bate, P. (2000) Synthesing research and practice: using the action research approach in health care settings, *Social Policy and Administration*, **34**(4), 478–493.

Baum, F. (1995) Researching Public Health: Behind the Qualitative–Quantitative Methodological Debate, *Social Science and Medicine*, **40**(4), 459–468.

Bell, J. (1999) *Doing your research project: a guide for first time researchers in education and social science*, 2nd edn. Open University Press, Buckingham.

Benner, P. (1984) *From Novice to Expert: excellence and power in clinical nursing practice*. Addison Wesley, Menlo Park, California.

Black, N. (1994) Why we need qualitative research. *Journal of Epidemiology and Community Health*, **48**, 425–426.

Bliss, J. (1998) District nurses' and social workers' understanding of each other's role. *British Journal of Community Nursing*, **3**, 330–336.

Bliss, J. (2000) Palliative Care in the Community. *British Journal of Community Nursing*, **5**, 390–395.

Bliss, J., Cowley, S. & While, A. (2000) Interprofessional working in palliative care in the community: a review of the literature. *Journal of Interprofessional Care*, **14**, 281–290.

Bliss, J. & While, A. (2003) Decision-making in palliative and continuing care in the community: an analysis of the published literature with reference to the context of UK care provision. *International Journal of Nursing Studies*, **40**, 881–888.

Brink, P.J. & Wood, M.J. (1994) *Basic steps in planning nursing research: from question to proposal*. Jones & Bartlett, Boston.

Chambers, R. (1994) The Origins and Practice of Participatory Rural Appraisal. *World Development*, **22**(7), 953–969.

Coghlan, D. & Brannick, T. (2001) *Doing Action Research in Your Organisation*. Sage, London.

Cotter, A. & Smith, P. (1998) Epilogue: setting new research agendas. In: *Nursing Research: Setting New Agendas* P. Smith (ed). Arnold, Hodder Headlines, London. pp. 212–228.

Cowley, S., Bliss, J., Mathew, A. & McVey, G. (2002) *Investigation of the impact of different service configurations on the effectiveness of palliative care and multi-professional collaboration*. King's College, London.

Crichton, N. (1990) The importance of statistics in research design. *Complementary Medical Research*, **4**(2), 42–49.

Czuber-Dochan, W., Mcbride, L. & Wilson, J. (1997) Exploring the concepts of research through the media. In: *Research mindedness for practice* P. Smith (ed). Churchill Livingstone, Edinburgh.

Daly, J., Macdonald, I & Willis, E. (1992) *Researching health: designs, dilemmas, disciplines*. Tavistock/Routledge, London.

Denzin, N. (1989) Strategies of multiple triangulation. In: *The Research Act: a theoretical introduction to sociological methods*. McGraw-Hill, New York. pp. 234–247.

Department of Health (Research and Development Division) (1991) *Research for Health*. HMSO, London.

Department of Health (1992) *Health of the Nation: A Strategy for England*. DoH, London.

Department of Health (1993) *Report of the Taskforce on the Strategy for Research in Nursing, Midwifery and Health Visiting*. DoH, London.

Department of Health (1997a) *Research and Development: Towards an Evidence-based Health Service*. DoH, London.

Department of Health (1997b) *The New NHS: Modern, Dependable*. DoH, London.

Department of Health (1998) *A First Class Service: Quality in the New NHS*. DoH, Leeds.

Department of Health (1999a) *Saving Lives: Our Healthier Nation*. DoH, London.

Department of Health (1999b) *Clinical Governance: Quality in the new NHS*. HSC 1999/065. DoH, Leeds.

Department of Health (1999c) *Health Impact Assessment: Report of a Methodological Seminar*. DoH, London.

Department of Health (2000a) The NHS Plan: a Plan for Investment, a Plan for Reform. DoH, London.

Department of Health (2000b) *Research and Development for a First Class Service*. DoH, London.

Department of Health (2001) Research governance: framework for health and social care. DoH, London.

Department of Health (2002a) *Shifting the Balance of Power: The Next Steps*. DoH, London.

Department of Health (2002b) *Liberating the Talents: Helping Primary Care Trusts and Nurses to Deliver the NHS Plan*. DoH, London.

Department of Health (2002c) *The Single Assessment Process for Older People*. DoH, London.

Department of Health (2003a) General Medical Services (GMS) Primary Care Contracting. DoH, London.

Department of Health (2003b) *Supplementary prescribing by nurses and pharmacists within the NHS in England: A guide for implementation*. DoH, London.

Department of Health (2004) *NHS Improvement Plan: Putting people at the heart of the public services*. DoH, London.

Dingwall, R. & Fox, S. (1986) Health visitors' and social workers' perceptions of child care problems. In: *Research in Preventive Community Nursing Care: Fifteen Studies in Health Visiting* A. While (ed). Wiley, Chichester.

Drummond, N. (2000) Quality of life with asthma: the existential and aesthetic. *Sociology of Health and Illness*, **22**(2), 235–253.

Everitt, A., Hardiker, P., Littlewood, J. & Mullender, A. (1992) *Applied Research for Better Practice*. Macmillan, Basingstoke. pp. 4–5.

Foundation of Nursing Studies (FoNS) (1996) *Reflection for Action*. FoNS, London.

Franks, V. & Smith, P. (2002) *Context, Continuity and Change: reassessing the nursing task*. Presentation to the Association for Psychoanalytic Psychotherapy in the NHS, Tavistock Clinic, London.

Gibbons, M., Limoges, C., Nowonty, H., Schwattzman, S., Scott, P. & Trow, M. (1994) *The new production of knowledge: The dynamics of science and research in contemporary societies*. Sage, London.

Gomm, R., Needham, G. & Bellman, A. (2000) *Evaluating Research in Health and Social Care*. Sage and the Open University, London.

Goodman, B. & Strange, F. (1997) Ethnomethodology. In: *Research mindedness for practice.* P. Smith (ed) Churchill Livingstone, Edinburgh. pp. 139–164.

Guba, E.G. & Lincoln, Y.S. (1989) *Fourth generation evaluation.* Sage, Newbury Park.

Guba, E.G. & Lincoln, Y.S. (1994) Competing Paradigms in Qualitative Research. In: *Handbook of Qualitative Research,* N.K. Denzin & Y.S. Lincoln (eds). Sage, Thousand Oaks, California. pp. 105–117.

Haase, J.E. & Myers, S.T. (1988) Reconciling paradigm assumptions of qualitative and quantitative research. *Western Journal of Nursing Research,* **10**(2), 128–137.

Hanlon, J. (1994) Ghost of the poll tax. *Red Pepper,* June: 33.

Harden, A. & Ogden, J. (1999) Young women's experiences of arranging and having abortions. *Sociology of Health and Illness,* **21**(4), 426–444.

Harper, M. & Hartman, M. (1997) Research Paradigms. In: *Research mindedness for practice* P. Smith (ed). Churchill Livingstone, Edinburgh. pp. 19–52.

Harris, A. (1993) Developing a research and development strategy for primary care. *British Medical Journal.* **306,** 189–192.

Hawksley, B., Carnwell, R. & Callwood, R. (2003) A literature review of the public health roles of health visitors and school nurses. *British Journal of Community Nursing,* **8**(10), 447–454.

Health Visitors Association (HVA) (1994) *Mix and Match.* HVA, London.

Health Visitors Association (HVA) (1995) *Weights and Measures.* HVA, London.

Holloway, I. & Wheeler, S. (2002) *Qualitative Research in Nursing,* 2nd edn. Blackwell Publishing, Oxford.

Howson, A. (1999) Cervical screening, compliance and moral obligation. *Sociology of Health and Illness,* **21**(4), 401–425.

James, T. (1999) *Chingford Hall Estate: Participatory Appraisal.* Unpublished Report, Community Health Project, Redbridge and Waltham Forest Health Authority.

James, T., Smith, P. & Gray, B. (2004) Emotions, evidence and practice: the struggle for effectiveness. In: *Shaping the Facts: evidence-based nursing and health care* (eds P. Smith *et al.*) Elsevier Science, Edinburgh.

Johnson, J., Smith, P. & Goldstone, L. (2001) *The MS Nurse specialist, A review and evalaution of the role, Part II Case Study.* Unpublished report/CD, The MS Trust, Spirella House, Letchworth.

Jolley, J. (1991) Using statistics. Computing in practice: information management and technology series. *Nursing Times,* **87**(25), 57–59.

Kendall, S. (1997) What do we mean by evidence? Implications for primary health care nursing. *Journal of Interprofessional Care,* **11**(1), 23–34.

Kitzinger, J. (1994) The Methodology of Focus Groups: the importance of interaction between research participants. *Sociology of Health and Illness,* **16**(1), 103–121.

Koch, T. (1994) Establishing rigour in qualitative research: the decision trail. *Journal of Advanced Nursing* **19,** 976–986.

Kuhn, T. (1970) *The Structure of Scientific Revolutions,* 2nd Edition. University of Chicago Press, Chicago.

Laming, H. (2003) *The Victoria Climbie Inquiry,* Report of an Inquiry, Departments of Health & Home Office, London.

Macaulay, A., Commanda, L., Freeman, W., Gibson, N., McCabe, M., Robbins, C. & Twohig, P. (1999) Participatory research maximises community and lay involvement. *British Medical Journal,* **319,** 774–778.

Macleod Clark, J. & Hockey, L. (1989) *Further research for nursing.* Scutari press, London.

Medawar, P. (1984) *The Limits of Science.* Oxford University Press, Oxford.

Melia, K. (1982) 'Tell it as it is': qualitative methodology and nursing research: understanding the student nurse's world. *Journal of Advanced Nursing,* **7,** 327–335.

Meyrick, J., Burke, S. & Speller, V. (2001) *Public Health Skills Audit 2001: A Short Report.* Health Development Agency, London.

Monkley-Poole, (1997) Research proposal writing and funding. In: *Research mindedness for practice* P. Smith (ed). Churchill Livingstone, Edinburgh.

Moore, R.A. (1995) *Heliobacter pylori and peptic ulcer – a systematic review of effectiveness and an overview of the economic benefits of implementing what is known to be effective.* Cortecs, Isleworth.

Morse, J.M. & Field, P.A. (1996) *Nursing research: the application of qualitative approaches,* 2nd edn. Chapman and Hall, London.

Mulhall, A. (1996) *Epidemiology Nursing and Healthcare: A new perspective.* Macmillan, London.

Oakley, A. (1992) *Social Support and Motherhood: the natural history of a research project.* Blackwell Publishers, Oxford.

Popay, J., Rogers, A. & Williams, G. (1998) Rationale and Standards for the Systematic Review of Qualitative Literature in Health Services Research. *Qualitative Health Research,* **8**(3), 341–351.

Pope, R., Graham, L. & Jones, P.C. (2004) Randomised controlled trials: illustrative case studies. In: *Shaping the Facts: evidence-based nursing and health care* (eds P. Smith *et al.*) Elsevier Science, Edinburgh.

Pound, P., Bury, M., Gompertz, P. & Ebrahim, S. (1995) Stroke patients' views on their admission to hospital. *British Medical Journal*, **311**, 18–22.

Punch, K.F. (2000) *Developing Effective Research Proposals*. Sage, London.

Rees, C. (1992) Practising research based teaching. *Nursing Times*, **88**(2), 55–57.

Royal College of Nursing (1982) *Promoting Research Mindedness*. RCN, London.

Royal College of Nursing (1993) *Ethics related to research in nursing*. RCN, London.

Saks, M. (2000) Introduction. p. 1 In: *Developing Research in Primary Care*. M. Saks, M. Williams & B. Hancock (eds). Radcliffe Medical Press, Abingdon.

Sandelowski, M. (1993) Rigor or rigor mortis: the problem of rigor in qualitative research. *Advances in Nursing Sciences*, **16**(2), 1–8.

Sapsford, R. & Abbott, P. (1998) *Research methods for nurses and the caring professions*. Open University Press, Buckingham.

Schön, D.A. (1987) *Educating the reflective practitioner*. Jossey Bass, San Francisco.

Silverman, D. (1993) *Interpreting Qualitative Data: methods for analysing talk, text and interaction*. Sage, London.

Silverman, D. (2001) *Interpreting Qualitative Data: methods for analysing talk and text and interaction*, 2nd ed. Sage, London.

Smart, T. (1997) Data Analysis. In: *Research Mindedness for Practice* P. Smith (ed). Churchill Livingstone, Edinburgh. pp. 77–114.

Smith, P. (1987) The relationship between quality of nursing care and the ward as a learning environment: developing a methodology. *Journal of Advanced Nursing*, **12**, 413–420.

Smith, P. (1989) Nurses' Emotional Labour, *Nursing Times*, **85**(47), 49–51.

Smith, P. (1991) The nursing process: raising the profile of emotional care in nurse training. *Journal of Advanced Nursing*, **16**, 74–81.

Smith, P. (ed) (1997) *Research Mindedness for Practice*. Churchill, Livingstone, Edinburgh.

Smith, P. (2004) Gathering Evidence: The New Production of Knowledge. In: *Shaping the Facts: Evidence-based nursing and health care* P. Smith, T. James, M. Lorentzon, and R. Pope, (eds). Elsevier Science, Edinburgh. pp. 111–138.

Smith, P., Schickler, P., Masterson, A., James, T., Jordan, G., Roth, C., Conroy, D., Emery, S. &

Lovegrove, M. (1998) *Our Healthier Nation: An Evaluation of Clinical Placements*, Unpublished Report. South Bank University, London. See also SW NHSE (1999) *Our Healthier Nation: Improving the Competence of the Workforce in Health Promotion*. South West NHSE, Bristol.

Smith, P., James, T., Lorentzon, M. and Pope, R. (eds) (2004) *Shaping the Facts: Evidence-based nursing and health care*. Elsevier Science, Edinburgh.

Smithies, J. & Adams, L. (1993) Walking the tightrope: Issues in evaluation and community participation for Health for All. In: *Healthy Cities: research and practice* J. Davis & M. Kelly (eds). Routledge, London.

Strauss, A. & Corbin, J. (1994) Grounded theory methodology: an overview. In: *Handbook of Qualitative Research* N.K. Denzin & Y.S. Lincoln (eds). Sage, Thousand Oaks, California. pp. 273–285.

Taylor, L. & Blair-Stevens, C. (2002) *Introducing health impact assessment (HIA): informing the decision-making process*. Health Development Agency, London.

The NHS and Community Care Act 1990. HMSO, London.

Vydelingum, V., Colliety, P., Hutchinson, K. & Smith, P. (2004) Mapping the Needs of the NHS Public Health Practitioner Workforce in PCTS. Surrey and Sussex Strategic Health Authority, unpublished report.

Walker, M.F., Gladman, J.R.F., Lincoln, N.B., Siemonsma, P. & Whiteley, T. (1999) Occupational therapy for stroke patients not admitted to hospital: a randomised controlled trial, *The Lancet*, **354**, 278–280.

Wanless, D. (2004) *Securing Good Health for the Whole Population, Population Health trends*, Treasury, London.

Watts, G. (1999) Cases in need of evaluations. *The Times Higher*, July 2nd, pp. 30–31.

Webb, C. (1992) The use of the first person in academic writing: objectivity, language and gatekeeping. *Journal of Advanced Nursing*, **17**, 747–752.

Wedderburn Tate, C. (1998) Charting a future for nursing research. In: *Nursing Research: Setting New Agendas* P. Smith (ed). Hodder Headline, London. pp. 8–29.

Journals

Journal of Interprofessional Care (2000) Special Issue on the New Collaboration, **14**(1).

Nursing Ethics: An International Journal for Health Care Professionals. Hodder Headline, London.

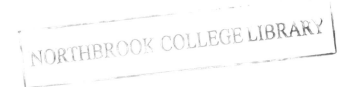
NORTHBROOK COLLEGE LIBRARY

Chapter 8 **Public Health Nursing – Health Visiting**

Frances Appleby and Marion Frost

Introduction

This chapter will explore a number of issues affecting registered specialist community public health nursing (health visiting) practice including the recommendation that health visitors develop a family-centred public health role (DoH 1999a). Legislation and reports, which specifically identify health visiting practice as pivotal to the government agenda for promoting the health of individuals, families and communities through public health approaches, will be examined. Specialist community public health nurses are responsible for identifying and organising services for defined populations that may include vulnerable individuals (NMC 2004). This process involves searching for actual and potential health needs, stimulating an awareness of health needs, influencing policies affecting health and facilitating activities that enhance health in a variety of settings. The extent to which health visitors are embracing this approach in their practice, the scope and opportunities for doing so and the potential constraints which inhibit such developments will be explored.

The development of health visiting

There is some debate about the nature of the work undertaken by the original practitioners who came to be known as health visitors (Dingwall 1977). Whilst much of their early focus was on the provision of health advice and assistance to mothers of young infants in response to the high infant mortality rates that were witnessed in the late 1800s, some were prominent in influencing policy decisions that aimed to reduce inequalities in health. There was also a missionary aspect to the service which grew out of the philanthropic endeavours of the middle classes and only gradually became organised by the state.

Overcrowding, poverty and high infant mortality in the nineteenth century prompted the emergence of voluntary movements aimed at improving the moral, social and hygienic welfare of the urban poor. One such organisation, the Ladies Sanitary Reform Association, was formed in Manchester and Salford in 1862 and this is generally acknowledged to be the start of health visiting. Respectable working women were appointed to go from door to door among the poorer classes of the population, to teach and help them as the opportunity offered (McCleary 1933). They were to teach hygiene and child welfare, mental and moral welfare, and provide social support.

Co-existing with the voluntary lady visitors at the turn of the century, women sanitary inspectors carried out public health work, despite the prevailing feeling of the time that this latter work was unsuitable for women. The women sanitary inspectors aimed to increase their marketability by combining inspection duties with home visiting; they opposed the separation of sanitary inspection and home visiting as jobs, fearing that the latter would be demoted as 'female work' with lower status and pay. Eventually however, this occurred and a lower level qualification was devised for health visitors, as they were increasingly known (Davies 1988; Robinson 1982).'

(Mason 1995)

However, before this demarcation occurred, overlap continued to exist in the work of some lady sanitary inspectors. One of their members, Margaret Llewellyn-Davies, identified the effects of social and economic deprivation on the health and well-being of families visited in London and Sheffield. As a consequence of her experiences she published a harrowing book detailing women's accounts of their childbirth and parenting experiences. These were instrumental in maternity and child welfare benefits being introduced into the National Insurance Act of 1911 (Billingham *et al.* 1996). Another example of sanitary inspectors seeking to influence the socio-economic environment of their clients is exemplified by the work of the Women's Public Health Officers Association (which later became the Health Visitors Association). They moved a number of resolutions on the need for improved maternity services at the Trades Union Congress (TUC) in the 1920s and 1930s which led to the TUC, jointly with the British Medical Association, drawing up a scheme in 1939 for a national maternity service (TUC 1981).

While these activities could be described as evidence that health visiting is firmly rooted in a public health approach, there is little doubt that during the first half of the twentieth century health visiting activity focused on maternal and child health from a more individualised perspective. Indeed, Blane (1989) argues that it was the assiduous work of the health visitors at this time that played a central role in reducing infant mortality. Ironically, although the dramatic reduction in infant and child deaths seemed to vindicate the work of health visitors it also raised questions about the continued need for the service which had, by 1918, become obligatory (Dingwall & Robinson 1993).

Under the National Health Service (NHS) Act 1946 the scope of health visiting broadened to include working with all age groups although still retaining a major focus on mothers and children:

'It shall be the duty of every local authority to make provision...for the visiting of persons in their homes by visitors, to be called health visitors, for the purpose of giving advice as to the care of young children, persons suffering from illness and expectant or nursing mothers...'

(NHS Act 1946, para 24 (1) cited in Abbott & Sapsford 1990)

While the Jameson report (MoH 1956) reiterated the 'family visitor' focus of health visiting with extended roles in the fields of mental health and the care of the older person, health visitors themselves felt they had a continued responsibility to raise public awareness of health needs as well as influence the public sphere of health policy (CETHV 1977; Mason 1995).

Principles of health visiting

In 1977, the Council for the Education and Training of Health Visitors (CETHV) formulated principles of professional practice based on a belief in the value of health which reflected the process of health visiting:

- The search for health needs
- The stimulation of an awareness of health needs
- The influence on policies affecting health
- The facilitation of health enhancing activities
                                            (CETHV 1997)

The principles both reinforced the public health nature of health visiting work (see Box 8.1) and provided a framework for the new public health agenda which began to emerge in the mid-1970s as part of the World Health Organization's global strategy (Lalonde 1974; also see Chapter 1). This in turn legitimised the broader public health approaches to which the profession had aspired over the years. However, in 1974 the health visiting service moved from the control of the local authority to be part of the NHS. General practitioners remained outside of this merger and the introduction of 'GP fundholding' under the NHS and Community Care Act 1990 enabled them to contract for health visiting services which included a maximum 10% public health role (Potrykus 1993). The focus of general practitioners on the medical model of service provision created tensions for many health visitors who became concerned about the emphasis placed on achieving measurable targets with the practice population (such as the uptake of child development checks and immunisations) at the expense of public health work in the community.

The publication of the Standing Nursing and Midwifery Advisory Committee Report (SNMAC 1995) reaffirmed the contribution of health visitors in 'championing' public health approaches through

---

Box 8.1 Principles of health visiting. (Sources: CETHV 1977; Twinn & Cowley 1992)

(1) *The search for health needs*
Health visitors work proactively in their search for acknowledged and potential health needs of individuals, families and communities using a partnership approach to collect both qualitative and quantitative data.

(2) *Stimulation of an awareness of health needs*
Having identified the health needs of the population health visitors seek to stimulate an awareness of inequalities such as poverty among individuals, families and communities. Awareness raising may involve work with the media, community groups, lay organisations, action, pressure- and self-help groups. Targets for awareness raising include clients, families, communities, health service managers, Primary Care Trusts (PCT) Boards, politicians and policy makers, and all those agencies whose activities impact on health.

(3) *Influences on policies affecting health*
Health visitors are assessors of health need who participate in the public health policy process by contributing nursing advice. They may seek to influence policies which impact on health at many levels, for example through pressure groups and consumer organisations. Targets for political pressure include local councillors and MPs and PCTs.

(4) *The facilitation of health-enhancing activities*
Health visitors acknowledge that individuals may find it difficult to adopt a healthy lifestyle because of their circumstances and therefore, in keeping with the principle of influencing policies, health visitors seek to facilitate healthy lifestyles for individuals by contributing towards changing the conditions in which people live. They will also assist the development of group or community activities that aim to develop personal confidence, knowledge and self-esteem in order to enable people to adopt health-enhancing behaviours and to make informed lifestyle choices.

---

individual and community health promotion. The connection between health visiting and public health was further highlighted in the UKCC proposals for the education of specialist community nursing practitioners (UKCC 1994) in which the title of health visiting was expanded to 'public health nursing – health visiting' in recognition of the broader function. More recently, the Labour Government's modernisation agenda for nursing, midwifery and health visiting has spelt out a need for health visitors to develop a role which includes both a family centred and public health element of practice (DoH 1999a, 1999b, 2001). This has been supported by the development of an educational training programme based on the principles of health visiting that prepares students, when qualified, to work at the individual, family, group or community level (NMC 2002a).

Modernising the role of the health visitor

Health visiting has a strong tradition of working with individuals, families and communities to offer health promotion and preventive health care to all age groups (DoH 2001). Findings from a systematic review of the effectiveness of domiciliary health visiting (Elkan *et al.* 2000; Robinson, 1999) suggest not only that a home visiting service to families with young children, similar to that provided by health visitors, can prove cost effective but also that it can enhance parenting skills and the quality of the home environment, ameliorate child behaviour problems and improve the detection and management of postnatal depression. The study acknowledged, however, that home visiting as a strategy is insufficient to bring about radical improvements in health and social outcomes without collaborative working with other disciplines and agencies in order to provide effective support.

Yet it is the very nature of the way in which health visitors work that has often made it difficult to define their activities and measure the long-term outcomes. In a climate of limited resources and ever-increasing demands on the service, the management emphasis in the NHS has been on short-term identifiable outcomes and immediately measurable outputs which has failed to take account of the longer-term benefits of health visiting activities.

With the election of a Labour government in 1997 this ethos appeared to have changed and the opportunity for health visitors to further develop their role in the promotion of health and prevention of ill health for individuals, families and communities was acknowledged. The publication of a number of significant documents set out a new health agenda in which health visitors were identified as having a pivotal role (Acheson 1998; DoH 1999a, 1999b, 2001; Home Office 1998). Health visitors were encouraged to modernise their role supported by the development of facilitative management structures which would enable practice to further develop in response to policy directives. The Government's strategy for health, with its focus on health promotion, preventive care and reducing inequalities in health, placed public health and primary health care centre stage.

Significantly at this time several major government reports identified that the role of the health visitor was key to advancing this agenda. The first of these, a consultation paper, *Supporting Families* (Home Office 1998) outlined a number of proposals for strengthening family life including activities already being carried out by many health visitors such as weaning groups, sleep clinics, behaviour management clinics and early relationship groups and an enhancement of the role to promote the health of the schoolchild and teenager. The document also referred to the Sure Start programme which has been developed to improve the lives of young children and their families in areas of greatest need. As Cowley and Houston

(1999) pointed out the Home Office was responding to clear evidence that support for all families would reduce inequalities and lead to improvements in public health and community stability in the long term.

Following this, the Acheson Report (1998) similarly identified a need for high priority to be given to the health of families with children as well as reducing income inequalities and improving the living standards of poor households. It specifically recommended that health visitors should further develop their role in providing social and emotional support for parents and their children in disadvantaged circumstances. The report identified the need to target the least well off in society in order to reduce health inequalities and, very importantly, considered that improving the health of women and children would have the most influential effect on the health of future generations.

Subsequently, in line with the government's 'joined up thinking' policy, *Saving Lives: Our Healthier Nation* (DoH 1999a) set out a plan for improving the health of everyone but particularly the health of the worst off in society. The report identified health visitors as public health practitioners who would be pivotal to the achievement of the strategy, working in collaboration with local agencies, local communities and primary care trusts. Health visitors were encouraged to respond effectively to the Government's agenda through developing 'a family-centred public health role, working with individuals, families and communities to improve health and tackle health inequality' (DoH 1999a, p. 132).

This role would include developing family health plans in partnership with individuals and families plus initiating and developing outreach programmes based on examples such as Home Start, New Pin and 'community mothers'. Health visitors would be expected to address health needs of groups such as homeless people and to help local communities identify and address their own health needs. The report specifically outlined that a team led by the health visitor would provide a range of health improvement activities including (DoH 1999a, p. 133):

- Child health programmes
- Parenting support and education including support to Sure Start, parenting groups and home visits
- Developing support networks in communities, for example, tackling social isolation in older people
- Support and advice for breastfeeding mothers and women at risk of postnatal depression
- Health promotion programmes to target cancer, coronary heart disease and stroke, accidents and mental health
- Advice on family relationships and support to vulnerable children and their families

Building on the above, the Department of Health published a strategy for nursing, midwifery and health visiting to respond positively to the modernisation agenda (DoH 1999b) which re-stated the components of the modern role for health visitors as previously outlined. In addition it placed greater emphasis on a leadership role for health visitors leading teams of nurses, nursery nurses and community workers working in partnership with local communities and vulnerable groups to identify and tackle their own health needs.

It was evident from these recommendations that whilst an important component of the health visitor's role would still be supporting families with young children they would also be expected to seek opportunities to work with other groups in the community. The publication of the *Health Visitor Practice Development Resource Pack* (DoH 2001) offered a framework and guidance for practitioners, their colleagues and managers to develop the modern way of working with families and communities, to work to common priorities such as national service frameworks. Furthermore it recognised that health visitors had always been trained as public health workers and suggested that they needed to refocus their professional practice from routine task orientated activities to respond to priorities identified through community health needs assessment. However, as

Dingwall and Robinson (1993) warn, starting from this perspective, which is frequently based on an epidemiological approach to data collection, may lead to professionals determining health care provision without consultation with service users as required by Labour government policy.

Delivering improvements in the health of the population is central to the Government's plan for modernising the NHS (DoH 2002a, 2003a, 2004a) and is discussed in more detail in Chapters 1 and 3. Nurses, midwives and health visitors are required to be at the forefront of change in order to improve health and health care for clients and local communities (DoH 2002b, 2003a). Achieving the national targets to reduce the gap in infant mortality across social groups and raise life expectancy in the most disadvantaged areas faster than elsewhere, requires co-ordination at government level, local strategic partnerships, participation of local people and innovation by front line staff (DoH 2003b). The National Service Framework for Children, Young People and Maternity Services sets out a clear role for all those working with children to deliver a high quality service for children, young people their parents or carers (DfEE & DoH 2004).

As part of the modernisation programme, the Government has also recognised the need to secure public protection through improved professional self-regulation that is more open, responsive and accountable (DoH 1999a). The professional body, the Nursing and Midwifery Council (NMC), had been required by law to develop a new simplified register as part of their function to protect the public. Following lengthy consultation, three parts were agreed to include nursing, midwifery and specialist community public health nursing (SCPHN) (see Chapter 20). Commencing on 1st August 2004, all health visitors on Part 11 of the UKCC register have automatically been transferred to the new register with the current title of Registered Specialist Community Public Health Nursing (Health Visiting) (NMC 2004).

This loss of registration for the health visiting profession is in direct conflict with the Government's decision in 1999 to maintain separate registration for health visitors and has had a demoralising effect on the profession. While initially this endorsement of the unique and distinct nature of health visiting practice appeared to be further confirmed by contemporary government policy, the subsequent Nursing and Midwifery Order 2001 removed all mention of health visiting which is now subsumed under the umbrella of specialist community public health nursing. However, as Brocklehurst (2004a) suggests, health visiting has the ability to respond and adapt to political and professional change. The way forward appears to lie in recognising the opportunities available, forming strategic alliances with other agencies and supporting local communities in identifying and developing their own services (Brocklehurst 2004b).

Dilemmas for health visiting practice

The requirement for health visitors to work in new ways to respond to the changing context of health care has been clearly spelt out by the Department of Health (DoH 1999b, 2002b). However, there are a number of dilemmas for health visiting practice that need to be examined in relation to their contribution to supporting the developing public health agenda.

First, the uniqueness of health visiting practice has been recognised for its provision of a universal, non-stigmatising service to the well population, particularly families with children aged under five years (CETHV 1977; Home Office 1998). This has provided the opportunity to work with clients to identify and prioritise the health needs of a local population, taking into account the user perspective as required by current government policy (DoH 2002b). However, with a steady decline in the health visiting workforce over the past 15 years it is doubtful whether these policy expectations are continuing to be met (Cowley 2003). Targeting of services and selective visiting may lead to a failure to identify vulnerable families who are least able to access services. Robinson (1999, p. 18) argues that 'without universalist surveillance it is not possible to identify those in need of a greater health visiting input since

the bulk of health and social problems occur in the large number of people who are not especially high risk rather than in the few who are high risk'.

The government emphasis on targeting of services creates dilemmas for the health visiting profession particularly in relation to health promotion, health surveillance and child protection. Dingwall and Robinson (1993) suggest that developing the health visiting service on a contractual basis in response to expressed need changes the nature of health surveillance with, for example, children being seen only at clinics where inadequacies of parenting may be difficult to identify. Opportunities for family health promotion and ill health prevention may be further eroded by the use of questionnaires to review the developmental progress of children unless targeted at those with known low dependency needs (Clarke *et al.* 2004). In order to reduce inequalities in health, Dingwall and Robinson argue that home visiting should be viewed as a 'valid instrument of social policy' which advocates for those excluded from political decision making through age or other factors.

The pressure for the provision of a more targeted health visiting service has also led some primary care trusts to introduce the use of screening tools in an attempt to identify those most at risk. While some practitioners may find these tools a useful aid in practice, questions arise as to whether the level of risk is, or should be, determined by professionals or clients, particularly where the vulnerable are involved. In addition, concerns have been expressed about the sensitivity of such tools in accurately identifying risk factors and the continuing relevance of identified factors which may change over time (Elkan *et al.* 2000). It is therefore crucial that health visitors use any such tool in conjunction with professional judgement, continually reviewing the factors identified and ensuring protection for children and vulnerable adults in line with government policy such as *Every Child Matters: Next Steps* (DoH 2004b) and the *National Service Framework for Children, Young People and Maternity Services* (DfEE & DoH 2004).

Nevertheless, the identification of actual and potential health needs is a cornerstone of the public health approach and remains fundamental to the planning of health care interventions in the modern NHS. In response to this health visitors must continue to use their well established skills in caseload analysis and community profiling combined with their knowledge of local communities, and as part of their leadership role, raise awareness and influence primary care trust decisions about the development of appropriate health care interventions and services to meet the needs of the local population. Key issues may arise from the results of such data collection that could be in variance with central government targets and local health improvement plans.

Caseload analysis (Hunt 1982; Sheldrake & Rowbotham 2000) provides health visitors with important information about the local population and the factors that impact on their lives which may not be revealed in the local public health report. Whilst mortality and morbidity rates provide a vital overview of the health of the community they may not identify those health issues which most concern individuals, nor do they necessarily identify relevant variables. For example, the Director of Public Health's report may identify a high incidence of accidents amongst the under fives. Yet it is the health visitor's records which could show the links between maternal depression and accidents, or the fact that accidents occur most frequently where families are poorly accommodated or where there is a lack of play facilities. Health visitor records may also identify families who are becoming isolated because of racial harassment or fear of crime.

Furthermore, caseload and workload analysis provides an opportunity for health visitors to review work patterns to provide evidence for research-based practice and to evaluate their own practice. Information gathered should be critically analysed, acknowledging both its strengths and weakness, and used to support primary care trusts in the implementation of local public health action plans and in commissioning relevant services. However, the collection of this data is problematic and where staffing shortages occur data collection and analysis may be incomplete.

At a time when the role of the health visitor has been validated as fundamental to advancing the public health agenda, questions must be asked about the extent to which the reality of practice reflects this expectation. This view is expressed in a report written by the Office for Public Management (2000), which notes that the uniqueness of the profession's contribution to the public health agenda lies in its potential rather than in contemporary practice. Smith's (2004) study identified isolation in practice, GP attachment and reactive casework practice as inhibitors to developing a broader public health role as demonstrated in the following conceptual framework.

A framework for health visiting practice

The adaptation of a typology proposed by Beattie (1991) provides a useful framework for identifying different aspects of the health visitor's role. In Beattie's typology (Figure 8.1) a basic premise is that effective public health interventions demand the application of an eclectic approach that combines activities at both the individual and collective level. These activities may be either expert led (authoritative) or undertaken in partnership with clients (negotiated). The concept of collective activities includes alerting politicians and policy makers to significant environmental influences and social circumstances which may make it difficult for individuals, families and communities to adopt or experience healthier lifestyles despite health advice and client awareness.

This collective response to changing the environment, in which individuals seek to achieve health, has been referred to as 'making the healthier choice the easier choice' a phrase coined by Milio in 1986. This reflects an acknowledgement that whilst individuals have a personal responsibility for maintaining their own health there maybe internal and/or external constraints which make this difficult or even impossible to achieve. Thus there is a need for interventions by government and other relevant agencies aimed at minimising these constraints and strengthening the resources of individuals, families and

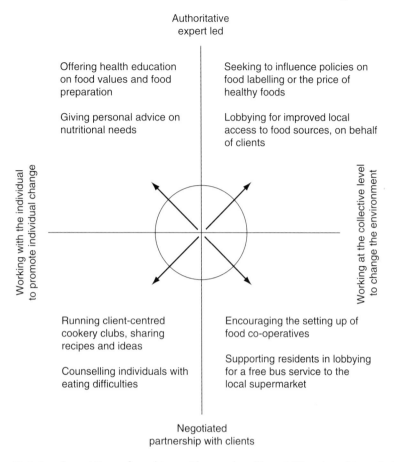

Figure 8.1 Beattie's typology. Ways of working with people with nutritional problems (adapted) (1991)

communities so that they are better equipped to resist breakdown and meet their own health needs.

In seeking to develop initiatives aimed at meeting health needs, the health visitor is expected to work in collaboration with other relevant agencies across the state, private and voluntary sectors.

Examples of public health activities in health visiting practice which reflect the above model

The following examples of health visiting practice demonstrate how the core functions of the modern health visiting service identified in the Health Visitor Practice Development Resource Pack (www.innovate.had.online.org.uk) incorpor-

ate the public health role of the health visitor (see Box 8.2).

Practice examples

Example one
Health visitors in the Birkby area of Huddersfield worked collaboratively with the oral dental health department, interpreters and local health educators to plan a public health campaign aimed at improving child oral health, targeting the South Asian population in particular (Andrew 2004). Evidence for developing the initiative was identified through population profiling. The campaign included a health promotion event to give advice to clients about the correct use of feeding bottles and beakers, to raise awareness of causes of dental decay and to

> **Box 8.2   Health visitor practice development resource pack. (Source: DoH 2001)**
>
> A public health approach for health visiting practice means:
>
> - Tackling the causes of ill health, not just responding to the consequences
> - Looking at health needs across the whole population rather than only responding to the needs of the individual
> - Planning work on the basis of local need, evidence and national health priorities rather than custom and practice
> - Working within the framework of the local HimP and considering what your team can do with others to achieve HimP goals
> - Using the live information you have about local community needs and strengths into the HimP development process
> - Working with other agencies and sectors to plan services and promote well-being
> - Finding out which population groups have significant health needs and targeting resources to address these
> - Taking action to make healthy choices easy choices
> - Leading or joining a multi-disciplinary team rather than working alone or in a uni-disciplinary team
> - Influencing policies that affect health locally and nationally
> - Finding meaningful ways to evaluate the impact of your work

encourage pro-active use of dental services. This example fits with the top left quadrant of the adaptation of Beattie's model (giving health education advice to individuals, an authoritative, individual approach) and the top right quadrant (an authoritative, collective approach in relation to population profiling).

Example two

Health visitors in south London (New Addington Health Visitors 1993) started a cookery club at which mothers could learn to prepare a cheap nutritious meal whilst their children were cared for and then shared the meal for which they made a small financial contribution. This activity provided opportunities for a break from the children, social contact and support and health education as well as a low cost meal. In the adaptation of Beattie's model this example fits in the bottom left quadrant (negotiated partnership with clients and working with the individual to promote change).

Example three

Health Promotion England in partnership with the Department of Trade and Industry launched the 'Avoiding slips, trips and broken hips' campaign to help prevent older people falling in the home (Carlin 2002). Interventions by health visitors and other members of the primary health care team involved giving advice supported by leaflets, encouraging physical exercise to improve balance, making the home environment safer and analysing accident statistics. Using the adaptation of Beattie's model the above example would fit in the top and bottom left quadrant (authoritative and negotiated partnership with individuals to promote change) plus the top right quadrant (use by health visitors of accident statistics to influence practice development, an authoritative, collective approach).

Example four

The Home Play project in Sheffield was a skill mix parent support initiative developed by health visitors to improve confidence and self-esteem in families with young children (Brown 1997). Drawing on community development approaches local families were consulted about their health needs and identified concerns around social isolation, child behaviour problems and poor quality local play facilities. Working with other statutory and voluntary agencies, health visitors and nursery nurses provided a home visiting programme in partnership with clients, developed social networks through facilitating toddler groups, produced information leaflets about play resources for children and organised a 12 week course about learning through play. This example fits with all four quadrants of the model (health workers provided expert advice to clients in response to negotiated health concerns, and worked collectively with clients and other agencies to change the environment).

Changing to a 'family-centred public health' approach to practice

Whilst the concept of a 'family-centred public health' role has never been clearly defined by the Government, the continuum in the *Health Visitor Practice Development Resource Pack* (DoH 2001, p. 13) endorses the view that several levels of practice are involved including individual, group and community interventions. As part of the programme of reform the Department of Health funded four pilot sites to explore changes in service delivery leading to a public health approach to practice. Practitioners in all four pilot sites identified current working practice as being at the individual and group level rather than at the community level (Rowe 2002). Brocklehurst (2004b, p. 215) reported that while most health visitors believed that practice had to change, many lacked skills in public health work including 'community development, partnership working, project management, team leadership, research and evaluation'. Programmes of support and development were therefore required to enable change to occur and for practitioners to work with the community to meet identified needs.

According to Forester (2004) the move from individual interventions to a community development approach to practice requires organisational support, strong leadership, effective team working, partnership working with communities and other agencies and the ability to work with multiple agendas. Expecting practitioners to work at a community level as well as provide expert family support may be unrealistic. The Stockport model of health visiting has developed over many years with three distinct components: generic primary care health visiting, first parent visitor programme and community development

workers. This tripartite model has been strengthened as part of the modernisation programme (Swann & Brocklehurst 2004) and findings that have emerged in changing health visiting practice include:

- The need for consistent and visionary leadership
- Consultation with all concerned in the change process
- Strong support from management
- Support with appropriate training enabling health visitors to provide high quality family support and leadership in community development
- Close partnership working between the NHS, local authority and voluntary sector

Brocklehurst (2004b) further suggests that Sure Start programmes have proved to be enablers of change for health visiting practice in the pilot sites. Sure Start programmes operate in the most disadvantaged areas of the country and are designed to promote the health and educational development of pre-school children as well as strengthen families and communities, thus enabling children to achieve their full potential and eradicate child poverty (DfEE 2001). There is significant opportunity for the expertise and skill of health visitors to work with other disciplines and agencies to reduce the problems of social exclusion among vulnerable children and their families by identifying needs and ensuring that appropriate services are in place. The Chief Nursing Officer's review (DoH 2004c) recognises that whilst health visitors are a central component of integrated children's services their public health role needs to be more clearly articulated within Sure Start programmes to ensure vulnerable children have access to their services.

A practice-based example of a Sure Start initiative is the Millmead Estate trailblazer project set up three years ago in Thanet (Rehal & Langley 2004). The Sure Start team consists of a multi-agency, multi-skilled group of individuals with either a health professional background, community development knowledge, educational or social work expertise, led by a director with a health visiting background. To minimise conflict between team members from different agencies principles of respect including a willingness to listen to each other, an open attitude, valuing of each other, and encouraging development as individuals have been required of all those involved in the programme. This new way of working has involved the breaking down of professional boundaries and working alongside families, allowing them to set the agenda. Evaluation of the project shows that it is welcomed by local people and has enabled personal growth both for clients and staff.

Another enabler of change that has arisen from the pilot sites is that of corporate working which involves health visitors sharing caseloads and workloads and using a team approach to working. Brocklehurst and Adams (2004) found that the strengths of this method of working included clients having more choice and access to a greater range of skills whilst practitioners felt supported and kept up to date through sharing knowledge and skills. However, a key risk associated with this model of practice, which needs to be addressed, is the potential for lack of continuity of service provision.

As well as corporate working, leading teams of workers with differing levels of skills as identified in the strategy *Making a Difference* (DoH 1999b) is becoming more commonplace in health visiting practice. Teams of health visitors, nursery nurses, staff nurses, health care assistants and administrative officers work together within a primary care setting, pooling their skills and knowledge in order to provide the most effective care for the practice population and community in which they work. This team approach to the delivery of health care is increasingly becoming the model of choice for health visiting practice, particularly where staff shortages are evident. Accountability is a key issue in this model of care as outlined in the code of professional conduct (NMC 2002b).

The way forward

There is an urgent need for health visitors to re-evaluate their contribution to the public health agenda and seek out new ways of working that more effectively support collective as well as individual approaches to health care. The government

has clearly identified that all nurses, midwives and health visitors are required to change existing practice and plan services, with others, in new ways looking at the whole system and the pathway of care (DoH 2002b; see also Chapter 1). Services are to be based on need with service users and the public being central to the planning and development process. Working in isolation, as identified by Smith (2004), is no longer a viable option. Whilst geographical constraints or unsuitable premises have in the past inhibited collaborative working, organisational and managerial structures must be developed that support staff in changing practice and developing new roles.

Developing skills in partnership with the wider public health workforce and using opportunities to lead and influence change are essential components of specialist community public health practice. Health visitors need to have the confidence to value their expertise and contribution to supporting families, mothers and children, a key theme of government policy outlined in *Tackling Health Inequalities: A Programme for Action* and essential for improving the nation's health and well-being (DoH 2003b).

Lowenhoff (2004), a nurse consultant in parental and child mental health, argues strongly for a universal service that builds relationships with clients, supporting families in a pro-active way in order to promote health, prevent ill health and reduce inequalities in health. Health visitors leading teams of community staff nurses, nursery nurses and administrative officers need to work with consultants in public health medicine, general practitioners, midwives, mental health services, social workers, community development workers, health promotion specialists, benefits advisors, nursery school workers and others from the state, voluntary and private sectors. The provision of innovative, accessible services that promote positive parenting, engaging communities as well as individuals, is vital for addressing the underlying determinants of health. The development of children's trusts bringing together health, social and education services in order to secure integrated commissioning of services has been designed to facilitate this process (DoH 2004b).

Health visitors have much to contribute to an agenda that involves breaking down health and social care boundaries, a task which, for many, is part of everyday practice. Dealing with the long-term underlying causes of health inequalities such as poverty and poor housing has always been part of health visiting practice. Health visitors have well developed negotiation and advocacy skills that can be used in working with differing age groups to influence service provision, gain access to appropriate resources and make a difference to people's lives (Rogers 2003). They need to develop their leadership role, embracing opportunities to become representatives on the professional executive committee and acting on ideas based on best available evidence that meet the needs of local people (DoH 2002b).

The use of current best evidence to support health care decision making underpins clinical governance and accountability in practice. The systematic review of research evidence on the effectiveness of domiciliary health visiting is of significance in the move towards evidence-based practice and the consequence of health visiting practice on the health outcomes for clients and communities (Elkan *et al.* 2000). However, Wanless (2004) warns of the general lack of evidence about the cost effectiveness of public health interventions which has led to the development of a wide range of initiatives with unclear objectives and limited evaluation of outcomes. Evaluation in situations where outcomes evolve over a period of time (such as public health work) is a complex process as it is difficult to prove that any change is due to a particular intervention (Houston 2003).

Salvage (1998) suggests that there is an inappropriate range of resources and a lack of will to use evidence-based practice. Health visitors must therefore have access to databases and training, allocating time to search for good quality information. They must develop the skills and the will to change practice based on the findings of research. As the emphasis increases on health informatics and the application of information technology within the educational preparation of health visitors and the work setting, such challenges should be overcome. Education and training, including continuing professional development,

must prepare practitioners appropriately for their new roles to enable the future generation of registered specialist community public health nurses (health visitors) to contribute effectively to the changing public health agenda.

Conclusion

This chapter has explored the need for specialist community public health nurses (health visitors) to participate pro-actively in public health provision at the individual, family and community level working collaboratively with public, private and non-statutory agencies to promote health and prevent ill health across all age ranges in different settings. Valuing health and treating it as a positive resource has always been central to health visiting practice.

The requirement to modernise practice has been clearly identified in government policy. Health visitors must value their knowledge and skills, confront the dilemmas in practice, and have the confidence to seek opportunities to plan, develop and lead new approaches to practice in consultation with the public. To enable this process, supportive management and organisational structures need to be developed that facilitate advancing practice.

Health visitors can take pride in the fact that the principles of health visiting practice have been used to underpin the new standards for specialist community public health nursing practice and influence the public health agenda. In searching for actual and potential health needs, health visitors must be pro-active in advocating for resources and environments that support the health needs of individuals, families and communities, and through influencing policies and facilitating health enhancing activities, enable healthy choices to become a reality.

Equally importantly, new ways of measuring the effectiveness of specialist community public health nursing practice must be found, based on a realisation that public health activities aim to produce long-term benefits to society. Measuring the number of activities achieved excludes opportunities for developing imaginative and strategic public health approaches identified as essential for promoting the health of society. As the Office for Public Management (2000, p. 40) said, health visiting must be 'measured not by the activity it undertakes but by the difference it makes.'

References

Abbott, P. & Sapsford, R. (1990) *Family Gender and Welfare. D211 (Units 10 & 11).* Open University Press, Milton Keynes.

Acheson, D. (1998) *Independent Inquiry into Inequalities in Health Report.* The Stationery Office, London.

Andrew, L. (2004) Beakers for bottles – a health visitor oral health campaign. *Community Practitioner,* 77(1), 18–22.

Beattie, A. (1991) Knowledge and control in health promotion: a test case for social policy and social theory. In: *The Sociology of the Health Service* (J. Gabe, M. Calnan & M. Bury eds). Routledge, London.

Billingham, K., Morrell, J. & Billingham, C. (1996) Reflections on the History of Health Visiting. *British Journal of Community Health Care Nursing,* 1(7), 386–392.

Blane, D. (1989) Preventive Medicine and Public Health: England and Wales 1870–1914. In: *Readings for a New Public Health,* (C. Martin & D. McQueen eds). Edinburgh University Press, Edinburgh.

Brocklehurst, N. (2004a) The new health visiting: thriving at the edge of chaos. *Community Practitioner,* 77(4), 135–139.

Brocklehurst, N. (2004b) Is health visiting 'fully engaged' in its own future well-being? *Community Practitioner,* 77(6), 214–218.

Brocklehurst, N. & Adams, C. (2004) Embodying modernization: corporate working. *Community Practitioner,* 77(8), 292–296.

Brown, I. (1997) A skill mix parent support initiative in health visiting: an evaluation study. *Community Practitioner,* 70(9), 339–343.

Carlin, H. (2002) Slips, trips and broken hips. *Community Practitioner,* 75(3), 85–86.

Clarke, M., Hague, D., Mortimer, B. & Thompson, S. (2004) Should every three year old receive a routine review? *Community Practitioner,* 77(3), 101–104.

CETHV (1977) *An Investigation into the Principles of Health Visiting.* Council for the Education and Training of Health Visitors, London.

Cowley, S. (2003) Modernising health visiting education: potential, problems and progress. *Community Practitioner,* 76(11), 418–422.

Cowley, S. & Houston, A. (1999) *Health Visiting and School Nursing: The Croydon Story.* King's College London, London.

Davies, C. (1988) The health visitor as mother's friend: a woman's place in public health, 1900–1914. *The Social History of Medicine,* 1, 38–57.

DfEE (2001) *Sure Start: A guide to planning and delivering your programme.* Department for Education & Employment, London.

DfEE & DoH (2004) *National Service Framework for Children, Young People and Maternity Services.* The Stationery Office, London.

DoH (1999a) *Saving Lives: Our Healthier Nation.* Department of Health, London.

DoH (1999b) *Making a Difference: A Strategy for Nursing, Midwifery and Health Visiting.* Department of Health, London.

DoH (2001) *Health visitor development resource pack.* Department of Health, London.

DoH (2002a) *Delivering the NHS Plan, Next steps on Investment, Next Steps on Reform.* Department of Health, London.

DoH (2002b) *Liberating the Talents Helping Primary Care Trusts and Nurses to Deliver the NHS Plan.* Department of Health, London.

DoH (2003a) *Liberating the Public Health Talents of Community Practitioners and Health Visitors.* Department of Health, London.

DoH (2003b) *Tackling Health Inequalities; A Programme for Action.* Department of Health, London.

DoH (2004a) *The NHS Improvement Plan.* Department of Health, London.

DoH (2004b) *Every Child Matters: Next Steps.* Department of Health, London.

DoH (2004c) *The Chief Nursing Officer's review of the nursing, midwifery and health visiting contribution to children and young people.* Department of Health, London.

Dingwall, R. (1977) *The Social Organisation of Health Visitor Training.* Croom Helm, London.

Dingwall, R. & Robinson, K.M. (1993) Policing the family? Health visiting and the public surveillance of private behaviour. In: *Health & Wellbeing: A Reader* (A. Beattie, M. Gott, L. Jones & M. Sidell eds). Macmillan, London.

Elkan, R., Kendrick, D., Hewitt, M., Robinson, J.J.A., Tolley, K., Blair, M., *et al.* (2000) The effectiveness of domiciliary health visiting: a systematic review of international studies and a selective review of the British literature. *Health Technol. Assess.* 4(13).

Forester, S. (2004) Adopting community development approaches. *Community Practitioner,* 77(4), 140–145.

Home Office (1998) *Supporting Families*. The Stationery Office, London.

Houston, A. (2003) Sure Start: the example of one approach to evaluation. *Community Practitioner*, **76**(8), 294–298.

Hunt, M. (1982) New Approaches in Health Visiting: Caseload Profiles an alternative to the Neighbourhood Study. *Health Visitor*, **55**(11), 606–607.

Lalonde, M. (1974) *A New Perspective on the Health of Canadians*. Minister of Supply and Services Information Canada, Ottowa.

Lowenhoff, C. (2004) Have Talents: need liberating. *Community Practitioner*, **77**(1), 23–25.

Mason, C. (1995) Towards Public Health Nursing. In: *Community Health Care Nursing*, (D. Sines ed). Blackwell Science, Oxford.

McCleary, G.F. (1933) *The Early History of the Infant Welfare Movement*. HK Lewis and Co, London.

Milio, N. (1986) *Promoting Health through Public Policy*. Canadian Public Health Association, Ottowa.

MOH (1956) *An Inquiry into Health Visiting (The Jameson Committee)*. HMSO, London.

New Addington Health Visitors (1993) *The Cooking Club*. Croydon Community Health, Croydon.

NMC (2002a) *Requirements for Pre-registration Health Visitor Programmes*. Nursing and Midwifery Council, London.

NMC (2002b) *Code of Professional Conduct*. Nursing and Midwifery Council, London.

NMC (2004) *Standards of Proficiency for Specialist Community Public Health Nurses*. Nursing and Midwifery Council, London.

Office for Public Management (2000) *Leading the Future*. TG Scott, London.

Potrykus, C. (1993) Public health role cut as GP contracts start to bite. *Health Visitor*, **66**(6), 188–189.

Rehal, F. & Langley, H. (2004) Ensuring a Sure Start. *Community Practitioner*, **77**(5), 168–171.

Robinson, J. (1982) *An Evaluation of Health Visiting*. CETHV, London.

Robinson, J. (1999) Domiciliary Health Visiting a systematic review. *Community Practitioner*, **72**(2), 15–18.

Rogers, E. (2003) Health visitors and older people: 'thinking out of the box'. *Community Practitioner*, **76**(10), 381–385.

Rowe, A. (2002) Using a 'whole systems' approach to change in service delivery. *Community Practitioner*, **75**(3), 91–93.

Salvage, J. (1998) Evidence-based practice: a mixture of motives? *Nursing Times*, **94**(23), 61–64.

Sheldrake, D. & Robotham, D. (2000) Skills in health visiting. In: *Health Visiting: Specialist and Higher Level Practice*. (A. Robotham & D. Sheldrake eds) Churchill Livingstone, London.

Smith, M. (2004) Health visiting: the public health role. *Journal of Advanced Nursing*, **45**(1), 17–25.

SNMAC (1995) *Making It Happen*. Department of Health, London.

Swann, B. & Brocklehurst, N. (2004) Three in one: the Stockport model of health visiting. *Community Practitioner*, **77**(7), 251–256.

TUC (1981) *Women's Health at Risk*. Trades Union Congress, London.

Twinn, S. & Cowley, S. (1992) *The Principles of Health Visiting: a re-examination*. Health Visitors Association, London.

UKCC (1994) *The future of professional practice: the Council's standards for education and practice following registration*. United Kingdom Central Council for Nursing, Midwifery and Health Visiting, London.

Wanless, D. (2004) *Securing Good Health for the Whole Population*. Treasury, London.

Introduction

General practice nursing is the fastest growing community health care nursing discipline and the number of nurses working in general practice in England has trebled over the past fifteen years (Waller 2000). Practice nursing has emerged as a high profile career opportunity and offers a range of opportunities for nurses who enjoy patient contact, wish to work autonomously but within a team, caring not just for individuals but also for families and communities within the wider primary and social care context. This chapter will briefly review the historical development of practice nursing and then consider the developing role of the practice nurse, particularly since 1997. The impact of health policies on the role of practice nurses, with particular emphasis on the new General Medical Services (GMS) contract (NHS Confederation/BMA 2003), extended, supplementary and non-medical prescribing for nurses, the introduction of skill mix in general practice and the leadership and management skills necessary for specialist practitioners at both a practice and strategic level will also be discussed. The following section will be structured around the three roles identified in *Liberating the Talents* (DoH 2002). These are:

- First contact – the expansion of the role of practice nurses in seeing patients with undifferentiated conditions and the skills necessary for effective history taking and management
- Public health – the range of the role from individual interventions through screening programmes, immunisation programmes to health needs assessment and practice profiling and development plans
- Chronic disease management and continuing care – reflecting the continuing growth of chronic disease and change in emphasis in light of policy and clinical practice initiatives

Throughout this discussion the role of the practice nurse in engaging user and patient involvement and promoting patient empowerment and self-management will be emphasised. The next section will focus on clinical governance and how contemporary practice nurses need to be equipped with skills and knowledge to ensure quality assurance. These skills will be achieved through a range of different activities, including supporting staff in new skill mix teams, assessing competence, developing user involvement strategies, use of audit for quality assurance and compliance with standards derived from National Service Frameworks (NSF) and the Healthcare Commission (which has incorporated the Commission for Audit and Inspection (CHAI)). Consideration will also be given to linkages with the Quality and Outcomes Framework (QOF), uptake of clinical supervision of practice nurses, working with the PCT in its monitoring role as well as collaborative working with respect to the development of protocols, guidelines and care pathways in clinical care. The final section will consider the future of general practice and practice nursing.

Historical development

The first practice nurse was employed in 1913 but it was not until 1966 that changes in regulations in the doctor's charter enabled GPs to employ nurses as part of their ancillary staff. This anomaly, in considering nurses as part of ancillary staff, had a detrimental effect on the development of the role as nurses were often denied opportunities for professional development through lack of funding and subsequently often led to relative professional isolation. The changes incorporated within the GP contract (DoH 1989), implemented in 1990, had a large impact on the numbers of practice nurses employed as the contract advocated a change from the focus of general practice as being curative and reactive to one of being preventive and proactive.

Practice nurses, throughout the 1990s, developed expertise in chronic disease management and health promotion. However, this rapid expansion highlighted the existence of a fragmented approach to education and training for the profession. Despite this, practice nurses developed their own informal networks to support and disseminate good practice and, through the Royal College of Nursing (RCN) practice nurse forum, lobbied for specialist practitioner recognition from the United Kingdom Central Council (UKCC). This was achieved in 1994 and approved by the Department of Health in 1995 and, subsequently, practice nursing became one of eight recognised community nursing specialist practitioner programmes (UKCC 1994). A much wider range of continuing professional development programmes are now available for practice nurses. The advent of continuing professional development has been further assisted to some extent by primary care trusts (PCTs) who have responsibility for clinical governance for all GP practices within the PCT area. This has meant that the continuing professional development needs of practice nurses have now been incorporated into education commissioning in partnership with strategic health authorities and their local universities.

However, the majority of practice nurses are employed by GPs who maintain independent contractor status within the health service with the consequent classification of practices as small businesses. This has both advantages and disadvantages. Freedom from a hierarchical nursing structure has allowed many nurses a significant level of autonomy, but alongside this is the potential for lack of professional supervision and development as well as participation in the network of support that usually comes from belonging to a larger organisation. Nurses looking to work in general practice should be aware that the direct employer/employee relationship may mean the practice nurse may have to negotiate her own contract, conditions of service and study time to meet professional development needs.

The developing role of the practice nurse

The role of the practice nurse can be extremely broad and span the complete age range of the practice population. The variety of service provided by practice nurses can range from tasks such as dressings, suture removal and venepuncture through to nurse-led chronic disease management programmes and first contact consultations where the nurse sees patients with minor illness and undifferentiated conditions. The degree of specialisation of the nurse will depend on the size of the practice, the support of the GP partners and the health needs of the practice population. However, current health policy supports expansion of nursing roles and many new services are being designed and developed with practice nurses adopting the lead role (Prime 2003). All practice nurses need to be able to function as part of a team but also work autonomously, managing the nursing workload and governance aspects linked to their role. They are also required to work effectively on an interpersonal level with patients, members of the wider health care team and other agencies and are, therefore, required to possess a broad range of clinical knowledge and skills as well as being cognisant of the context within which general practice and the PCT function.

Impact of policy on general practice and practice nursing

The drive to modernise general practice probably started with the implementation of the 1990 GP contract (DoH 1989). How GPs chose to implement the contract was in effect left to them but this resulted in some areas being poorly served by GPs as the result of varying levels of service provision, leaving unmet needs within the community. The introduction of GP fundholding for some practices in 1990 also had a mixed impact (DOH 1990). Throughout the 1990s a number of government initiatives introduced opportunities for new service developments and innovation in the way in which general practice was delivered within the UK. One such driver related to the establishment of personal medical services (PMS) contracts (McKeon 1997). The introduction of personal medical services in 1997 reflected a growing consensus that the nationally negotiated general medical services system for contracting with GPs was too bureaucratic and did not always encourage GPs to innovate or contribute to the overall improvement of health and health care. The intended benefits and outcomes of PMS were:

- To provide faster, more convenient and accessible services for local patients
- To extend primary care services for populations that had not previously received their full share of such services
- To give health care professionals more opportunity to use their skills to the full
- To offer more flexible employment opportunities in general practice
- To reduce the bureaucracy in administering the GMS fees and allowances regime
- To inform national policy formulation

PMS providers could be individual GPs, a practice, a PCT or a group of practitioners including GPs and nurses. Fundholding, and subsequently the PMS contract, enabled practices to exert greater control over their substantive budgets provided they were able to demonstrate how resources would be utilised to improve services to meet the identified needs of the registered practice population and increase facilities for disadvantaged groups such as the homeless and individuals with mental health needs. The implementation of the PMS contract also provided significant opportunities to raise the profile of practice nurses who undertook the provision of a variety of nursing-led services that utilised a considerable diversity of advanced practitioner roles and competencies. The nature of PMS schemes varies widely and evaluating their impact is complex. A more extensive discussion of these innovative contracts is provided in Lewis *et al.* (2001).

Throughout the 1990s primary care services assumed a much higher priority following the realisation that many services currently provided in hospitals could be provided more effectively in primary and community care settings. This, coupled with shorter hospital stays and a reduc-

tion in hospital beds (Woodcock 2004) necessitated a formal review of the primary care workforce and of the context of care within which practice nurses function. With the change of government in 1997 the pace of change accelerated. The new government set out their vision in 'The New NHS: Modern, Dependable (DoH 1997). A policy shift was proposed away from the quasi market advocated by the previous government towards a more equitable system of care provision. Primary care groups (PCG) were instituted in April 2000 to take on the commissioning role previously undertaken by health authorities. PCGs offered clinicians (GPs and community nurses) the opportunity to serve on the PCG executive board and thus facilitated their involvement in executive and strategic decision making.

The move to the community continued with the publication of policies such as *Shifting the Balance of Power* (DoH 2001a), which advocated that more services currently provided in secondary care should move to primary care settings. One specific example of such changes related to chronic disease management within the primary care sector through the development of new services such as intermediate care teams, stroke rehabilitation schemes and other services which were provided to focus care outside of acute hospital settings.

Further government polices such as *A First Class Service* (DoH 1998) determined how clinical governance would be operationalised. Clinical governance has had a major impact on service delivery in general practice with particular regard to the implementation of a range of national service frameworks (NSFs) (e.g. for mental health, coronary heart disease, care of the older person, diabetes) which have set national standards for specialist care planning and delivery (much of which relates to primary care). Practice nurses have had to ensure that services are structured to meet not only the needs of patients but also the standards embedded in the NSFs. Primary care organisations have also been required to develop stringent mechanisms to ensure that they provide a high quality service that meets externally evaluated standards (e.g. such as those demanded by CHAI). Alongside the clinical governance framework, the government published *Saving Lives – Our Healthier Nation* (DoH 1999c). This policy document set out four key priority areas of cardiovascular disease, mental illness, cancer and accidents that were deemed to represent major challenges for effective delivery of health care services, for investment in health gain/improvement and for prevention and reduced mortality. This strategy has influenced the way services are prioritised and delivered in general practice.

However, by far the most influential policy for primary care has been the NHS Plan which was published in 2000 (DoH 2000). This set out the government's health care strategy for the next ten years. Access targets for general practice were set within the plan which exerted a major influence on performance. These targets advised that by 2004 patients could expect to see a health care professional within 24 hours or a GP within 48 hours of their request. Many practices have had to review their appointment systems to ensure they have been able to meet these targets. One impact has been that many practice nurses are fulfilling new roles such as triaging patients, undertaking telephone consultations or offering first contact services (see later section in this chapter on 'First contact').

Labour government policy has focused on modernising the health service and many initiatives have been developed to support this. Drivers for change have been the impact of the European Working Time Directive (DoH 2003) which has reduced junior doctors' working hours and necessitated new ways of providing services, the new consultants' contract and the new GMS contract (which commenced in April 2004) and more recently *Agenda for Change* (DoH 2004b). *Agenda for Change* is predominantly about pay modernisation for NHS trust employees, the opportunity to review roles, to redesign services and to reward staff performance/competence. Currently, *Agenda for Change* does not apply to practice nurses employed by GP practices but it is expected that the good employment practice highlighted in the new GMS contract will encourage GPs to adopt the scheme for universal application.

There have also been a number of other documents that have influenced the context of practice nursing delivery. *Making a Difference* (DoH 1999a) highlighted ten key roles for nurses that offered them opportunities to expand their roles, to undertake complete consultations with patients and to be able to instigate investigations without needing to refer to other health care practitioners. Alongside these changes in practice has been the introduction of new primary care services such as walk in centres, minor injury centres and more recently, changes in the out of hours services as PCTs have taken over responsibility from GP practices for providing out of hours care. The role that nurses play in leading and delivering such services is likely to become more prominent in the future.

The opportunities for nurses to expand their roles have been strengthened by changes in legislation to allow nurses to become extended and supplementary prescribers. In 1992 legislation was passed that gave nurses the legal right to prescribe and prescribing by certain groups of nurses began on October 3 1994.

The second Crown report (DoH 1999b) set out a proposed new framework for the prescribing, supply and administration of medicines. It recommended the introduction of two distinct categories of nurse prescribers: independent and dependent. Independent prescribers are defined as the person responsible for the initial assessment of patients with undiagnosed conditions and for decisions about the clinical management required including prescribing. The 'dependent' prescriber (altered to supplementary prescribers in the NHS Plan (DoH 2000) is defined as the person who is responsible for the continuing care of patients who have been clinically assessed by an independent practitioner. The continuing care could also include prescribing which is informed by clinical guidelines and is consistent with individual treatment plans. It was further proposed that dependent prescribers could be involved in continuing established treatments by issuing repeat prescriptions, with authority to adjust the dose or dosage form according to the patient's needs. These significant recommendations have had a major impact on the development of the scope of professional practice of nurses and other registered health professionals and the number of nurses able to prescribe medicines within the NHS has increased dramatically over the past decade. It has been a key feature of the Government's drive toward a health service which aims to empower patients by placing them at the centre of service provision, incorporating shared decision making in treatment options which includes increased choice as to where services may be accessed. The ability to complete an episode of care by providing the patient with the appropriate prescribed medication is vital in enabling nurses to provide a comprehensive, holistic package of care.

Furthermore, this initiative has increased the level of collaboration and cohesiveness exhibited within the primary care team.

An additional component of the practice nurse role when dealing with patients attending with minor illnesses is to advise patients on the rationale for the management of the presenting complaint. Advice on self-care together with interventions that encourage patient empowerment frames the central element of the nurses' role when dealing with these conditions. Exploration of patient's expectations and understanding of the nature and cause of their illness allows for a greater acceptance of a plan of treatment that may not fulfil initial expectations of the interaction. Although there may initially be difficulties in practice nurses accessing the necessary medical supervision to gain competence, practice nurses are likely to be able to manage care more independently within supplementary prescribing legislation.

The new GMS contract

Historically, GPs were contracted to the NHS to provide medical services for a registered population according to non-negotiable terms defined within the 'Terms and Conditions of Service' which included 24-hour responsibility for patients 365 days per year. From 1st April 2004, primary care organisations (PCO) were placed under a new duty to secure the provision of primary medical services. This provided greater flexibility over how and from whom these services were commissioned and included for the first time the potential to utilise alternative providers such as the voluntary sector, commercial providers, NHS trusts, other PCTs, and allowed for direct PCT provision of services as well as GMS and PMS contracts. The new commissioning arrangements were designed to support an expansion of primary care capacity, including delivery of a wider range of services. The underpinning concept was to introduce new mechanisms to afford practices greater control over the range of services that they provided alongside rewarding an increase in the quality of that service.

The new GMS contract (NHS Confederation/BMA 2003) preserves the status of existing practices as incumbent providers who maintain an obligation to provide those core services deemed essential, such as the management of patients who are ill, or believe themselves to be ill, and the management of individuals with chronic disease or terminal illnesses. Furthermore practices will have a preferential right to provide additional services but may opt out of such provision in accordance with fixed UK-wide rules.

Three groups of enhanced services, that is, essential or additional services (see Box 9.1) delivered to a higher standard, or services not provided through essential or additional services may also be commissioned by PCOs as appropriate to meet local health need. These three groups are directed, national and local enhanced services.

Directed enhanced services must be commissioned by each PCO but will not always be

---

Box 9.1 Additional services in the new GMS contract

- Cervical screening
- Contraceptive services
- Vaccinations and immunisations
- Childhood vaccinations and immunisations
- Child health surveillance
- Maternity services (excluding intra-partum care)
- Minor surgery procedures of curettage, cautery, cryocautery of warts and verrucae and skin lesions

provided by every practice. These services include childhood immunisations, influenza immunisations in the over 65 and 'at risk groups', minor surgery above that included as an additional service and services for violent patients, have nationally developed specifications and costs. As there is no requirement for all national enhanced services (Box 9.2) to be provided within a PCT area, it is possible that such national benchmarking might be considered as only a guide by the PCO. Any other enhanced service that a PCO wished to agree with a practice or other provider would be classed as a local enhanced service.

The new GMS contract is the biggest change to occur in NHS general practice since its inception (NHS confederation/BMA 2003). Although list-based general practice remains at the heart of the new contract, it is an NHS contract between the PCO and the practice, not the individual GP. This radical shift allows, for the first time, for nurses, and others, to become partners within a practice rather than employees. This remodelling will situate practice nurses in a compelling position to manage and influence the development of general practice and consequently enhance their strategic role within primary care organisations. For example, where GPs choose to opt out of providing services, it is now possible for practice nurses to become the providers of additional, enhanced and out of hours services by holding a contract with their local primary care organisation.

Box 9.2   National enhanced services

- Anti-coagulant monitoring
- Provision of near-patient testing
- Specialist care of patients with depression
- Services for patients who are alcohol misusers
- Fitting of intra-uterine devices
- Services for patients who are drug misusers
- More specialised services for patients with multiple sclerosis
- Intra-partum care
- Provision of immediate and first response care
- Minor injury services
- Enhanced care of the homeless
- More specialised sexual health services

The framework of the new GMS contract has an inbuilt duty of clinical governance weaving through a new quality and outcomes framework (QOF) based on current best available evidence. The QOF is a voluntary system designed to encourage and reward high quality care and management through participation in an annual quality improvement cycle. The framework covers four domains: clinical, organisational, additional service and patient experience which contain a series of areas with quality standards defined by key indicators. Achievement against each indicator will earn the practice points that convert into a monetary value. Additional points are available to reward improved access and breadth of care.

However, in order to ensure that resources are targeted at areas where both morbidity and contractor achievement are greatest in order to assist in the reduction of health inequalities, QOF clinical domain payments will be adjusted by practice disease prevalence as recorded by practice data and relative to national prevalence. The aim of this adjustment is to deliver a more equitable distribution of quality rewards in the light of the different workloads that contractors will face in delivering the same amount of quality points. Verification of achievement will be via the introduction of the Quality and Outcomes Framework Management and Analysis System (QMAS) and annual review visits by a team of assessors.

The disease categories incorporated within the clinical indicators are those previously identified as a national priority where evidence exists of the health benefits to be gained from enhancement of service provision and where the principal responsibility for ongoing management resides with the primary care team (see Box 9.3). However, it is on the shoulders of practice nurses that the demands of the new contract will fall. Already practice nurses provide, on the whole, the bulk of any chronic disease management services within primary care and the complex needs of individuals with co-morbidities have been well documented (NatPact 2004). It is the intention that the focus within the clinical standards of the new contract on the active management of chronic

---

Box 9.3 The new GMS contract clinical domain disease areas

- Coronary heart disease including left ventricular dysfunction
- Stroke and transient ischaemic attacks
- Hypertension
- Hypothyroidism
- Diabetes
- Mental health
- Chronic obstructive pulmonary disease
- Asthma
- Epilepsy
- Cancer

---

diseases will demonstrate a significant benefit for such individuals who are often, but not always, older members of the practice population. The development of accurate registers of patients who experience chronic disease has, over time, allowed for an increasingly structured approach to the provision of services. The range of indicators contained within the clinical domain of the contract is intended to ensure that consistent standards of appropriate intervention are provided across practice populations.

Practice nurses are ideally placed to deliver the clinical standards within the clinical domain by taking the lead on the management within practice of the ten identified disease areas. It is imperative, therefore, that practice nurses continue to develop specialist skills in these areas and ensure that they fully engage with the opportunities currently being presented by the development of emerging positions such as nurses with specialist interests (NwSI) in areas such as heart failure and diabetes within primary care organisations.

The next section moves on to consider the role of the practice nurse within the context of the *Liberating the Talents* (DoH 2002) areas of first contact, public health and continuing care/chronic disease management.

First contact

On a typical day in the NHS, one million people contact their GP (DOH/RCN 2003). In order to meet this demand, care should be provided by the professional who is best able to deliver the required service as part of an integrated team. Consequently, clinical roles are being re-designed, and many practice nurses are now providing first contact services in general practice. This can take a variety of forms from telephone triage to providing a nurse-led minor illness service. The level of clinical autonomy and the range and scope of clinical conditions individual practitioners are able to manage will remain dependent on their experience and the depth and breadth of their knowledge. In developing this area of professional practice, the nurse must be acutely aware of her accountability and acknowledge the limits of her competence (NMC 2002). The role requires nurses to be skilled in consultation skills and accurate history taking with advanced clinical examination and decision making skills. The nurse undertaking this service must be aware of the legal and professional frameworks within which care is offered. However, evidence from a number of studies demonstrates that nurses are able to provide care to patients with minor illness or undifferentiated conditions at least as effectively as GPs (Shum *et al.* 2000) and nurses also bring a different emphasis to the consultation as they tend to have a greater holistic focus and incorporate health promotion in the consultation to enable patients to self-manage their conditions in future.

It has been estimated that 70% of GP consultations could be closed by a nurse with appropriate first contact training (personal communication). The Government, through the National Health Service University (NHSU) is currently piloting a course to educate first contact practitioners although it focuses on a broad range of health care practitioners rather than just nurses. It is anticipated that these practitioners will generate new models of service provision to meet the health care needs of the 21st century.

Public health

Public health, and by implication the health of the nation, has assumed increasing importance over the past ten years. Public health can be described as:

'...a collective view of the health needs and health care of a population rather than an emphasis on an individual perspective. A central component of this collective approach is an emphasis on a partnership at all stages and levels of the public health process. This means partnership with communities and clients within them as well as partnerships across and between professional groups. Teamwork is an essential prerequisite to effective public health work'

(RCN 1994:1)

The RCN (1994) describe public health as involving more than medical care and including:

- Socio-environmental measures to create the conditions for people to attain and maintain health
- Health promotion to encourage individual responsibility for healthy lifestyles

From these descriptions it can be seen that components of public health feature highly in practice nursing workloads. The RCN describe four levels of public health intervention:

- Government policy – sanitation and hygiene, action to reduce poverty, air pollution and road accidents etc.
- Health service measures – immunisation programmes, commissioning services for health improvement, information systems and methods of evaluation
- Action at a local level – involvement and participation of communities – community assessment and community health profiling by community nurses and community development work
- Individually focused health promotion e.g. one to one or with groups

Practice nurses are certainly involved in the latter three levels particularly as much greater emphasis is now placed on engaging patients and users through individual management plans but also in identifying needs, planning and evaluating services.

Practice nurses are involved with both individual consultations aimed at improving individuals' health and also with identifying and implementing population-based approaches to improving health.

The *Health of the Nation* was published in 1992 (DoH 1992) and was the Government's first attempt at producing a strategy for health as well as health services. However, its focus was on the individual's responsibility for improving their health status and did not take account of other influences, often outside of the individual's control, that may impact on their health.

The change in government in 1997 introduced policies that recognised the role of health inequalities in determining health status. Health inequalities were made a key priority for the NHS in the Priorities and Planning Framework for 2003–6. This means that PCTs will take the lead locally in driving forward health inequalities work in the NHS, working closely with NHS trusts, local authorities and other partners to take concerted action on public health and illness prevention, health services and the wider determinants of health such as housing, transport and education. Key NHS interventions will relate to improving life expectancy by ensuring that prevention and treatment for cancer and coronary heart disease (CHD) reach those in greatest need or with poorest health outcomes, including disadvantaged groups and ethnic groups with high prevalence rates.

Practice nurses are actively involved in delivering programmes to meet NSF standards but also have a role in helping to develop the practice profile so that the practice team is conversant with the characteristics of the practice population and how services can best be targeted. There is also a need to increase smoking cessation and reduce excessive winter deaths by increasing influenza immunisation uptake. Practice nurses are actively involved in both these areas and often design and implement innovative schemes targeted at those patients with chronic needs who are hard to reach.

A second key intervention relates to improving infant mortality rates. Again the practice nurse is involved in many initiatives, such as family planning services that are accessible to young people with a view to reducing teenage pregnancy, focusing on improving nutrition in women of childbearing age through well women services, promoting and educating patients about immunisation programmes and working collaboratively with other primary health care team members such as midwives, health visitors and public health nurses who will be engaged in a number of other approaches aimed at improving infant mortality.

Effective consultations are the key to fulfilling a successful practice nursing service. However, there are many areas of discrete knowledge that are necessary in order to work sucessfully with patients to enable efficient and effective management of their conditions and health promotion is a key skill. Whilst there are many excellent textbooks that introduce the reader to theories and models of health promotion (for example Naidoo & Wills 1998, 2000) it is important to consider the application of health promotion to practice. Practice nurses who come directly from an acute nursing background may have to appraise not only how their consultation skills may have to be adapted but also their approach to health promotion. Because of time constraints in acute settings health promotion may only have been practised as a peripheral activity, for example providing a leaflet for the patient as he leaves the ward. In general practice much of the practice nurse's role will focus on health promoting activities. This may entail working with the patient in primary prevention, for example the giving of childhood immunisation or travel vaccinations and health advice. In secondary prevention the role may involve screening for cervical cancer or hypertension. In tertiary prevention many practice nurses are involved with chronic disease management where activity is focused on assisting patients to attain the best quality of life within the constraints of the disease. In addition, practice nurses need to consistently utilise opportunistic health promotion (Doyle & Thomas 1996; Wilson *et al*. 1992). In order to do this they need to have an understanding of how to influence patient attitudes and behaviour at an individual level. This requires nurses to possess an awareness of cognitive psychological theories if attitudes and behaviour are to be addressed. However, this needs to be applied in the context of other structural factors such as poverty, socio-economic status, inequalities and opportunities

which may significantly limit an individual's ability to make a healthy choice.

Becker's Health Belief Model (1974) provides a useful framework to assist in the identification of various factors that influence health beliefs. The model identifies that behaviour change will follow when the person has evaluated the feasibility and benefits of change against the costs. This evaluation may include their susceptibility to the disease, illness or injury and its severity. These individual perceptions may be influenced by modifying factors such as demographic variables (age, gender, ethnicity), sociopsychological variables (personality, social class, peer and reference pressure) and structural variables (knowledge of the disease, prior contact with the disease). Patients may also be prompted to seek advice following 'cues to action' which may be anything from newspaper reports (seeking help following 'contraceptive pill scare stories') to the illness of a family member or friend. Some idea of these influences elicited during the consultation will help the nurse to see how the patient may weigh up the positive and negative outcomes of behaviour change. Becker's model (1974) has also been expanded to include Bandura's (1977) concept of self efficacy which suggest that for behavioural change to take place, an individual:

- Must have an incentive to change
- Must feel threatened by their current behaviour
- Must feel a change would be beneficial in some way and have few adverse consequences
- Must feel competent to carry out the change (Naidoo & Wills 2000)

During consultations it is often helpful to use a problem solving approach, working with the patient to assess their health needs, prioritising with them the issues that are most important. It is here that the nurse is likely to introduce information that may challenge beliefs although care must be taken that the information is tailored to that particular patient. Use of Prochaska and Diclemente's (1984) transtheoretical model of change is helpful in trying to understand how ready a patient is to accept change. However, one limitation is that it focuses on the psychology of the individual whereas the person's ability to change is also influenced by social factors. Integration of such disparate factors before moving on to implement an agreed plan demonstrates significant nursing expertise. Practice nurses have the advantage of often being able to implement health-promoting activities over a period of time and therefore knowledge of a staged educational approach is essential. Models such as that described by Ewles and Simnett (2003) help to structure such an approach but it is essential that this is accompanied by robust record keeping that clearly articulates the process and progress for evaluation. An example of patients who might benefit from this approach are those who have been newly diagnosed with a chronic disease such as asthma. Occasionally shock or anxiety at the time of diagnosis may limit the patient's ability to take in information and the nurse must prioritise essential information and subsequently build on this to encourage patient self-management over the ensuing weeks and months. Accordingly, practice nurses need a thorough understanding of health promotion, health psychology and how to support behaviour change in order to accomplish effective relationships with patients.

As well as working with patients on an individual level the nurse will need to work collaboratively with other members of the primary care team. The practice, as part of the primary care trust, will have to demonstrate how it is responding to the local health targets set by the PCT Board in the Local Development Plan (LDP). There are two-way links between all of these and the next section describes how the practice nurse contributes to the assessment of health needs for the practice population. However, the practice nurse will discover many opportunities for health promotion and, in so doing, broaden her role, for example through involvement in the review of protocols or guidelines. The modernisation agency offers a useful step by step guide to developing protocols which are valuable in identifying key priorities for the practice and enabling consistently evidence-based approaches to care and disease management.

Alternatively the nurse may recognise a health need that would be more effectively met by instituting group work such as a smoking cessation group or after school asthma club for children. Obviously developments such as these depend on priority, time, commitment and the provision of appropriate premises.

Health needs assessment

Needs assessment has been an integral part of government policy since 1990 (DoH 1990). This means that practices need to develop collaborative strategies for developing the practice profile and analysing collected data in order to target particular health issues within the practice and, subsequently, inform the PCT strategic plan. Practice nurses are an integral part of the practice team and require a range of knowledge and skills to assist in the development of the profile (for further information see the chapters on needs assessment and specialist community public health nursing). Linked with this will be the key targets identified at national and strategic health authority levels. Mechanisms are in place to transcribe information from local practice health assessments to the PCT and then to the strategic health authority and vice versa with the aim of providing a 'larger picture'. Part of the practice nurse's role will be to collaborate in the development of practice profiles and to develop skills in presentation and influencing in order to articulate the identified needs. This is vital in ensuring that the practice nurse's voice is heard at PCT level where decision making about strategy and deployment of resources takes place. Community nursing is usually represented at the PCT's professional executive committee which is the conduit forum between the trust board and its clinical employees.

A practice profile can be defined as a collection of data that identifies characteristics of the practice and its population in the context of the environment in which it is situated. Practice profiles should be a collaborative exercise incorporating all those who care for the practice population. It should set the practice in context giving key demographic, socio-economic and geographical information, as these factors are known to influence health. Health visitors and community nurses who work within the local community are usually able to offer interesting insights into the functioning of the local community and likewise, ancillary staff who are likely to live locally. Other forms of useful practice data may include:

- Age/sex characteristics of the practice population
- Ethnic and cultural mix of the practice population
- Numbers of potentially vulnerable people registered e.g. travelling families, refugees, homeless people and families
- Chronic disease registers
- Prescribing patterns
- Consultation patterns
- Complaints
- Hospital referral and discharge patterns
- Outcomes of audits undertaken

However, the collection of data is fairly meaningless without further analysis and identification of the priorities of the LDP and local targets. Practices will be expected to identify how they are working towards targets set in the LDP, NSFs and QOF but at the same time it is vital that the local needs of the practice and its population arise from the profile and are responded to effectively.

One of the challenges is how to incorporate a public perspective into the profiling process. Without this, need will only be defined from a professional perspective which Bradshaw (1972) identifies as 'normative needs'. Normative needs reflect the judgement of the health care professional which may be different from that of their client. Practices have instituted a number of mechanisms to incorporate a patient perspective into planning such as patient councils or participation groups as part of their development strategies. This offers patients a formal opportunity to contribute to how services are developed and delivered. Obviously there are always critics of this approach who would say that this is only a vocal minority who get their views across in this way. However current government policy identifies the need to seek out patient opinion and collaborate with the public at all levels (DoH 2004c) and the inclusion of patient experience in the quality framework of the new contract represents an opportunity for practices to obtain systematic feedback from their patients about the services they provide as well as how they are provided. This data can subsequently be used to inform practice service development plans and service redesign. However, achieving integration of patients' perspectives in a general practice setting will be challenging, not least that patients may fear being critical of the service in case they are removed from the practice list. This will stimulate staff to think creatively about how patient's views are represented.

Once the data arising from the profile has been analysed and discussed within the practice team, decisions regarding prioritisation of service needs, resourcing such needs and responses to new developments will be required. It is likely that there will be conflicting demands from different professionals and groups of clients. Mental health issues are a good example of this as members of the practice team may well have differing views on how the practice should focus its resources. For example, the health visitor may perceive postnatal depression as being of primary concern whereas the district nurse may have more contact with patients with Alzheimer's disease and their carers, and consider their support to be a more pressing priority. Similarly the practice nurse may find that she is often identifying individuals with depression during new patient consultations and believes there is a need for better service provision in this area. The GP may also be more concerned that he has to manage greater numbers of patients with chronic enduring mental illness and may feel poorly supported in their management. All of these issues are real and important and on occasions it may be feasible to address them all. However, the more likely scenario is that the problems must be prioritised and in order reinforce these decisions, accurate data will be needed to support bids wherever a case is being made for more resources.

Chronic disease management

Managing chronic disease is a key component of the practice nurse's workload in general practice and this is likely to increase since chronic disease is regarded as the biggest problem facing the health care system with 60% of adults in England reporting a chronic health problem (NatPaCT 2004). Chronic disease can be described as those which current medical interventions can only control not cure. The data in Box 9.4 give some indication of the size and spread of chronic disease.

Many people with chronic illness have more than one chronic condition and 26% of these individuals in the UK have three or more problems. Most of these people are cared for by the primary health care team. However, health care professionals need to be aware that they often have complex medication regimes and may be under a number of different specialists as well as their general practitioner, that the burden of the disease may impact on their ability to function independently and they may have many social needs which may isolate them from their family or other support networks. Often the problems caused by the non-life-threatening aspects of their illness cause them the greatest problems; frequently the psychological aspects of their care are poorly understood and they may have co-morbidities such as depression.

Research has demonstrated that many people with chronic disease do not feel that health care professionals understand the impact that having a chronic illness has on their lives and focus just on the physical and medical management of the disease and pay lip service to patient empowerment (Paterson 2001; Thorne *et al.* 2000). Currently the government is piloting a number of schemes to change the way chronic disease is viewed and managed by patients and health care professionals (Evercare, Kaiser Permanente Expert Patient programme – see NatPaCT website and Matrix Reasearch and consultancy/Modernisation Agency 2004). Much chronic disease management takes place in general practice and accounts for about 80% of all GP consultations (British Household Panel Survey 2002 cited in NatPaCT 2004) but concerns about the quality of some of that care have been raised by the Audit Commission (2002) which found that quality of care was variable, with poor co-ordination between hospital and community and little integration between health and social care agencies. Currently, 50% of bed day use is accounted for by only 2.7% of medical conditions most of which are chronic diseases (HES data 2002 cited in NatPaCT 2004). Of the eleven leading causes of hospital bed use in the UK, eight are due to conditions which need not have caused admission if community and primary care services were strengthened (NatPaCT 2004). Other evidence (Campbell *et al.* 2001) shows that routine day to day care of chronic diseases could be improved, for example, one study showed that only 49% of patients with diabetes had their eyes routinely examined for retinal damage and only 47% of eligible patients had been prescribed beta blockers after a myocardial infarction (Seddon *et al.* 2001). Patients with chronic disease are twice as likely to be admitted to hospital and stay there disproportionately longer and the new approach to managing chronic disease reflects the need to address these issues.

Figure 9.1 shows three levels of care for people with chronic illness. Most practice nurses will be involved with patients at levels one and two. There is interesting evidence to suggest that supported self-care can be a highly effective means of improving the care of chronic disease (NatPaCT 2004). However, self-management encompasses more than the provision of

---

Box 9.4 The size and spread of chronic disease. (Source: NatPaCT 2004)

The UK has a total population of 59 million. Common chronic diseases include:

- *Diabetes mellitus* – current estimates put the number of people with diabetes at 1.3 million with potentially another million undiagnosed
- *Chronic obstructive pulmonary disease* – affecting 600 000 people
- *Asthma* – affecting 3.7 m adults and 1.5 m children
- *Arthritis* – affecting 8.5 m in the UK
- *Epilepsy* – affecting 400 000 people in England and Wales (1998)
- *Mental ill health* – affecting 1 in 6 of the population including 1 in 10 children
- *8.8 m people* have a *long-term illness* that severely limits their day to day ability to cope

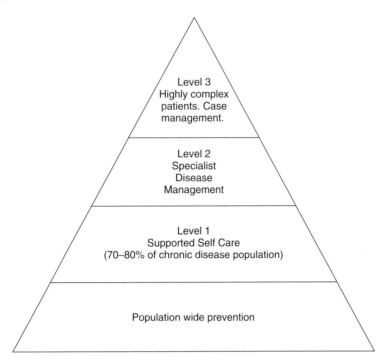

Figure 9.1   Three levels of care for people with chronic illness. (Source: *Chronic Disease Management: a compendium of information*. NatPact 2004)

information to patients, and the future will see a range of strategies designed to support patients and their carers in the ongoing management of their illness. Practice nurses are likely to be one of the key health care professionals involved in the education of patients and carers regarding self-management of their illness, supporting them in developing an understanding of the disease process and its potential impact, how to manage medication and other treatments and how and when to seek health care. In order to do this practice nurses need to be knowledgeable about common chronic diseases, the psychological impact on patients and families and how to take this into account when planning a learning programme with the patient as well as awareness of the range of other support services available. The expert patient programme (DoH 2001b) is one example of a new initiative aimed at empowering patients to take control of their disease and their lives.

The main providers of supported care are primary care teams but this is wider than just general practice and includes, among others, community nurses, physiotherapists, opticians, pharmacists, dieticians and podiatrists. In order for care to be co-ordinated and evidence-based, primary care teams will need to work in partnership with patients to ensure that there is:

- Registration of a population of patients for whom primary care teams identify problems, co-ordinate care and help support their condition – this will be enhanced when electronic patient records allow for better information and easier access to this information and is linked in with the requirements of the QOF
- Recall of people to ensure they get the care they need by using prompts and reminders
- Regular reviews of patients to ensure they receive the best evidence-based care and are supported to manage their care

The standards established within the National Service Frameworks have started the process of ensuring an evidence-based approach to the care and management of coronary heart disease and diabetes. The Quality and Outcomes Framework in the new GMS/PMS contracts, which targets ten significant chronic diseases, is likely to be influential in further improving care.

Some practice nurses will be involved in disease specific case management and may run designated disease clinics within general practice. However, for a minority of patients with severe or unstable forms of disease there is evidence that specialist input can make a difference especially with respect to reducing hospital admissions. Practice nurses therefore need to have strong links with specialist services to ensure patients are referred appropriately, although many patients will make their own contact if they are sufficiently aware of signs of deterioration in their condition. Examples of responsive specialist services that have been shown to improve patient outcomes are for chronic obstructive pulmonary disease, asthma, heart failure, depression and diabetes (NatPaCT 2004).

For those patients who have highly complex needs and who are often intensive users of the health services, case management is being introduced. This means identifying patients who are deemed to be at risk of deterioration, often by reviewing those who are frequently admitted to hospital or frequently attend accident and emergency departments. The US Evercare project, which targets the frail and elderly and those with complex conditions, has shown good outcomes in terms of reduced admission rates and patient satisfaction and similar schemes are being rolled out across PCTs (Evercare 2004).

Overall the future of chronic disease management has been modelled on the chronic care model, Figure 9.2, (Wagner *et al.* 1999). With respect to the development of this model, many initiatives are taking place or being planned for the future (see Figure 9.3).

Systems for accountability and responsibility

Systems for accountability and responsibility are enshrined within the concept of clinical governance. Clinical governance was introduced with the aim of developing a nationwide coherent approach to quality in the NHS and to reduce the incidence of unacceptable variation in

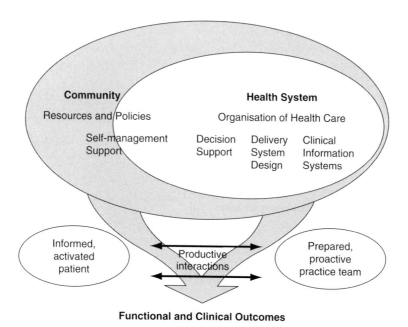

Figure 9.2 The Chronic Care model

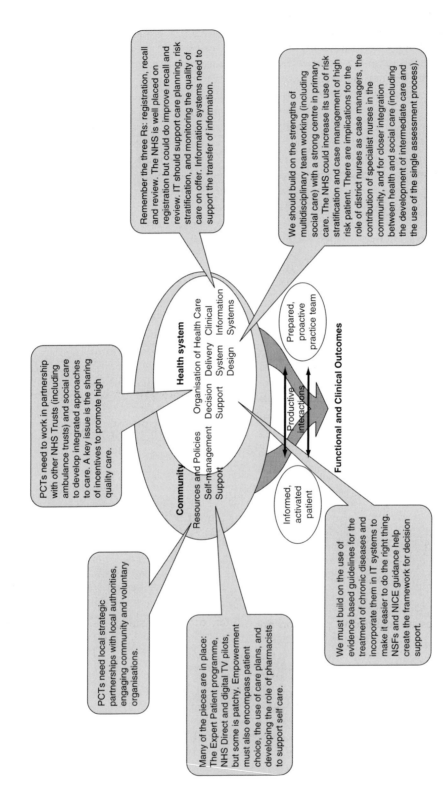

Figure 9.3 Planned initiatives for the Chronic Care model. Source: NatPact 2004

performance and practice (DoH 1997). Clinical governance is an umbrella term that provides a framework for a number of different approaches aimed at improving quality. McSherry and Pearce (2002) summarise it as a system or systems that manage risk and monitor clinical quality through an organisation. These systems are underpinned by a drive towards increased collaborative working matched by an increased emphasis on individual accountability. There are three main areas within the clinical governance framework:

- Quality improvement
- Risk management/management of performance
- Systems for accountability and responsibility

Practice nurses need to have a good understanding of these key areas. They will be involved in a range of quality improvement mechanisms such as auditing and collection of data to demonstrate achievement of standards in the NSFs and QOF. A key challenge in general practice is the introduction of skill mix into practice nursing teams with a subsequent renegotiation of professional roles. The development of specialist practitioner roles alongside the expansion of nursing roles has meant that practices are employing a wider range of staff with a diversity of qualifications and skill. This has included the introduction of health care assistants (HCA) into general practice to fill the void created by the metamorphosis of professional practitioners. This is in common with the NHS generally where, between 1999 and 2002, the number of registered nurses within the workforce increased by 12% in England while the number of health care assistants rose by 46% (O'Dowd 2004). It has been suggested that HCAs could cover 12.5% of nurses' current workload and, subsequently, current structures of health care provision are under examination. Consultation regarding the regulation of this expanding and highly varied role has been undertaken across the UK regarding potential regulation of this expanding and highly varied role (DoH 2004a). This progressive level of skill mix within the primary care team, which includes HCAs and less skilled nurses, raises issues of accountability. Specialist practitioner practice nurses need to possess leadership and team management skills ensuring that staff to whom work is delegated are both competent to undertake the work and recognise their own accountability.

However, a general practice team study undertaken by Savage and Moore (2004) found the meaning of accountability to be both elusive and ambiguous. This raises concerns of risk as patient safety must be paramount. Ongoing programmes of continuing professional development need to be in place to ensure competence, safety and evidence-based practice but the team leaders must also assume responsibility for the ongoing assessment of competence which, as Hatchett (2003) identifies, is an area that has been poorly addressed in nursing. All staff are required to have personal development plans (PDP) and therefore appraisal skills are essential for those in team leader roles. If *Agenda for Change* is operationalised in general practice this will be linked to achievement within the knowledge and skills framework and pay progression. The development of protocols and care pathways, providing this is undertaken as a collaborative activity, is one way of guiding and standardising practice and ensuring clarity for all staff involved in providing care. This process is supported by the use and application of national guidelines sponsored by the National Institute for Clinical Excellence (NICE) and other organisations such as the Scottish Intercollegiate Guidelines Network (SIGN), British Hypertension Society etc. A range of decision making tools (such as Prodigy www.prodigy.nhs.uk) are also available online which can easily be accessed in practices. As the use of the internet becomes even more widespread it is likely that many more online facilities/software packages will be deployed by practice staff during consultations. These will either be used to enhance the effectiveness of face-to-face consultations or may be applied through the use of telemedicine and video-conferencing, enabling the practice to communicate directly with off-site specialists, diagnosticians and therapists.

The future

The pace of change in the health service is so rapid that it is difficult to predict what the future holds for practice nursing. However, services provided in primary care settings are bound to increase and the future will see more nurses and other health care professionals and ancillary staff working in these settings to support new developments. At present, the Nursing and Midwifery Council is consulting on changes to specialist practitioner educational preparation and feedback will not be until November 2004. Skills that the specialist practitioner of the future are likely to require will include an excellent understanding and application of leadership and management skills to support a changing skill mix and opportunities for service redesign and the need for innovative approaches to service delivery. This will be alongside patient focused management of a broad range of chronic diseases and expansion of roles into first contact services often overlapping with services provided by nurse practitioners. At the time of writing the new GMS contract is only just being implemented, however, much of the practice nursing service provision will be focused on meeting the requirements of the contract and QOF by continually developing professional clinical practice.

References

Audit Commission (2002) *A Focus on General Practice in England*. www.audit-commission.gov.uk

Bandura, A. (1977) *Social Learning Theory*. Prentice Hall: Englewood Cliffs.

Becker, M.H. (ed) (1974) *The Health Belief Model and Personal Health Behaviour*. Slack, New Jersey.

Bradshaw, J. (1972) The Concept of Need. *New Society*, **30**, 640–643.

Campbell, S.M., Hann, M., Hacker, J., Burns, C., Oliver, D., Thapar, A., *et al.* (2001) Identifying predictors of high quality care in English General Practice: observational study. *BMJ*, **323**, 784–787.

Department of Health (1989) *General Practice in the National Health Service: the 1990 GP Contract*. HMSO, London.

Department of Health (1990) *NHS and Community Care Act*. Department of Health, London.

Department of Health (1992) *The Health of the Nation – a Strategy for Health in England*. Department of Health, London.

Department of Health (1997) *The New NHS: Modern, Dependable*. Department of Health, London.

Department of Health (1998) *A First Class Service: Quality in the New NHS*. Department of Health, London.

Department of Health (1999a) *Making a Difference: Strengthening the Nursing, Midwifery and Health Visiting Contribution to Health and Healthcare*. Department of Health, London.

Department of Health (Crown Report) (1999b) *Review of Prescribing, Supply and Administration of Medicines: Final report*. Department of Health, London.

Department of Health (1999c) *Saving Lives – Our Healthier Nation*. Department of Health, London.

Department of Health (2000) *NHS Plan*. Department of Health, London.

Department of Health (2001a) *Shifting the Balance of Power within the NHS – Securing Delivery*. Department of Health, London.

Department of Health (2001b) *The Expert Patient – a new approach to chronic disease management for the 21st century*. Department of Health, London.

Department of Health (2002) *Liberating the Talents*. Department of Health, London.

Department of Health (2003) *Protecting Staff, Delivering Services: Implementing the European working Time Directive for Doctors in Training*. Department of Health, London.

Department of Health (2004a) *Enhancing Public Protection: Proposals for the Statutory Regulation of Health Care Support Staff in England and Wales*. Department of Health, London.

Department of Health (2004b) *Agenda for Change – proposed agreement*. Department of Health, London.

Department of Health (2004c) *The NHS Improvement Plan: Putting People at the Heart of Public Services*. Department of Health, London.

Department of Health/Royal College of Nursing (2003) *Freedom to Practice: Dispelling the Myths*. Department of Health, London.

Doyle, Y. & Thomas, P. (1996) Promoting health through primary care: challenges in taking a strategic approach, *Health Education Journal*, **55**, 3–10.

Evercare (2004) *Implementing the Evercare Programme – Interim Report*. February 28. Available from www.natpact.nhs.uk

Ewles, L. & Simnett, I. (2003) *Promoting Health – a Practical Guide*. 5th edn. Balliere Tindall, New York.

Hatchett, R. (2003) *Nurse Led Clinic – Practice Issues*. Routledge, London.

Lewis, R., Gillam, S. & Jenkins, C. (2001) *Personal Medical Services – Modernising Primary Care?* King's Fund, London.

Matrix Research and Consultancy/Modernisation Agency (2004) *Learning Distillation of Chronic Disease*

Management Programmes in the UK (available www. natpact.nhs.uk)

McKeon, A. (1997) *A Guide to Personal Medical Services Pilots under the NHS (Primary Care) Act 199*. Department of Health, London.

McSherry, R. & Pearce, P. (eds) (2002) *Clinical Governance: a guide to implementation for health care professionals*. Blackwell Science, Oxford.

Naidoo, J. & Wills, J. (1998) *Practising Health Promotion: Dilemmas and Challenges*. Balliere Tindall, London.

Naidoo, J. & Wills, J. (2000) *Health Promotion: foundations for practice*. 2nd edn. Balliere Tindall, London.

NatPaCT (2004) *Chronic Disease Management – a Compendium of Information*. Available from www. natpact.nhs.uk

NHS Confederation/BMA (2003) *The GMS Contract – Investing in General Practice*. NHS Confederation. www.nhsconfed.org/gmscontract

NMC (2002) *Code of Conduct*. Nursing and Midwifery Council, London.

O'Dowd, A. (2004) Developing the HCA role, *Nursing Times*, **100**(25), 22–24.

Paterson, B. (2001) Myth of Empowerment in Chronic Illness. *Journal of Advanced Nursing*, **34**(3), 574–581.

Prime, L. (ed) (2003) Making a Difference, *Practice Nurse*, **26**(6), 29–34.

Prochaska, J.O. & DiClemente, C. (1984) *The Transtheoretical Approach: Crossing Traditional Foundations of Change*. Don Jones/Irwin, Harnewood IL.

RCN (1994) *Public Health: Nursing Rises to the Challenge*. Royal College of Nurses, London.

Savage, J. & Moore, L. (2004) *Interpreting Accountability – an Ethnographic Study of Practice Nurses, Accountability and Multidisciplinary Team Decision-making in the Context of Clinical Governance*. RCN Institute, London.

Seddon, M.E., Marshall, M.N., Campbell, S.M. & Roland, M.O. (2001) Systematic Review of Studies of Quality of Clinical Care in General Practice in the UK, Australia and New Zealand. *Quality Health Care*, **10**(3), 152–158.

Shum, C., Humphreys, A., Wheeler, D., Cochrane, M.A., Skoda, S. & Clement, S. (2000) Nurse management of minor illness in general practice: multicentre randomised controlled trial. *British Medical Journal*, **320**, 1038–1043.

Thorne, S., Nyhlin, K.T. & Paterson, B. (2000) Attitudes toward patient expertise in chronic illness. *International Journal of Nursing Studies*, **37**, 303–311.

UKCC (1994) *The Future of Professional Practice: the Council's Standards for Education and Practice Following Registration*. United Kingdom Central Council, London.

Wagner, E.H., Schaefer, J., Von Korff, M. & Austin, B. (1999) A survey of leading chronic disease management programs: are they consistent with the literature? *Managing Care Quality*, **7**, 56–66.

Waller, J. (2000) What do practice nurses do? *Nursing Times*, **96**(34), 31.

Wilson, A., McDonald, P., Hayes, L. & Cooney, J. (1992) Health promotion in the general practice consultation: a minute makes all the difference. *British Medical Journal*, **304**, 227–230.

Woodcock, A. (2004) *NHS loses 2000 beds*. www. scotsman.com

Introduction

Since the last edition of this book (2001), there has been an astonishing amount of change within the National Health Service and in primary care. The publications produced regularly by the Department of Health have already had, and will continue to have, a profound effect on community nursing and the role of the district nurse.

At the time of writing there is some uncertainty as to the future of the familiar title of 'district nurse' but there can be no doubt regarding the future role. There exists a clear vision and a determination that the district nurse of the future shall deliver a flexible, high quality and forward thinking service that works in partnership with diverse communities to place the patient at the centre of care delivery.

The aims of the district nurse are multi-faceted: to prevent ill health and to keep people healthy thus avoiding the need for medical care; to provide support for those living with chronic disease so that they are able to remain at home; to treat curable problems and to provide nursing care to those whose needs are acute and complex; to offer palliative and terminal care to those who require it so that they may die in accordance with their wishes.

The fulfilment of these aims represents a major task and one that makes complex demands on the role of the district nurse. To meet such demands the role must be redefined, especially if the district nurse of the future is to make a real difference to people's lives.

Historical origins

District nurses can trace the roots of their role back to the nineteenth century. The earliest mention of nurses being specifically prepared to work in the community was in 1848. These nurses were trained by the Society of St John to care for the sick poor in their own homes. Prior to this period earlier references had been made to home-based visiting to 'the sick' by members of religious orders. The person attributed as being the founder of district nursing was William Rathbone who provided the first fully trained hospital nurse, Mrs Robinson, to work with the sick poor in Liverpool in 1859 (Murray & Irven 1948). The philanthropic movement of the nineteenth century formed the basis of social reform leading to public welfare and eventually the inception of the NHS, though it took many years to achieve. District nurses together with health visitors were a part of that movement (Ross 1990).

In a pamphlet written by Florence Nightingale, part of which was contained in a letter addressed to The Times newspaper and subsequently published on April 14th 1876, Miss Nightingale wrote in some detail her expectations of a district nurse, the manner of her training and the organisation of her life. The letter continued with a colourful account of the work of a district nurse giving examples of the type of situations encountered in the course of her daily work.

> 'To patients living up five or six pairs of stairs in Soho and St. Giles' the district nurse has often to go; the water-tap is below the pavement in a cellar; the dust heap in the basement, and sometimes below it; no dustpan or tins for fetching water. This is the room the nurse has to clean and purify. And she does it. These are the very triumphs of her art. The ultimate object is to nurse all sick at home'.

The intention of this letter was to heighten public awareness of the need to train nurses to care for the sick poor and to secure support for the nurses' training. Miss Nightingale's letter ended with a final comment,

'but the object of the Association is: to give first-rate nursing to the sick poor at home (which they never have had). And this costs money'.

The sick nurse, as she was called, was concerned not only with the immediate nursing needs of the patient but also with the wider issues affecting patients and their families' or carers' health and welfare within the context of contemporary issues. In 1859 some of those issues were poor sanitation, unemployment, overcrowding and a lack of education (Ridgely Seymer 1954, p. 313).

Thus it can be seen that from their earliest origins district nurses have been concerned with meeting not only the nursing needs of the individual but also with caring for the whole person and for the carer's needs. Furthermore, district nurses acknowledge the significance of the environment in which the individual lives as well as acquiring an awareness of the wider factors influencing that individual's well-being.

At the present time the district nurse remains the main provider of professional nursing care in peoples' homes (Audit Commission 1999). From such humble beginnings in the service to the 'sick poor' the contemporary district nurse practitioner has become firmly established in the role of provider for a home-based universal nursing service.

The changing role of the district nurse

Since the 1970s the role of the district nurse has continued to receive attention. A number of policy documents have been issued which emphasise the valuable contribution made by community nurses in the delivery of health and social care in the community and in improving peoples' health (DoH 1992a, 1997, 1999a, 1999b; NHSME 1993). More recently The NHS Plan (DoH 2000), *Liberating the Talents* (DoH 2002) and the *NHS Improvement Plan* (DoH 2004) clearly place district nurses and other community nurses in new flexible roles that are critical in enabling individuals to be supported at home and in

spearheading community-based health provision to improve the public's health. As part of the primary health care team the district nurse can be seen to be at the interface of health and social care delivery, undertaking a vital and increasingly complex role (Figure 10.1).

Community nursing has been constantly developing and changing in response to government policy and to the changing needs of the communities served. In line with these changes the role of the district nurse will need to evolve and expand still further. Traditionally, the caseload of the district nurse has largely comprised the chronic sick, older people and the terminally ill. However, this does not take account of the work required when caring for people with complex and multiple needs. The present workload of the district nurse encompasses a whole range of activities (Figure 10.1), which involve taking professional and managerial responsibility for the provision of appropriate pathways of nursing care and treatment through acute, chronic and terminal illness.

The district nurse provides a service which is accessible and meets the highly individual and complex needs of patients and carers in an effective and responsive way (DoH 1999b; ENB 1991). Advanced nursing care is formulated within a holistic framework to be delivered in the home setting. It is based on a knowledge of the individual's physical, psychological and social needs and may involve the application of both technical and specialist skills.

District nursing has been a demand-led and highly responsive service which is determined by the referrals that it receives. However, the lack of control over the number of referrals and whether such referrals are appropriate has implications for the management of the nurse's workload. There is a constant need to re-organise and delegate visits to patients especially when the amount of time spent can be unpredictable, as in those cases of high dependency where terminal illness is involved.

District nurses will continue to be professionally responsible and accountable for the quality of care provided by the district nursing team. They are pivotal in assessing the needs of individuals and

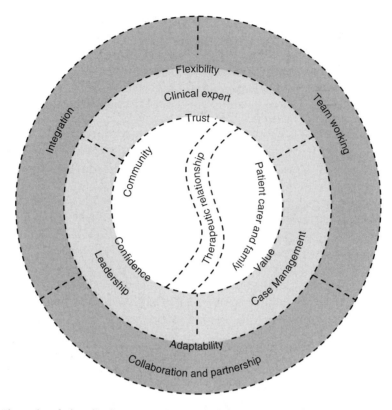

Figure 10.1 The role of the district nurse. Core principles: trust, confidence value. Key roles: clinical expert, case management, leadership. Key characteristics: adaptability, flexibility, collaboration and partnership, integration, team working. The broken circles: movement between each area. □, core principles; ▨, key roles; ▩, key characteristics

their carers and in leading and managing a multi-skilled team of nurses able to work collaboratively with a multiplicity of agencies (statutory, voluntary and private) in order to deliver care to a defined population. However, they will need to broaden their scope of practice to manage the burden of chronic disease and to fulfil the public health role of maintaining people at home. In order to maintain this central role in primary care it is important that the district nurse, as the expert in the assessment and identification of nursing and health needs, is clear about what it is possible to offer in terms of health care (Figure 10.1). The district nurse is accountable and responsible for maintaining a high level of clinical proficiency in order to ensure effective and safe delivery of advanced technical care by the nursing team in the community.

However, it is the context of care in which the district nurse functions which has changed most significantly in the past two decades. It will continue to change as government policy emphasises the provision of care either in the community, at home or as close as possible to people's homes, (DoH 2002, 2004a). The shift from secondary to primary care has changed the emphasis of nursing need in the community. This change is reflected in the increasing number of frail older people and those with chronic disability and disease who are now being cared for at home. There is a growing demand on the district nursing service from the significant number of people requiring complex nursing care who are being discharged from hospital earlier because of the need for hospital beds. At the same time there is a developing need for high technological care, intermediate care and rehabilitation for the increasing number of people with complex or terminal illnesses who are being cared for within their own homes.

The district nurse must, therefore, create opportunities to expand and further develop her role by building on the considerable body of knowledge and skill derived from the experience of many years of caring for individuals in the community. District nurses have come a long way from their initial roots but what remains true is the variety encountered in their daily work and the need to be able to respond appropriately to each and every situation in a competent and professional manner. From 1848 until the present day, the district nurse has always been concerned with the holistic needs of the patient – not simply their physical and nursing care needs but also their psychological, environmental, financial and social care needs.

Whilst it is clear that the district nurse has the necessary knowledge and skills to lead a team of nurses who are able to deliver the Government's modernisation agenda it is evident that traditional methods of working will need to change. Nevertheless, it is important to have a professional identity. The more flexible approach to meeting the needs of the community will require a balance of skills between those of the generic primary care nurse and those of the primary care workers. The full range of skills offered by the primary workforce will continue to be needed to provide competent and effective care. In this way the needs of the patient will be met and there will be continuing motivation to recruit and retain staff for future practice nurses, district nurses, health visitors and school nurses, all of whom have a role that is meaningful to the public.

Beside the necessary core competencies specific skills will also be required to respond to local needs and priorities. Inevitably there will be variations across the country: district nursing in city centres such as London and Manchester will be different from that in rural areas such as Cornwall and Yorkshire.

There are concerns that the number of district nurses is not increasing sufficiently to meet the demands made on them. The public at large is now better informed. Patients want to have more care at home and spend less time in hospital particularly in the light of increasing prevalence of hospital acquired infections. This adds to the demands made on the district nursing team. District nurses will be obliged to change their practice but they will need the support of their organisation to do so effectively. The challenge for them is to how to make their voices heard so that they can be part of the implementation of future change. It can be done by:

- Taking the initiative and informing their organisations of the needs and priorities of their communities rather than waiting to be told what to do
- Seizing this opportunity to redefine their role as district nurses for the future
- Obtaining more user involvement
- Organising a service that is responsive to the needs of the people for whom it is intended

The goal for the district nurse should be to provide services at a point that maximises access for people and provides greater flexibility (DoH 2004a), so that being able to go to a district nurse or a pharmacist rather than the GP is a viable option.

Health needs assessment and profiling

The development of primary care trusts (DoH 1997) has extended the base of primary care from general practice to a broader responsibility for the health needs of local communities where social services and health care teams work together to provide integrated services (Gerrish 1997). Earlier, Cain *et al.* (1995) supported the notion that commissioning of health care is dependent on detailed information of the local community which should include data on both health and social needs for effective planning and financial distribution. In this process it is the duty of the district nurse to inform the commissioners of services about local health needs by providing a practice profile that acts as an indicator to identify health deficits. This involvement with the commissioners of service represents a vital part of the district nurse's role as an advocate for patients' needs.

In order to provide relevant information district nurses need to consider the following questions regarding their community: who lives in this community, what are their needs, what sort of service do they prefer and who is to provide it? Once the community needs have been identified district nurses can determine how the required services might best be provided. It might well involve enlisting the help of other professionals. District nurses need to know that if they have a vision for the future it is possible, with appropriate support, to take the opportunity and move forward. The public expects high quality, improved services, choice and convenience (DoH 2004a) and local services need to reflect and be appropriate to local circumstances. It is here that district nurses can be instrumental in highlighting a variety of needs for help such as with language, literacy and mobility; or with access to more personalised health care, for instance in severely deprived areas where the need is great, or for commuter populations where convenience is important to minimise disruption to working lives.

It is imperative that district nurses draw upon their skills of population profiling in order to identify the nature of the populations with whom they work. Their concern must be not just with the health needs but with the constituents of a given population, its ethnicity and diversity in terms of age range and gender. Equally important are the public health concerns: housing, unemployment and the numbers of people with chronic diseases. This source of data will provide evidence for the planning of services to meet the needs of a particular population.

The district nurse, whilst fulfilling a duty in informing the commissioners of services of local needs and priorities, has a key role in the process. The representation should include liaison with social services, the general public, general practice and other branches of community nursing. Whilst the assessment of an individual's nursing needs remains central to the work of the district nurse a consideration of the needs of the wider population is of equal importance. District nurses find themselves in a unique position working in partnership with patients on a day to day basis

which enables them to advise the service commissioners of the needs of both patients and carers (Wall 1998). The close relationships that develop over weeks or even years between district nurses and patients and their families builds a confidence and trust that enables patients to express their needs.

The district nurse with concerns not only for the immediate environment but also for the broader picture is equally well-placed to identify normative needs as described by Bradshaw in 1992. These may then be considered further and incorporated within the context of the local practice community health profile. This type of profile reflects the needs of a defined population and is a useful source of data collated from a variety of sources. Information is gathered from sources such as caseload profiles from district nurses, health visitors and, most importantly, user surveys. Collaboration amongst the professionals working in the community to compile such a profile is essential if the wealth of experience derived from direct contact with the service users is to be drawn together. The profile combines quantitative data, such as demographic information, epidemiological data and indicators of deprivation with qualitative data such as the information from district nurses' caseloads and general practitioners' visiting patterns and surgeries (Wright 1997). An analysis and identification of the population can then be drawn up on the basis of the collated data.

The district nurse by virtue of involvement with other professionals and with the public is ideally placed to ensure that the profiles are truly representative and meaningful so that resources can be allocated appropriately. An advantage of profiling the population in this way is that it provides a valuable, comprehensive snapshot view of the population needs for health care at a given time. A comparison between the service provisions and identified health care needs serves to highlight any mismatches. However, the limitation is the length of time taken between completing the profile and responding to identified needs. It also provides a 'picture' of the effectiveness of existing services which not only highlights deficiencies but also offers the potential for change in practice and service development.

There has been an impressive growth in services provided effectively in the community. The growing number of primary and community clinics offering services to patients has the potential to reduce the need for a hospital visit. Over 70% of patients' contact with the NHS is now at home or in primary and community care facilities, a proportion set to increase significantly (DoH 2004a).

Clinical governance

Quality remains a focal point of health care delivery (DoH 1999b) and as the government clearly states in the document *Making a Difference*, 'Clinical governance is at the centre of our plans for quality improvement' (DoH 1999b, p. 44). The government's aim is to 'improve the overall standard of clinical care, to reduce unacceptable variations in practice and to ensure patient care is based on the most up-to-date evidence', (DoH 1999b, p. 44). The range of activities related to clinical governance cover five main elements: audit, research and development, risk management, quality initiatives and clinical effectiveness activities. All of these elements require movement and change both at an individual and organisational level.

Further advances in clinical practice have placed greater demands upon nurses to provide safe, effective care. Whilst this may be exciting and challenging, district nurses need to be supported to ensure that they remain clinically competent and confident in the care they are providing as well as being accountable for their practice. As a team leader the district nurse has prime responsibility for the care carried out by all members of the district nursing team.

In order to ensure the success of clinical governance and provide an environment in which clinical excellence may be vigorously adopted, professionals will be required to sustain their professional development and professional practice. The principles of clinical governance correspond with the requirements of the Code of Professional Conduct (NMC 2002). The objectives of clinical governance place the responsibility

for active participation at an individual practitioner level as well as at organisational level (DoH 1997).

There is an abundance of literature concerning change and managing change at an individual and organisational level. A key issue that emerges from the literature is the need to support people working through the process of change. The role of the district nurse is fundamental in the facilitation of change within the team whilst maintaining motivation and high standards of clinical care (Carnall 1995; Chin & Benne 1985; Clarke 1994; Lovatt 1999; Senior 1997; Taylor 1997). Within this context, clinical supervision is a necessary and important element in providing the support needed by district nurses not only to maintain their clinical standards but also to uphold them in their role as leaders of a team (DoH 1999b).

Clinical supervision in nursing is an effective means of attaining clinical excellence and strengthening the experience of interpersonal relationships. The term itself encompasses a range of strategies including mentorship, peer review and upholding professional standards (Butterworth *et al.* 1996). Although clinical supervision has been part of nursing practice since 1993 with the publication of *A Vision for the Future* (NHSME 1993), there has as yet been a lack of research to determine the effectiveness of clinical supervision. However, what is clear is that there are three important components for clinical supervision in practice. First is the need for a sharp separation between clinical supervision and a management appraisal system. Second, participation in clinical supervision should remain a fundamental part of district nursing practice and third is the need to establish a contract or formal agreement between the supervisor and the supervisee.

Evidence-based practice demands that patients' care is based on the most up-to-date evidence of what is known to be effective, (DoH 1999b, p. 44). It requires that practitioners need continuously to develop their information and research appraisal skills so they can use the best available evidence to support their practice (DoH 1999b). Within this context the district nurse needs to consider three elements: that practice is based on the best evidence available to her that will meet the patients' needs; that practice operates within a framework of reflection, evaluation and audit of outcomes; that knowledge of achieved effectiveness is disseminated to other practitioners. These elements together reflect the duty of the nurse under the Code of Professional Conduct to ensure that each individual receives care based on current evidence (NMC 2002).

What is equally clear from the literature is that patients as the recipients of care are integral to the clinical decision making process. When the district nurse makes a decision regarding a patient's clinical care, not only should that decision be based on the best evidence available but it should also be made in consultation with the patient and the carers so that it best suits the patient and the carers' needs. Patients who have a chronic disease, such as diabetes or multiple sclerosis, accrue a wealth of expertise in managing their own condition. The inclusion of the patients' and the carers' experiences will ensure that the expertise of the district nursing team and of other involved professionals is complemented by the expertise of the patients and the carers. The active involvement of patients in this process is central to the whole endeavour of clinical effectiveness, patient empowerment and evidence-based practice.

Risk management is another key aspect of clinical governance that district nurses must make integral to their work. It comprises the management of all aspects of clinical risk by ensuring that there are mechanisms in place to establish safe practice, which in turn safeguards the patients (DoH 1999b). Risk may be defined as the potential for an unwanted or unexpected outcome, for example injury to a patient or patient dissatisfaction and unhappiness in the form of a complaint. Risk management by definition is the systematic identification, assessment and reduction of risk to patients and staff (DoH 1999b). When things go wrong there is often finger-pointing and blame attribution instead of support and guidance for staff. For risk management to operate successfully there needs to be a culture of openness where incidents can be reported without fear of associated disciplinary action and where lessons can be learned and mistakes and problems such as poor clinical performance can be dealt with constructively.

The introduction of adverse incident reporting or significant event auditing systems is fundamental to the clinical risk management process. It offers the opportunity to review incidents and claims at an early stage. Where trends and similarities from incidents can be identified there may be opportunities to highlight organisational and communication problems which permit remedial action to be taken to prevent recurrence.

Managing chronic disease through population management and a geographical perspective

In Great Britain, 17.5 million adults may be living with a chronic disease. It is also likely that up to 75% of people aged over 75 years have a chronic disease, a figure which continues to rise (DoH 2004b). Within every strategic health authority there will be specialist 'demonstrator sites' that provide advice, care and treatment for people with chronic disease (late 2004). These sites will introduce active management of high risk patients and provide coordinated care within a 'whole systems approach' to enable people with chronic disease to keep healthy for longer. The organisation of such sites will be in the hands of primary health care professionals, both nurses and doctors who will be employed by the primary care trust. Their specialist knowledge will be used to effect a reduction of hospital admissions and GP waiting times. Currently, 80% of GP visits relate to chronic conditions – a situation that should be improved by the operation of the sites.

Recent management of selected chronic conditions has been through the introduction of National Service Frameworks (NSF) together with the associated activity of the NHS Modernisation Agency. As yet the NHS has no agreed model for managing all chronic disease: although underpinned by the best available international evidence the focus remains on single diseases or groups. Older people in particular often have multiple pathology where a general principles or generic approach to chronic disease management would be more applicable. The intention is that patients should have access to a wider range of services in primary care, including services near their workplace. More care is to be provided closer to home or in the home itself. Appropriate support could enable many people to learn how to be active participants in their own care, permitting them to live with and manage their condition as an expert patient. With regular monitoring of the condition and support to make any necessary changes to lifestyle, complications might well be avoided, deterioration slowed and the development of further complications might even be prevented.

Patients considered to be at a higher risk are to be provided with proactive support from a multidisciplinary team under the leadership of a district nurse. The aim is that patients will be enabled to make use of reliably researched protocols and pathways to manage their diseases themselves and avoid complications. To achieve this, good information technology will be required, with patient registers, shared electronic health records and care planning.

For people with more than one chronic condition there is the potential for care to be complex, involving integrated health and social care agencies working together. Such situations would require a personalised case management approach that would be entirely suited to a district nurse in the role of key worker actively managing and coordinating the care.

People with complex long-term conditions are to be supported locally by a 'community matron': a district nurse with specialist knowledge who could support these patients in such a way that they would be able to minimise the impact of the disease on their lives. The community matron would help them to manage their conditions in ways that suited them, anticipating problems and helping to avoid complications in order to maximise their health and assist them to live longer. These illnesses that people live with for the rest of their lives such as diabetes, asthma, arthritis, depression or heart disease, can be controlled but not cured.

Case management has always been a major part of the district nurse's role. However, district nurses are now being required to extend their physical and clinical assessment skills to include extended and supplementary prescribing in order to provide more comprehensive care in the community. The projected outcome is for fewer emergency admissions to hospital and the consequent trauma for patients and families. Teaching people to cope and to manage their diseases is a more productive use of resources and would enable them to take greater control of their own treatment. In this way they would be able to spend more time at home with their families and friends and have an enhanced quality of life. District nurses are able to monitor and manage high blood pressure and high cholesterol rates in patients with heart disease which could mean that fewer of these patients would require heart surgery; effective physiotherapy for patients with arthritis could delay the need for joint replacements (DoH 2004a).

District nurses are expert at assessing nursing care needs and have much experience of collaborating with local GPs and other members of the wider primary care team. They already occupy a familiar point of contact for other health care professionals so that they would be ideally placed to instigate joint responsibility for developing personal care plans. In this way the best possible care would be delivered to patients and their families and problems for the patients could be anticipated or dealt with before reaching a deterioration in health and hospitalisation.

By 2008 the Department of Health will adopt this model of care with 3000 community matrons (district nurses) using case management techniques to care for around 250 000 patients with complex needs. The single assessment process and better care coordination will be essential to achieve this aim. Effective social care services working together with health care services will be of critical importance when meeting the needs of people with long term conditions. For such people, who are often frail and old, it may be difficult to be at home coping with medication and trying to keep warm, well nourished and hydrated without support, particularly if they are alone, under stress, recently bereaved or have lost confidence in their ability to manage on their own. It is in such cases that district nurses can be so effective in targeting resources and coordinating community based personalised health and social care so that stressful and disruptive admission to hospital can be prevented. (DoH 2004a).

Nurse consultants and community matrons

The concept of the 'nurse consultant' was introduced in the Government's nursing strategy *Making a Difference*, (DoH 1999b). The *NHS Improvement Plan* (DoH 2004a) makes reference to 3000 community matrons whose role would be to improve the quality of life for thousands of patients living with distressing and incurable conditions. It would also be their responsibility to care for an ageing population with more complex and chronic conditions. At the same time these new posts would be structured to provide a stronger professional leadership. The areas of responsibility would be:

- Expert practice
- Professional leadership and consultancy
- Education and development
- Practice and service development linked to research

The inclusion of a clinical component would be expected to attract district nurses and those working as specialist nurses for older people to take up these new roles. Further education and development of professional skills will be an essential element of the roles. Areas such as health assessment, illness monitoring and pharmacology will need to be strengthened. Effective communication skills will be critical for engagement with patients and their families and liaison with patient support teams. An ability to facilitate and coordinate care will be essential together with the ability to develop service networks. The aim is to ensure that the care thus provided is patient-centred and is focused on attaining maximum independence, comfort and quality of life in the least invasive manner in the most appropriate setting.

Specific responses for older people

A model of community nursing care that has been imported from the USA, the Evercare Model (Evercare 2003), is being implemented across a number of primary care trusts. The service currently provides a proactive assessment and treatment service for older people considered to be at high risk of hospital admission. Key workers, many of whom are district nurses, together with a significant number of nurses from the acute sector, are responsible for the coordination of the service and the care of the patients. District nurses may need to expand their physical and clinical assessment skills in order to provide care within the model and also to extend their scope of practice to include prescribing. Their specialist community nursing knowledge places district nurses in a position to take the lead, identifying 'high risk' patients in their communities and managing and monitoring caseloads appropriately to prevent acute exacerbations or problems. This model of care targets the specific needs of the vulnerable older person who is at risk of admission or readmission to hospital and should effectively reduce the number of people needing to be admitted to care homes for the older person (Evercare 2003).

The era of the patient as the passive recipient of care is changing. It is being replaced by a partnership approach in which patients are empowered through information to contribute ideas that can help in their treatment and care. Linked to this is the expert patient programme (DoH 2001), introduced in the White Paper *Saving Lives: Our Healthier Nation* (DoH 1999a) and further developed in *The NHS Plan* (DoH 2000). These expert patients are people with the confidence, skills, information and knowledge to play a central role in the management of living with a chronic disease and to minimise the impact of the disease on their lives. The programme is designed to empower patients to manage their own health care and to listen to themselves and their symptoms. With the support of a district nursing team, and a range of other health and social care professionals in the community as appropriate, the programme can be made effective. The rationale for this programme is that patients understand their disease better than health care professionals because they have acquired skills from their experiences of coping with their own chronic condition. This, of course, is also closely linked to the series of National Service Frameworks that have relevance for expert patient programmes (CHD, mental health, older people, NHS cancer plan, diabetes, long-term health conditions).

GMS contract and nurses with specialist interests

The new contract (DoH 2004b) is designed to provide demonstrable benefits to GPs, other primary care professionals, the NHS and patients. It seeks to reward practices for higher quality care and to improve professionals' working lives thereby ensuring that patients benefit from a wider range of services in the community. Practices will have greater freedom to decide how to design their services to meet local need and GPs will be able to choose to opt out of providing specific and out of hours services. The transfer of responsibility for such provision to the primary care trust creates the opportunity for district nurses and other community nurses to fill these gaps by becoming the providers of such 'additional services'. The opportunities are boundless for those with a creative mind and specialist knowledge and skills. They include working in minor injury units, or with the ambulance service to prevent unnecessary journeys to the accident and emergency department, or in urology and continence, dermatology and tissue viability services, depending on local need.

It has always been the practice of district nurses to extend their knowledge and clinical practice in response to patient need, creating a service that provides additional expertise in areas such as diabetes, dermatology, tissue viability and respiratory disease and with older people in stroke care and falls prevention. A district nurse with a special interest working alongside other nurses, GPs and consultants could offer a specialist service to a whole primary care trust or a collection of practices. Such a service, operating within the framework of general practice in collaboration with general practice nurses, diabetes or tissue viability could support patients with chronic disease at home or provide clinic sessions, for example in diabetes or tissue viability. An effective and high quality health service needs both specialist and generalists (DoH 2003)

Extended and supplementary prescribing

There have been huge developments in prescribing by non-medical practitioners within the last three years. The inclusion of extended and supplementary prescribing in the future district nurse's role makes the separate chapter assigned to the topic in this book compulsory reading.

The *Report of the Advisory Group on Nurse Prescribing* (DoH 1989) recommended that the district nurse would be eligible to prescribe from a limited nursing formulary following the successful completion of a specific education programme. The legal framework for nurse prescribing came into being with the passing of The Medicines Products: Prescriptions by Nurses etc. Act 1992. However, it cannot be expected to take effect in isolation from other professional and service developments. The implementation of nurse prescribing has involved the collaborative efforts by community trusts, health authorities and primary care groups to develop local systems and structures for its long-term support, monitoring and development.

For the district nurse it is just the beginning of a learning process that will enhance the care and treatment of patients. The introduction of nurse prescribing has already had a significant impact on the district nurse's workload by speeding up the commencement of treatment as prescribed items are obtained more efficiently.

The legal independence of nurse prescribing has brought with it additional accountability for practice: it is the responsibility of each prescribing district nurse to ensure that practice and prescribing is underpinned by current evidence and demonstrated competence. The recent extension of prescribing rights of community nurses requires them to build upon the skills, knowledge and competencies developed in the early stages of nurse prescribing (Anderson 1999). District nurses have also increased their skills and knowledge with regard to clinical assessment which has enabled them to exclude abnormal pathophysiology, enhance their diagnostic skills and build upon their pharmacology knowledge base (Banning 1999; Luker *et al.* 1998; May 1998; Scowen 1995). Future progress will undoubtedly see further increases in the number of nurse prescribers and in the range of medicines available to them, with electronic prescribing improving the efficiency and quality of prescribing (DoH 2004a).

Nurse prescribing forms an integral part of the care and treatment provided by the district nurse and is an essential element of professional practice. It will form a key component of the district nurse's continuous professional development portfolio (DoH 1998, 1999b; Hinchcliff 1999).

Continuing professional development and lifelong learning

Change within the NHS is an ongoing and continuous process. The past decade has seen enormous changes both from government reforms and from actual evidenced health needs. In order to provide the best possible evidence-based care to clients the district nurse of the future will be required to maintain the highest possible professional practice. Continuous professional development will be a process of lifelong learning whereby health professionals continually seek to improve their knowledge and acquire new cognitive skills, values and attitudes in order to meet the needs of patients and the health service as competent practitioners. Practising nurses are currently required to maintain their registration with the Nursing and Midwifery Council (NMC) and must demonstrate engagement in continuous professional development as an integral part of the registration renewal process (NMC 2002).

Primary health care teams and district nurses should look to the future and identify the skills and knowledge that will be required in the years ahead so that they can meet the challenges of a broader based policy and plan their research and development.

There will need to be a considerable shift, both within professional organisations and in the higher education sector, towards a culture that supports lifelong learning. For professional organisations the dilemma will be how to guide district nurses away from a defensive stance where change is always seen as a threat, towards the adoption of a more creative and proactive approach. This will mean that educational establishments will have to provide a flexible approach to educational preparation that is responsive to current developments.

With all the changes that future district nurses face, the need to equip them with the appropriate educational preparation will be demanding. What is certain is that different models will be required across the country which are responsive to local need. This could be more problematic for educational establishments that service several diverse workforce development confederations but easier for those that only have to relate to one. It will therefore be essential to work collaboratively with workforce development confederations and primary care trusts to develop a coherent and manageable programme that prepares practitioners for the enormous variety of opportunities that are available in primary health care.

The 'traditional' work of a district nurse will still be required, but alongside this is the need to develop a new proactive approach to the management of chronic disease and to develop the public health aspect of the work. Collaboration with general practice nurses and nurses in the acute care setting will be imperative as more complex care is being devolved to primary care settings. Although some patients will be able to attend the GP practice, there are significant numbers who will need to be managed in the home environment where standards of care will need to be the same. District nurses of the future will need different skills to manage patients effectively within the new models of service provision. In accordance with the knowledge and skills framework (DoH 2004c) within the *Agenda for Change* (NHS Modernisation Agency 2004), staff will be supported to fulfil their potential, with the NHS University and skills escalator helping staff to develop throughout their careers. The Agenda for Change programme is a job evaluation-based process that rewards increased knowledge and skills and provides real incentives for staff and managers to change existing patterns of working and embrace new ones.

It is anticipated that learning will be multi-focused with work and practice based learning, supported by university teaching and distance learning approaches. The focus of learning will be on contemporary practice in line with government policy and will involve contributions to programme delivery from nurse consultants, community matrons, nurses with special interests and expert patients in both primary and secondary care. Students will need the support of their employing trust, of the university and of the work-based mentor in a tripartite agreement. Education, training and learning will need to be more flexible, for example, based on transferable, competency based modules that have common learning and inter-professional outcomes agreed between higher education institutions and the NHS.

Conclusion

The Government has established a challenging agenda for change in primary care. The emergence of nurse consultants and community matrons in the community will provide the highest professional goal achievable by clinically based nurses. It should boost recruitment and foster retention of like-minded nurses who aspire to excellence in their profession.

District nurses are committed not only to helping people with chronic disease live more satisfying lives but also to being more actively involved in promoting the nation's health. The second Wanless report (2004) shows that the health of the population of England is not as good as that of other comparable countries. The factors that contribute to poor health include relatively high levels of smoking (27% of the adult population) and obesity, in conjunction with low levels of physical activity and low consumption of fresh fruit and vegetables (DoH 2004a). Heart disease and strokes, mental illness, accidents, injuries and cancers have the greatest impact on the health of the population. In developed countries such as the UK the key risk factors for these diseases are smoking, high blood pressure, alcohol, high cholesterol and obesity. If we are to improve our standards of health, the focus must be not simply on treatment but also on prevention and the prioritisation of preventative public health measures (White Paper – *Choosing Health: Making Healthy Choices Easier*, DoH 2004d).

Balanced against this is the need to provide care at home for people with complex needs, frail older people, and those with acute needs as well as those requiring palliative and terminal care.

This chapter has only touched on the role of the district nurse in the support of those patients and families requiring palliative and terminal care. The uncomfortable fact is that everyone will die. There is a need to ensure that all people at the end of their lives, regardless of diagnosis, will be given a choice of where they wish to die and how they wish to be treated.

All these challenges will lead to great changes in the traditional ways of working but exciting opportunities lie ahead. Primary care trusts are set on improving their respective populations' health and for patients this will be through access to the knowledge and skills of a community matron. The nursing community may not be keen on this title, but it is just that – a title, one from the past that is recognised by the public. It is associated with a figure of authority and influence, competence and compassion, who is in charge of patient care and in whom patients can have complete confidence.

As the NHS becomes ever more patient-focused with patient choice and involvement, district nurses need to respond to the challenges with enthusiasm and creativity. They should seize this opportunity to make a difference to people's lives and to become the experts in managing chronic disease. The employing organisation must consider the strategic purpose of district nursing and how it interfaces with other health and social services. There needs to be a greater clarification of the services it provides. The development of quality standards and pathways of care within a community framework will ensure that these services are effective, evidence-based and open to audit. It is important to appraise what is already being carried out effectively and what is still needed to enhance patient care. By becoming more vocal and assertive and by getting involved, district nurses and community specialists can be effective in the move for change.

Central to this vision of the future is the need for the district nurse to retain that element of the role which is held in such high esteem by patients and carers, namely their trust and confidence and the value they place on being treated with humanity and kindness, underpinned by effective teamwork, integration, collaboration and partnership (Audit Commission 1999, Hill 2000).

References

Anderson, P. (1999) Looking at the road ahead for nurse prescribing. *Nurse Prescriber Community*, December, pp. 35–36.

Audit Commission (1999) *First Assessment: a review of District Nursing services in England and Wales.* Audit Commission, London.

Banning, M. (1999) Nurse Prescribing – Education, education, education. In: M. Jones (ed) *Nurse Prescribing – Politics to Practice*, Bailliere Tindall, Royal College of Nursing, London.

Bradshaw, J. (1992) The concept of social need. *New Society*, **30**, 640–643.

Butterworth, T., Bishop, V. & Carson, J. (1996) First steps towards evaluating clinical supervision in nursing and health visiting. Theory, policy and practice development. A review. *Journal of Clinical Nursing*, **5**(2), 127–132.

Cain, P., Hyde, V. & Howkins, E. (1995) *Community Nursing, Dimensions and Dilemmas.* Arnold, London.

Carnall, C. (1995) *Managing Change in Organisations*, Prentice Hall, Toronto.

Chin, R. & Benne, K. (1985) General strategies for effecting changes in human systems, In: *The Planning of Change*, 4th edn, W. Bennis, K. Benne & R. Chin, (eds) Holt, Reinhart and Winston, New York, pp. 22–23.

Clarke, L. (1994) *The Essence of Change*, Prentice Hall, New York.

Department of Health (1989) *Report of the Advisory Group on Nurse Prescribing*, DoH, London.

Department of Health (1992) *The Health of the Nation: A Strategy of Health for England.* DoH, London.

Department of Health (1997) *The New NHS: Modern, Dependable.* DoH, London.

Department of Health (1998) *A First Class Service: Quality in the New NHS.* DoH, Leeds.

Department of Health (1999a) *Saving Lives: Our Healthier Nation.* DoH, London.

Department of Health (1999b) *Making a Difference: Strengthening the Nursing, Midwifery and Health Visiting Contribution to Health and Healthcare.* DoH, London.

Department of Health (2000) *The NHS Plan. A plan for investment. A plan for reform.* DoH, London.

Department of Health (2001) *The Expert Patient: A New Approach to Chronic Disease Management for the 21st Century.* DoH, London.

Department of Health (2002) *Liberating the Talents. Helping Primary Care Trusts and Nurses to Deliver the NHS Plan.* DoH, London.

Department of Health (2002) *Chronic Disease Management and Self-care. National Service Frameworks. A practical guide to implementation in primary care.* DoH, London.

Department of Health (2003) *Practitioners with Special Interest in Primary Care.* DoH, London.

Department of Health (2004a) *The NHS Improvement Plan. Putting People at the Heart of Public Services.* DoH, London.

Department of Health (2004b) *Investing in General Practice. The New General Medical Services (GMS) Contract.* DoH, London.

Department of Health (2004c) *The NHS Knowledge and Skills Framework (NHS KSF) and the Development Review Process.* The Stationery Office, London.

Department of Health (2004d) *Choosing Health: Making Healthy Choices Easier.* DoH, London.

English National Board (1991) *Criteria and guidelines for taught practice placements for district nurse students.* Circular 1991/05/MB. English National Board, London.

Evercare (2003) *Adapting the Evercare Programme for the National Health Service.* Evercare.

Gerrish, K. (1997) An evaluation of integrated nursing teams in Sheffield, (unpublished report submitted to Community Health Sheffield NHS Trust), Sheffield Hallam University, Sheffield.

Hill, J. (2000) Many Challenges. *Nursing Management.* **6**(9), 29.

Hinchcliff, S. (1999) *Lifelong learning for nursing.* Presentation given at ICN Centenary Conference London.

Lovatt, M. (1999) Implementing change in practice. *Journal of Community Nursing*, **13**(2).

Luker, K., Hogg, C., Austin, L., Ferguson, B. & Smith, K. (1998) Decision making: the context of Nurse Prescribing. *Journal of Advanced Nursing*, **27**, 657–665.

May, V. (1998) Ready or not. *Journal of Community Nursing*, **12**(3), 4, 6, 8.

Murray, E.J. & Irven, I.D. (1948) *District Nursing*. Bailliere Tindall and Cox, London.

NHSME (1993) *New World New Opportunities*. The Stationery Office, London.

NHS Modernisation Agency (2004) *Agenda for Change*. NHS Modernisation Agency, London.

NMC (2002) *Code of Professional Conduct*. Nursing and Midwifery Council, London.

Ridgely Seymer, L. (1954) *Selected Writings of Florence Nightingale*, Macmillan, New York.

Ross, F. (1990) *Key Issues in District Nursing. Paper two*, District Nursing Association, UK.

Scowen, P. (1995) Why community nurses need to know their pharmacology, *Professional Care of Mother and Child*, **5**(1), 2, 4.

Senior, B. (1997) *Organisational Change*. Pitman Publications, London.

Taylor, B.M. (1997) Analysis of job-share as a process of change. *Journal of Nursing Management*, **5**, 223–227.

Wall, A. (1998) From paper to practice. *Health Service Journal*, 19 February, pp. 28–29.

Wanless, D. (2004) *Securing Good Health for the Whole Population. Final Report*. The Stationery Office, London.

Wright, S.M. (1997) Profiling in community nursing, *Clinical Effectiveness in Nursing*, **1**, 166–168.

Chapter 11 **Community Children's Nursing**

Mark Whiting

Introduction

Quality has been at the top of the health service agenda since the major reform of the NHS heralded in the late 1980s by the Conservative Government in its key White Papers *Working for Patients* (DoH 1989a) and *Caring for People* (DoH 1989b). With the incoming Labour Government in 1997 the commitment to deliver high quality services remained a key target against which the Government has asked that its performance be judged. The words 'quality', 'audit', 'targets' and 'standards' continue to occur with quite startling regularity in almost any contemporary article one reads on almost any health care subject! With the launch in 1997 of the White Paper *The New NHS: Modern, Dependable* (DoH 1997a) the NHS was presented with a whole raft of new jargon and a range of initiatives which were destined to drive and direct the 'quality' agenda for many years to come. Arguably the most prominent and sustained theme to arise within the current social policy framework is the concept of 'clinical governance', with both the Department of Health and the United Kingdom Central Council for Nursing, Midwifery and Health Visiting recognising the key role that nurses have to play in delivering on this aspect of the quality agenda (DoH 1999; UKCC 1999). Clinical governance has provided the cornerstone of the 'Performance Framework' within which the component parts of the NHS have become accountable for the quality and standards of the services that they provide. During the late 1990s, this was supported by three key developments (DoH 1998):

- The establishment of a National Institute for Clinical Excellence (NICE), responsible for the development and dissemination of evidence-based clinical guidelines to underpin the delivery of practice

- The development of a series of National Services Frameworks (NSFs) through which National standards for services delivery would be set
- The creation of a Commission for Health Improvement (CHI – now superseded by the Healthcare Commission) which was to provide independent monitoring of local health services delivery in order to assure and improve clinical quality

The notion of clinical governance remains central to the delivery of high quality services and has been defined as:

'a framework through which NHS organisations are accountable for continuously improving the quality of their services and safeguarding high standards of care by creating an environment in which excellence in clinical care will flourish'.

(NHSE 1999, p. 6)

For community children's nurses (CCNs), the need to demonstrate that their services are 'delivering on the quality agenda' has never been more important. Whilst there is strong support of the view that nursing care really does make a difference to people's lives (DoH 1999, 2002a, 2004a), it is imperative that community children's nurses both develop the necessary tools and use every possible opportunity to explicitly communicate the specific differences which they believe that they can make to the lives of children and their families. If CCNs are to fulfil their potential within a primary care led NHS, then it is imperative that alongside other nurses and health visitors working within primary care they are able to articulate clearly the particular skills and knowledge that they bring to their work:

'Our objective is to liberate the talents and skills of all the workforce so that every patient gets the right care in the right place at the right time.'

(DoH 2002b, p. 34)

This chapter is concerned with the achievement of excellence in practice. It is focused upon the work of nurses who are providing care to children and families in community settings. It will provide, through an exploration of both published and unpublished data sources, a systematic examination of a range of strategies that have been utilised in order to demonstrate the attainment of 'quality' in service provision. Although much of the literature to which reference will be made predates the current health care policy strategy, as stated above, the clinical governance 'performance framework' provides an overarching context to much of that policy. Of more specific relevance to children is the recently published *Children's National Services Framework* (NSF) (DoH/DfES 2004a, b, c) incorporating a range of standards against which children's health services provision might be judged. The NSF will form a key part of the cross-departmental 'Change for Children – Every Child Matters' implementation programme which is itself at the heart of the Children Act.

From an historical perspective, the development of community children's nursing predates the inception of the NHS by around sixty years and can be traced back to the closing decades of the eighteenth century (Hunt & Whiting, 1999; Whiting, 2000). At this time, the Medical Committee of the Hospital for Sick Children, Great Ormond Street considered that the establishment of a team of 'skilled Nurses for Children for services outside its walls' would address the specific needs of parents and children alike (The Hospital for Sick Children 1880). It was not, however, until the pioneering work of John Bowlby (1951) and James Robertson (1958) that a more specific rationale was offered in support of the development of such services. This particular rationale, based on a belief that community care might provide psychological advantages over hospital care for the child and family (and supported in the Ministry of Health's seminal review of hospital services for children, the Platt Report of 1959) has been the driving force behind much of the my own involvement in community children's nursing (see Box 11.1).

On reflection, however, it is clear that the high quality service, which I firmly believed I was delivering, simply did not have the necessary evidence base that I had always considered to be fundamental to the achievement of excellence in my own practice. Within the remainder of this chapter, I will endeavour, therefore, to demonstrate that some significant strides have been made in providing that 'missing' evidence and at the same time, hopefully allow some of my own 'ghosts' to be laid to rest.

Quality

The Oxford English Dictionary defines quality as a 'degree of excellence, relative nature or kind or character' and the Royal College of Nursing publication *Standards of Care: a framework for quality* offers some additional insight, suggesting that 'Quality of care begins and ends with the patient's experience of the service' (RCN 1989). John Reid, Secretary of State for Health, in the foreword launching the Children's National Services Framework stated:

[This framework] 'advocates a shift with services being designed and delivered around the needs of the child. Services are child centred and look at the whole child – not just the illness or the problem...'

(DoH/DfES 2004a, p. 2)

John Øvretveit, who has written widely on many aspects of management and organisation within the health services, suggests that there are three dimensions to quality: client quality, professional quality and service quality (Øvretveit 1992):

- *'Client Quality*: Clients' views of the extent to which the service gives them what they want and expect.' In terms of community children's nursing, this clearly relates to the perceptions of both children and their families, working in 'partnership' with the nursing team (Casey 1995; Gould 1996; Taylor 2000)

Box 11.1

During my career as a practitioner, manager or lecturer in community children's nursing services, I received many enquiries (often from people whom I did not know or had never met) asking about quality, audit and standards.

The conversations would run something like:

'Could you send me a copy of your audit tool?'
MW – 'We haven't actually got an audit tool as such.'
'When did you last audit your teams work then?'
MW – 'Never!'
'Well, what quality indicators do you use then?'
MW 'None!'
*'Well, I wonder then if you could tell me if anybody has published anything on audit
in community children's nursing services?'*
MW – 'Help!'
'Do you think you could send me a copy of your standards then, or clinical guidelines?'
MW – 'Help!!'

I had been so wrapped up in my own beliefs about community children's nursing that rather than get down to the business of developing the necessary tools to support my own opinions, I simply brushed the issue to one side. I firmly believed that my own practice was founded upon research-based evidence (whenever I could find any) but more often than not, there simply was no evidence. During the late 1980s and early 1990s community children's nursing was developing at such a pace – supported by a succession of Government imperatives to reduce the length of hospital stay for children – that there was hardly time to catch ones breath let alone subject that practice to rigorous audit!

- *'Professional Quality*: Professionals' judgement of the extent to which the service meets clients' needs as assessed by professionals', including both the CCNs themselves and those with whom they come into professional contact
- *'Service Quality*: Meeting client requirements at the lowest cost to the organisation, or meeting the needs of those most in need of the service at the lowest cost and within prescribed directives'

These three dimensions of quality are very closely intertwined. It is important, however, to recognise that when looking at indicators which are focused primarily within the *service* dimension of quality or at those that are based upon *professional* assessments of quality, the ultimate aim ought to be to optimise the quality of the *client's experience* of that service. This is fundamental to the whole philosophical underpinnings of clinical governance and is clearly at the heart of the children's National Services Framework:

'This is a ten year plan: by 2014 we expect health, social and educational services to have met the standards set in this document. Inequalities will be reduced, so that all children and young people have access to the services they need, no matter where they live or where they come from. Staff from all sectors need to work together so that the services they provide join up across health, social care and education, and offer the best possible solution for children and their families'.

(DoH/DfES 2004a, p. 2 – Foreword by Dr John Reid, Secretary of State for Health)

As indicated above, considerable energy has been expended in recent years both in seeking to improve quality and in developing the means to demonstrate improvement. In relation to the provision of child health services, Action for Sick Children, formerly the National Association for the Welfare of Children in Hospital (NAWCH), has been at the forefront of this activity. Publications such as the *NAWCH Charter* (1984), the *NAWCH Quality checklist: Caring for Children in Hospital* (1987) and the *NAWCH Quality review, Setting Standards for Children in Health Care* (1989) set the agenda for much of that which was to follow in later policy statements from the Department of Health and Audit Commission (see below). During the 1990s, a refocusing of the campaigning voice of NAWCH towards the provision of services for children in all health care settings saw it re-launched as 'Action for Sick Children'. A whole series of publications followed, including *Health Services for Children and Young People* (Hogg 1996), *Emergency Health Services for Children and Young People* (Hogg 1997) and *Child Friendly Primary Health Care* (Hogg 1998), the last of which included a short checklist for CCN Services.

In the specific context of paediatric nursing, there have been a number of publications on the theme of 'standards', including documents from the Royal Hospital for Sick Children in Edinburgh (1987), the South West Thames Regional Health Authority (1990) and the Great Ormond Street Hospital for Children NHS Trust (1996). However, a review of each of these documents finds no more than a passing mention of any aspects of community care. For example, the South West Thames document identifies the following standard statement: 'On discharge the child will receive attention which is suited to his own and his family's special requirements' (1990, p. 10). However the standard's criteria for achievement make no mention of the potential contribution of a community children's nurse. In contrast, the Royal College of Nursing *Standards of Care: paediatric nursing* (RCN 1990, 1994) includes a specific requirement for districts to provide a paediatric community nursing service (CCN) as part of the standard for children being discharged from hospital. A number of CCN teams have developed their own local 'standards', though the Southampton based team is perhaps unique in having actually published their own document for wider consideration (Jefferson & Gow 1995).

From the broader social policy perspective, a number of documents have provided some guidance on the provision of community child health services. In the early 1990s, this included the Department of Health guidance on the *Welfare of Children and Young People in Hospital* (DoH 1991) and the Audit Commission's review of hospital services *Children First* (1993).

Although both documents were primarily concerned with hospital care, each drew attention to the need for appropriate follow-up of children following discharge. Unfortunately, neither provided any significant insight into what might constitute a 'quality service' in terms of CCN provision.

The publication of the Department of Health guidance on *Child Health in the Community* (NHSE 1996b) and the *Patients' Charter* (NHSE 1996a) provided a very clear opportunity for the Government to make unequivocal statements on quality in this area. Unfortunately, although both documents provided broad general guidance on some elements of CCN provision, they failed to offer any significant or consistent insight into what might constitute the components of a quality service. For instance whilst 'Child Health in the Community' recommended that 'services should be staffed by nurses who possess registration as a children's nurse and experience of community nursing' (NHSE 1996a, p. 61) the 'Children's charter' advised parents caring for a sick child at home 'if a CCN team has not been set up in your area, help will be from the district nursing team' (NHSE 1996b, p. 13).

It is hardly surprising therefore that when the House of Commons Health Select Committee undertook a major investigation of Child Health Services during 1996/7 significant concern was raised in relation to dramatic inconsistencies in CCN provision within the UK. The Committee made a series of recommendations, many of which arose from evidence provided to the Committee by both the Royal College of Nursing and a number of voluntary agencies (Box 11.2).

It is perhaps unfortunate that the Health Select Committee published its recommendation just as the Government was prorogued prior to the 1997 general election. However, in its response to the Committee's recommendations, the incoming Labour Government signalled a sea change in the approach that it intended to take in relation to the attainment of quality in health services and stated 'we do not accept that cost will be the only, or indeed the main driver in the move towards a community orientated service: quality and effectiveness are more important factors' (DoH 1997b, p. 19), a philosophy which was

---

Box 11.2 Examples of recommendations. (Source: House of Commons Health Select Committee, 1997)

Recommendation 9
The important thing at this stage is not the precise detail of administrative arrangements, but that sick children and their families should have access to an appropriate service. We therefore recommend the following:

- All children requiring nursing interventions should have easy access to a community children's nursing service, staffed by qualified children's nurses supplemented by those in training, in whatever setting in the community they are being nursed
- The service should be available 24 hours a day, seven days a week
- Every GP should have access to a named community children's nurse
- Information about the service should be easily available to all relevant health care professionals and voluntary organisations
- Co-ordination between agencies and professionals should be regarded as a necessary part of providing a good service

Recommendation 10
We further recommend that each health authority should be required to contract for a community children's nursing service. Health authorities should have flexibility in contracting subject to the overall requirement to provide a service along the lines we have set out above.

Box 11.3 Ten key roles for nurses. (Source: DoH 2000b)

- To order diagnostic investigations such as pathology tests and X-rays
- To make and receive referrals direct, e.g. to a therapist or pain consultant
- To admit and discharge patients for specified conditions and within agreed protocols
- To manage patient caseloads, e.g. for diabetes or rheumatology
- To run clinics, e.g. for ophthalmology or dermatology
- To prescribe medicines and treatments
- To carry out a wide range of resuscitation procedures including defibrillation
- To perform minor surgery and outpatient procedures
- To triage patients using the latest IT to the most appropriate health professional
- To take a lead in the way local health services are organised and in the way that they are run

---

strongly reiterated in the government's key statement on quality in the NHS 'A First Class Service: Quality in the New NHS' (DoH 1998) and at the heart of the *NHS Plan* (DoH 2000a).

The specific role which nurses might play in delivering that plan was outlined in a document which was published by the Chief Nursing Officer and distributed to every Registered Nurse in England. It included the identification of ten key roles that nurses might play in taking the *NHS Plan* forward (DoH 2000b, Box 11.3).

These ten key roles were given further emphasis within the Department of Health's key primary care nursing strategy document *Liberating the Talents* (DoH 2002a) which identified the three

activities of 'first contact', 'continuing care' and 'public health' as the core functions undertaken by community nurses. This was applied to the particular context of the care of children and young people in a detailed review published by the Chief Nursing Officer in 2004 (DoH 2004a). Each of these documents has continued to emphasise the need to ensure high quality, clinically effective, patient focussed services. In the remainder of this chapter, the clinical governance performance framework will be used as a basis for examining the extent to which these aspirations have been met within CCN services provision.

Monitoring and measuring quality and effectiveness

The clinical governance 'performance framework' is intended to 'support the drive for higher quality standards by ensuring that performance assessment is focused on the delivery of effective, appropriate and timely health services which meet local needs' (DoH 1998, p. 63). The framework consists of six areas of assessment:

- Patient and carer experience
- Fair access

- Health outcomes of NHS care
- Health improvement
- Efficiency
- Effective delivery of appropriate health care

Each of these areas will now be considered in turn within the specific context of community children's nursing.

Patient and carer experience: is community care what children and families really want?

The Department of Health has made it clear that 'the views and experiences of the people who use the NHS should form an important element of any assessment of its performance' (DoH 1998, p. 66). More evidence of the government's strong commitment to listening to the consumer voice is evident in the *NHS Plan*, offering 'a once in a lifetime opportunity for every member of public and NHS staff to have their say on the future of their health services.' (DoH 2000c). In developing the National Services Framework for children, there was an explicit commitment to consult with children and young people and their families, specifically to find out,

'What they think of the health and social care services we have now;

What is important to them from such services, and

What improvements could be made to services.'

(DoH/DfES 2004a, p. 10)

Many commentators, dating back to those who were responsible for the establishment of the first CCN service within the NHS (Gillett 1954), have suggested that by nursing children at home, it is possible to reduce the likelihood of occurrence of the adverse psychological reaction associated with hospitalisation. Indeed, almost every published 'mission statement' or set of 'aims and objectives' maintains that the CCN service will improve the psychological well-being of the child. Whilst this might appear to be quite logical, there is, in fact, very little evidence to support this contention. Indeed there is very little published material concerning either psychological evaluation of children receiving care in the community or the views of children

themselves. In addition, for those children who do require admission to hospital, much has been accomplished in addressing the psychological needs of both children and their parents. Undoubtedly the experience of Laura, the two year old who spent five days in hospital whilst undergoing repair of an umbilical hernia, so graphically displayed in the classic 1953 film by James Robertson can be confined to the pages of history! There is, however, a growing body of evidence that despite the improvements in the 'hospital experience' many parents would prefer care to be delivered in their own homes.

A number of CCN teams have carried out small scale family satisfaction surveys, many of which have asked parents' views, though it would appear that the views of children themselves have not been sought with quite the same rigour.

An independent review of 50 children receiving care from the service based at the North Middlesex Hospital found that all families considered the services to be helpful, 85% of parents were 'fully supportive' of the CCN services with 24% of families describing the service as 'vital' (Bosanquet *et al.* 1994).

Other surveys of parental satisfaction have been published from teams based in Greenwich, (While 1991, 1992), where 87.5% of a sample of 40 families expressed a preference for home care; Stockport (Marland 1994), where 95% of respondents preferred their child to be nursed at home and Tower Hamlets (Tatman *et al.* 1992), where in a sample of 35 families who had received care both in hospital and at home, 23 families felt that their child being in hospital was more stressful than their child being at home and only 2 families found home care more anxiety provoking. All 35 parents in the Tower Hamlets survey felt that their children were happier at home than in hospital.

In an evaluation of a sample of children receiving home enteral nutrition from Birmingham Children's Hospital (Holden 1991, p. 150), 34 out of 70 families reported 'spontaneously that their child appeared more happy and active', though it is unclear from this article what specific contribution, if any, CCN services made to the care of these children in the community, and the authors observed that twenty families reported that community nurses without paediatric training knew very little about paediatric nutrition but did provide helpful moral support in many instances.

Jennings (1994) undertook an evaluation of a recently established paediatric 'hospital at home' service in southern England. 96 parents were surveyed, of whom 96% thought that home care was better than hospital care from a 'social point of view' and 68% thought that home care was better from a 'medical point of view'.

Torr and Peter (1996) reported the results of ongoing satisfaction surveys undertaken with parents whose children had received support from the Paediatric Hospital at Home service in St Helens and Knowsley. Although a number of parents responding to an initial survey felt that too much responsibility had been placed on them, all 40 respondents felt that the service was 'good' with 39 able to list advantages of the service for themselves/their children.

A review of CCN services based in Basingstoke undertaken by the College of Health found that 90.5% of 106 parents responding to a postal questionnaire rated the service as 'good' or 'very good' (Smith *et al*. 1996). Follow up in-depth interviews with 21 families gave a strong endorsement of the service in terms of 'accessibility', 'confidence boosting skills', 'just being at home', 'linking between hospital and home' and 'involvement of the children' in their care.

The Basingstoke study mirrored many of the findings from the 'needs assessment' element of a small-scale study undertaken on behalf of the English National Board in 1994. In this study, by Cash *et al*. (1994), which formed part of a wider investigation of education of the clinical nursing experience of child branch students with CCN teams, six dimensions of parental need were identified as 'information, communication, support, advocacy, link-working and respect.' Cash and colleagues (1994) further identified that the skills that community children's nurses might be required to provide in response to these needs were technical skills, practical help, networking and advocacy skills and interpersonal/psychological skills. The extent to which the skills provided by

CCNs matched the perceived needs of parents were unfortunately not explored in any significant depth, though the clear message from the research was that the services provided by the CCN were very highly valued.

Proctor and colleagues (1998) undertook further research on behalf of the English National Board, and focused specifically on the educational and experiential preparation of the CCN. One element of this research involved detailed interviews with the parents of 40 children. Parents identified a number of key features of the CCN services provided to them including:

- Teaching skills
- Practical help
- Technical competence and clinical credibility
- 24 hour access to a nurse who knew the child and family
- Networking and problem solving skills
- Insight into the families skills and abilities (including learning abilities)
- Skills in interdependence and the sharing of care between nurse and family

The study clearly identified that in the absence of these skills, the burden of caring for children with complex needs within the community had the potential to overwhelm the families.

Further evidence of the demands placed on families by the responsibility of caring for children with complex needs are provided in a qualitative study of the experience of the parents of 21 children in Edinburgh as described by Whyte and colleagues in 1998. This study clearly illustrates the pressure felt by many parents when caring for children at home and although all of the children in this convenience sample were identified by members of the CCN team, significant gaps in provision identified by the parents included 'lack of coordination, need for help with benefits and more respite care as well as lack of information and ready access to information and services' (Whyte *et al*. 1998, p. 142).

In the late 1990s, Rosemary Thornes undertook a comprehensive review of 52 projects within the 'Programme of Pilot Projects for Children with Life Threatening Illnesses' (NHSE 1998a). Fifteen of these pilot projects researched and/or developed

CCN teams. Thornes concluded 'Without exception, surveys of parents show deep satisfaction with children's community services.' (p. 17). However, one of the larger studies undertaken within the overall programme (While *et al.* 1996) demonstrated very clearly the variability in provision of CCN services, with only 31 of a sample of 82 families in twelve district health authorities identifying that they had been seen by a CCN compared with 60 families who had been in contact with health visitors and 48 with district nurses.

However, it is not simply the actual provision of care itself which is important; it is the fact that whatever support that might be required is available as and when it is needed which facilitates the care of the children in the community. Parental perception of need is clearly very important here. This is demonstrated particularly well in a survey of parents of 100 children who had undergone day surgery at Yorkhill Hospital in Glasgow (Freeland & Munroe 1995). Fifty children were allocated to receive a home visit and fifty to receive a telephone follow-up. 48 out of 50 parents who received a post-operative home visit from a CCN said that they would not have been satisfied if the visit had been replaced with a follow-up telephone call. However, of the fifty parents who only received a telephone call, 74% were satisfied that this was adequate follow-up, with only thirteen parents expressing a preference for a home visit. This is an interesting finding, particularly when one considers that entire CCN services have been founded on the basis of following up children receiving day case surgery (such as in the Southampton based service described by Atwell & Gow 1985). 'Satisfaction' is clearly a complex phenomenon.

One of the areas of concern raised in several of the studies above relates to the issue of 'communication' between the CCN teams and the parents, particularly prior to the first visit. The Southampton 'standards' (Jefferson & Gow 1995) and an unpublished document from the Waltham Forest Paediatric Home Care Team (Sappa *et al.* 1990) have included specific standards relating to communication with parents, including the use of information leaflets. It is clear that when parents

are given the option to care for their child at home, the necessary framework of communication which will allow them to feel comfortable and well supported must be in place. However, as While (1992) found, communicating effectively with parents is something that CCNs seem to do very well indeed.

A number of studies have explored the need for effective communication between CCNs and fellow professionals (Bosanquet *et al.* 1994; Gow & Campbell 1996; Kelly *et al.* 1994; Sappa 1991; Smith *et al.* 1996; Tatman *et al.* 1992; While 1991). Many teams have made great efforts to address this issue, setting themselves very challenging targets for linking with and visiting general practices and primary health care teams, ensuring that GPs, health visitors and school nurses are notified of admissions and discharges from their caseloads and endeavouring to maintain links throughout an episode of care. Many have produced 'professional' information leaflets describing the services that they provide. As primary care trusts (PCTs) evolve the need to maintain sophisticated communication strategies between the CCN teams and the PCTs will be crucial. However, it would be wrong to underestimate the complexity of the task facing the CCN teams, given that many of them are likely to be providing services across three or more PCTs covering upwards of 50 different GPs (Whiting 1999).

In closing this discussion of the consumer perspective, it is important to acknowledge that the very great majority of evaluative research that has been undertaken in this area has focussed upon parental perception of the services. Only a small number of studies have sought to explore the opinions of children themselves (see for example the studies of Lauer & Camitta 1980 and Mulhern *et al.* 1983 in the USA and Jennings 1994; Smith *et al.* 1996 and While 1991, 1992 in the UK). However, in each of these small-scale studies, the response from children has been almost universally to express clear satisfaction with, and a definite preference for, home care.

The introduction of National Services Frameworks as a central component of the NHS Plan, has been accompanied by an explicit commitment to 'user involvement'. In respect of the Children's NSF, the development of the framework and the accompanying broader social policy framework of the Consultation Green Paper, 'Every Child Matters' (DfES 2003) and the government response to that consultation (DfES 2004) has involved a high level of engagement with both children and their parents. Community children's nursing teams will clearly need to demonstrate that the services they provide are the services that children and families want.

Fair access: Which children have access to CCN services?

The issue of fair access is complex, however, in terms of the provision of CCN services, it is possibly best expressed in a quote from the Health Select Committee (DoH 1997b),

'The overall intention must be to introduce as soon as possible a home nursing service provided by appropriately qualified staff and available to all children requiring home nursing and their families. For many years there has been such a service available to all adults in their own homes. We consider that as a matter of principle, sick children need and deserve no less.' (para. 49)

In the children's NSF, there is an explicit commitment that 'Inequalities will be reduced, so that all children and young people have access to the services they need, no matter where they live or where they come from.' (DoH/DfES 2004a, p. 2). The 'Ill child' module of the NSF is very specific about the need for consistent CCN services provision: 'Primary Care Trusts ensure that Community Children's Nursing Teams are available in each locality (as part of the Children's Community Teams) and are based on local need. Services are developed in an integrated way across the local health economy.' (DoH/DfES 2004b, p. 35).

The first NHS based CCN services were established in the 1950s (Gillet 1954; Lightwood 1956; Smellie 1956). In spite of the strong endorsement of both the Platt (Ministry of Health 1959) and Court (DHSS 1976) Reports – arguably the most influential reports on child health services in the first forty years of the NHS – by the end of 1988, there were still only 24 CCN teams (employing only 45 nurses) in the whole of England, with two services in Scotland and none at all in Northern Ireland or Wales (Whiting 1988). The 1990s, in particular, saw a dramatic growth in CCN provision both in terms of the numbers of teams and staff employed within those teams (RCN 2001), however, provision remains inconsistent, and, unlike the 'service for adults' referred to by the Health Select Committee (the district nursing service) there is no system for specifically monitoring service provision for children.

In evidence presented to the Health Select Committee by the Royal College of Nursing (RCN), and based upon the latest information available, it was suggested that CCN services were available in around half of the health authorities in England but that in only around 10% of the country was a service available 24 hours per day (RCN Paediatric Community Nurses Forum 1996). The RCN estimated that there were less than five hundred CCNs in the whole of the UK (compared to around 14 500 qualified nurse members of the district nursing service in England (NHSE 1996c). Some of the services described by the RCN in its evidence consisted of only one CCN providing a service across a whole community trust or district health authority, whereas other districts were served by a team of ten or more nurses. This clearly demonstrates significant inconsistency in provision. The Health Select Committee (DoH 1997b) concluded that there was 'no logical explanation for the disparities in provision' (p. xix) which this represents. It is, however, interesting to note that there has been much more service development in the large conurbations than in the more rural parts of the UK.

In the late 1960s, Robottom reviewed the provision of CCN services in Birmingham and suggested (with no specific rationale) a coverage of one nurse per 20 000 child population (Robottom 1969). A report based on questionnaire findings from 53 CCN services published in 1993 (Tatman & Woodroffe) noted a mean ratio of 4.9 nurses per 100 000 child population (approximately 1:20 000). The authors drew particular attention to their finding that there were 11 services of one whole time equivalent member or less and that larger and more well established services had a higher ratio of staff to child population.

In its evidence to the Health Select Committee, the RCN estimated that in order to provide a full range of services, a ratio of one nurse per 10 000 child population was required. The rationale behind this estimate was based upon four major assumptions:

- The first consideration is that the *skills required to confidently care for children with complex health needs at home are often quite sophisticated*. In consequence the level of support required by parents who choose to care for their child in the community is considerable (DoH 2000d; DoH 1997b; Whiting 1995).
- Balanced against this is the second assumption, which is that *parents will be taught to deliver much of the care to their own children* – in particular to children with complex and continuing care needs – this obviates, in many instances, the need for nurses to themselves provide 'hands-on' care on a day-by-day basis and is very much aligned with the philosophy of 'partnership' referred to earlier
- The third assumption is that the *demand for care in the community will increase*. This is a view supported by the Department of Health (NHSE 1996a), the British Paediatric Association (1993) and the Royal College of Nursing (1998). It is perhaps best illustrated by the growing population of children requiring long term respiratory support (ventilation) as identified by Jardine and Wallis (1998)
- The final strand of this argument establishes that *there is an agreed range of nursing care needs for which CCNs might provide*. This list draws upon research undertaken by the author in the late 1980s (Whiting 1988), that was included in the RCN evidence to the Health Select Committee and appears in slightly modified form within the Committee's Report:
  — Neonatal (and post-neonatal) care
  — Caring for children with acute paediatric nursing needs (Neill 2000a, b)

  — Supporting children undergoing planned surgery
  — Supporting children with long-term physical nursing needs
  — Follow-up of children who have required emergency treatment/care
  — Supporting the families of children with disability
  — Supporting families who are caring for children during the terminal phase of their lives

There are around 14 million children under the age of sixteen in the UK. Based upon the suggested ratio of one nurse per 10 000 children, this would require a working population of around 1400 CCNs, almost three times as many as were identified by the RCN in 1996. The most recent composite picture of CCN provision in the UK (RCN 2001) indicated wide variations in the size and composition of teams and the Children's NSF recognised that there remains a need for further development in CCN services in order to ensure that there is a sufficient pool of nurses to undertake the diversity of roles required of them. The 'ill child' module stated clearly 'Additional funding has been made available to increase capacity. Where these services are not in place locally, this funding can be used to develop them.' (DoH/DfES, 2004b, p. 35).

Health outcomes of NHS care: **Is home care safe?**

It is clearly essential that the provision of services to children and families in their own homes does not present additional clinical risks to those children. Any increases in morbidity (or mortality) represents an unacceptable tipping of the 'quality balance' away from community care. Indeed, it is important that home care should seek to 'reduce levels of disease, impairment and complications of treatment' (NHSE, 1998b, p. 64).

As noted earlier, it was the clear belief of many of the pioneers responsible for the development of CCN services in the UK that the provision of home nursing for children would reduce the potential psychological harm experienced by those children if they had remained in hospital for long periods. In addition, commentators on those early CCN services in particular suggested that they also offered the capacity to reduce the likelihood of hospital acquired infection (Atwell *et al*. 1973; Gillet 1954; Lightwood 1956). Although this would seem to have a sound logical basis, no specific research has been undertaken in this area to substantiate such claims. Unfortunately, research in this whole area of work is somewhat thin on the ground.

A number of small studies have looked at morbidity in babies discharged 'early' from Special Care Baby Units (e.g. Couriel & Davies 1988), children receiving home parenteral nutrition (e.g. Amarnath *et al*. 1987), youngsters with congenital dislocation of the hip (e.g. Joseph *et al*. 1982) and, more recently, children receiving home enteral nutrition in Birmingham (Holden *et al*. 1991). All have found home care to be safe when compared to hospital care, and have reported no significant deficit in clinical outcomes for children.

In 1985 Frates and colleagues published a retrospective review of the outcome of home ventilation in 54 children in Houston, Texas, USA. Over a twenty year period, seventeen children died including three as a result of disconnection from the ventilator. This group of technology dependant children clearly represent the very extreme of the range of complex medical and nursing needs for which home care and CCN provision might be appropriate. Bearing in mind the complexity of the children's needs, and considering that mortality in hospitalised long-term ventilator dependent children is a well recognised complication, the authors concluded 'Home mechanical ventilation may be a reasonably safe and cost-effective alternative to prolonged hospitalization for the ventilator-dependent child' (Frates *et al*. 1985, p. 850). In a recent statement on behalf of the UK Working Party on Paediatric Long Term Ventilation, Jardine and Wallis (1998) offered the following as the group's mission statement.

'The child with long term respiratory insufficiency who is stable medically can expect a better quality of life outside the environment of the acute hospital setting. Members are committed to measures which can facilitate this on a national basis.' (p. 762).

The technological support which is now available to support long-term ventilator dependent children at home has developed very significantly since the work of Frates and colleagues in the mid 1980s. Although there is no recent published data from the UK concerned specifically with the safety of home ventilation when compared to children receiving care in hospital, there is a strong belief that with strong case management and effective risk assessment strategies in place, the marginally increased risks associated with home care can be kept to an acceptable minimum (Jardine & Wallis 1998).

As the range of nursing needs for children who are being cared for in the community becomes ever greater, it is of crucial importance that services continue to demonstrate that potential morbidity amongst those children is minimised. In addition, although the absence of negative implications for children receiving care in the community is clearly an important factor, it is of equal importance that CCNs should demonstrate positive outcomes for the children in their care and not simply the absence of negative outcomes.

Health improvement: is it possible to identify positive clinical outcomes for children receiving services from CCNs?

As noted earlier, many CCN teams have set out to improve the psychological experience of children by facilitating the replacement of periods of hospital care with time at home (or in school or elsewhere). There is, however, very little published evidence to demonstrate improvements in the physical health of children by virtue of this change in the locus of care.

A number of possible indicators do exist. In 1992, the British Paediatric Association (BPA) published the second edition of the document 'Outcome measurements in child health'. In respect of two of the most common chronic diseases of children, the BPA offered the indicators in Box 11.4.

A number of small studies of CCN services have suggested improved compliance with asthma medication, and reduced incidence of readmission to hospital for children with asthma and diabetes, but the question of whether the

---
Box 11.4   Indicators for two of the most common chronic diseases of children. (British Paediatric Association 1992)

Asthma   *'The number of children admitted to hospital with a diagnosis of asthma remaining as in-patients for longer than 72 hours per 1000 population under 16 years of age.'*

Diabetes   *'The mean glycosylated haemoglobin value of the child diabetic population each year'*

          'The number of children with insulin dependent diabetes having a value of glycosylated haemoglobin more than 1.5 times the mean of the non-diabetic population as a proportion of all the children with insulin-dependent diabetes.'
---

children are actually clinically better or whether the CCN service simply provides an alternative method of care to admission to hospital remains unanswered. In addition, where CCNs have developed their practice in order to deal with populations of children experiencing specific diseases such as diabetes or asthma, other aspects of the child health services (such as specialist paediatricians or dedicated clinics for these children) have also developed alongside the 'specialist' CCN, and it is therefore very difficult indeed to demonstrate a clear 'cause and effect' relationship between CCN intervention and improved health of the children concerned.

In the team based in St George's Hospital, south London, a clinical nurse specialist (CNS) for children with diabetes was appointed in 1998. This appointment has allowed for the development of much closer titration of insulin doses as a result of improved home glucose monitoring. Glycosylated haemoglobin readings for a random sample of 10 out of the 72 children with diabetes on the CNSs caseload have shown a reduction from a mean of 9.2% to 8.74% between 1998 and 1999. Six of the ten children have shown a mean reduction of 1.2%, however three children have experienced a rise of

between 0.5 and 1.4% (two of these children are entering their pubertal growth spurt, during which glycaemic control is notoriously difficult, and the third child has recently developed an under-active thyroid gland which is recognised to affect glycaemic control). Whilst it would be tempting to suggest that a direct cause and effect relationship between the introduction of the CNS and the improvement in the health of the population of children with diabetes, it is important to acknowledge that other variables are also likely to have influenced events (Walker 2000).

Other possible indicators of health improvement might include: frequency of admission to hospital of children with cystic fibrosis, incidence of febrile neutropenia in children with acute lymphoblastic leukaemia, growth curves of children receiving TPN or gastrostomy feeding at home, global developmental progress in children who receive ventilator support in the community. All are worthy of further detailed investigation. In 2003, a comprehensive review of 'paediatric home care' was published by Parker and colleagues on behalf of the NHS research and development health technology assessment programme. Much of the focus of this very detailed review is related to the emergence of new health technologies in the context of more home based health care provision for children. The authors concluded 'despite increased provision, evidence about effectiveness, costs and impact remains elusive' (p. iii). Its recommendations were wide-ranging and advocated a clear need for an urgent and systematic review of many aspects of home care development, including community nursing provision for children (Parker *et al.* 2003).

Efficiency: can the question of resources and finance really be answered? Do CCNs prevent admission and facilitate discharge?

Many CCN teams have been established with a clear statement of intent that 'money will be saved' as a direct result of their work. The main argument behind such statements is based on the belief that, as a consequence of providing a nursing service to children in the community, children will spend less time in hospital. The average length of stay for all children in hospital

NORTHBROOK COLLEGE LIBRARY

in the UK has shown a steady and sustained decline over the last forty years (Audit Commission 1993). However, there is no evidence that this decline has been more marked in areas where CCNs are in place than in areas where no such services exist. Until very recently, this overall reduction in average length of stay has coincided with an equally steady increase in the numbers of children being admitted to hospital (Audit Commission 1993) – though it has been suggested that this year-on-year rise has now reached a plateau (DoH 2000d). Once again, there is no evidence to suggest that this increase has been any lower in areas with CCN services than those without.

Nationwide, over the last forty years, there has been a very significant overall reduction in the numbers of children's beds in hospital and the total number of children's wards. Between 1990 and 2000, there has been a reduction of approximately 12% of children's in-patient beds (DoH 2000d). However, it is not clear whether such bed reductions are greater in areas where CCN services have been established than in areas where they have not. A number of CCN services have, however, been introduced or expanded as part of an overall rationalisation or review of paediatric/child health services, as a consequence of which there has been an overall reduction in in-patient beds locally (for example in Haringey, Amersham, St Helens and Knowsley, Edgware and Nottingham). Dryden (1994) has suggested that over a ten year period, the facilitation of earlier discharge and prevention of some admissions arising from the work of the Nottingham CCN service has 'led to the closure of 16 beds.' It remains, however, an extremely complex task indeed to demonstrate a clear relationship between the availability of CCN services and the capacity to formally reduce in-patient bed provision.

Despite this, many commentators have argued that CCN availability keeps children out of hospital and a large number of studies have attempted to consider the potential monies that have been 'saved' by the introduction of a CCN service locally. Many have made claims of financial savings on the basis of multiplication of the numbers of 'bed-nights saved' by the actual cost of a hospital bed-night locally (for instance multiplying the cost of a hospital bed-night by the reduction in numbers of bed-nights occupied by children with femoral fractures who were nursed at home on traction). A summary of 11 studies published in both the UK and USA is included in Box 11.5.

Each of these studies is based upon the hypothetical realisation of savings from the reduction in occupied beds. However, simply keeping a child out of hospital does not necessarily result in an identifiable saving to the hospital and the use of this indicator to demonstrate financial savings significantly oversimplifies a very complex picture. The danger of using this methodology is perhaps best demonstrated in the study by Kahn who suggested in 1984 that four million dollars was saved over a four year period for ten children nursed at home rather than in hospital. Unfortunately the author offers no comment on how the transfer of these children to the community influenced expenditure on care in the local hospitals.

As Edwards (2000) observes such savings for the hospital ought not to be assumed because at least 80% of the cost per day arises from overheads which do not disappear simply because the patient has been transferred to the community.

'It is necessary to stop very large amounts of activity before a radiology room, anaesthetic team or trust manager can be dispensed with. Savings from the cost of nursing are similarly problematic. Even if there are 10–12 fewer patients it is still necessary to have two to three nurses on a night shift to make sure that patients are safe.'

(Edwards 2000, p. 28)

Parker and colleagues (2003) reviewed much of the literature on the economics of home care, including neonatal 'early discharge', oxygen dependent babies, children with newly diagnosed diabetes, home intravenous therapy and home haemodialysis. Although they found some

Box 11.5	Summary of 11 studies			
Author(s)	Date of Publication	Location	Estimated Saving	Detail
Bergman *et al.*	1965	Paddington, London, UK	'one third of equivalent hospital costs'	Estimated cost per case of $53.20 based on 237 referrals in 1963/4
Moldow *et al.*	1982	Minnesota, USA	$157 per day per child	Comparison of costs for two matched samples of 11 children dying at home or in hospital
Burr *et al.*	1983	Massachusetts, USA	$11 000 to $75 000 per year per child	Study of six ventilator-dependent children
Kahn	1984	Illinois, USA	$4 000 000 total	10 ventilator-dependent children over four year period
May	1984	Miami, USA	$200 per day per child	Study of 10 children receiving home IV therapy for an average of 18.2 days rather than in-hospital care
Atwell & Gow	1985	Southampton, UK	£215 000 total	Estimated saving based on reduced demand for in-patient stay by the provision CCN follow-up of day case patients
Brooten *et al.*	1986	Philadelphia, USA	$18 560 per infant	Based on facilitated early discharge of 39 very low birth weight infants discharged from SCBU on average 11 days earlier than a matched control sample
Couriel & Davies	1988	Manchester, UK	£250 000 total	Estimate based on reduced average length of stay in special care baby unit for 337 babies
While	1991	Greenwich, London, UK	£85 900 total	Based on an estimated saving in 1990 of 573 in-patient nights and 278 ward visits
Bosanquet *et al.*	1994	Haringey, UK	£245 000	'Minimum saving' based on avoidance of one admission per patient for 275 patients on CCN caseload with previous 'admission history'
Smith *et al.*	1996	Basingstoke, UK	£10 368 per annum	Based on home management of children with newly diagnosed diabetes compared with average eight-day diagnostic admission prior to 1991

evidence of financial savings for both health care providers and for the families of children with health problems, their overall view was that costing methods employed by many researchers were methodologically weak.

Avoiding admission and facilitating earlier discharge

As noted earlier, admission rates of children to UK hospitals increased steadily from the late 1950s up to the mid 1990s. However, as long ago as

1954, when the Paddington Home Care Team was established, it was estimated that as many as 30% of admissions could have been avoided if trained nursing and medical staff were available to care for the children at home (Lightwood 1956). It is interesting to note, therefore, that the provision of CCN services as an alternative to admission to hospital for acutely ill children is something that few CCN teams seem to provide, even though many claim that it is what they are seeking to do (Bosanquet *et al*. 1994; Fradd 1992; Smith *et al*. 1996; Tatman & Woodroffe 1993).

A notable exception to this is the BHB team who provide a '24 hour' visiting service. Part of the team's work involves the provision of a home visiting/nebuliser service for children with asthma. During 1999 the team undertook 325 'urgent call-out' visits to children with asthma, a service that is offered as an alternative to GP call out or accident and emergency attendance. As Hill observed in 1989, one of the most significant contributory diagnoses in the rising paediatric admission rate in recent years has been acute respiratory tract problems and in particular asthma. Without doubt, many of the children seen by the BHB team would have been admitted to hospital if the service had not been available (Green 2000).

To date, the major work of CCNs in avoiding admission is in the care of children with chronic illness, where quality might be considered in terms of reductions in *readmissions* for children with a range of problems including, for example, neonates being discharged early from special care baby units, or of children with asthma, diabetes, cystic fibrosis, congenital cardiac disease, nephrotic syndrome and cancer. For children with problems such as these, it might be possible to facilitate the avoidance of read-mission to hospital by a combination of activities including:

- The undertaking, in the community by nurses and parents, of technical care procedures which might otherwise require the child to be admitted to hospital
- Equipping parents with the necessary confidence, support mechanisms, equipment etc.

to allow them to care for their child at home at times when they might otherwise seek readmission
- Improving compliance with prescribed medical regimes and health behaviours

(See for example Whiting (1991) for a detailed examination of the role of the CCN in caring for a young child with asthma.)

It is, however very difficult indeed to quantify what doesn't happen, i.e. non-readmission. For CCNs to be able to demonstrate that they can make a difference in this regard, will, therefore require very careful and detailed analysis at both the individual and population level.

Facilitation of discharge is perhaps the area where CCNs might be considered to be having the greatest impact. A number of studies have described the success of CCNs in this area including:

- Neonates being discharged early from special care baby units (Hughes & Collins 1998; Sleath 1989)
- Early discharge or avoidance of admission altogether of children with newly diagnosed diabetes (McEvilly 1991)
- Home management of children with femoral fractures (Clayton 1997)
- Care of children with cystic fibrosis who require supplementary enteral feeding or who have acute respiratory tract infections (Sidey 1998)
- Caring for children who are dying at home (Beardsmore & Alder 1994; Farrell & Allen 1998)
- Provision of community follow-up to children who have undergone day surgery (Atwell & Gow 1985).

In order to achieve both reductions in admission and early discharge, it is absolutely vital that a comprehensive CCN service is available. In the final section of this chapter, consideration will be give to what might constitute such a service.

Effective delivery of appropriate health care
At the heart of the drive to improve quality within the 'New NHS' is the key role to be played by National Service Frameworks in defining,

driving and monitoring of standards for identified care groups (NHSE 1998b). Care should be 'Clinically effective, evidence-based, appropriate to need, timely, in line with agreed standards, provided according to best practice and delivered by appropriately trained and educated staff.' (DoH 1998, p. 64).

The children's NSF (DoH/DfES 2004a) sets out clearly what the Government is seeking to achieve for children over the next ten years:

- All children and young people achieving the best possible physical and emotional health and well-being, both in childhood and into adulthood
- Children, young people and families supported and able to make healthy choices in how they live their lives
- A measurable reduction in inequality of health outcomes for children and young people
- Integrated services that provide effective checks and more targeted support for children and young people who need it

The 11 Key standards of the National Services Framework are included in the Appendix.

In concluding this chapter, and based upon the forgoing examination of the extent to which CCNs are 'delivering on the quality agenda', the following list represents a series of standards against which CCN services might be monitored in determining whether children are receiving services that support these aspirations:

- When caring for a child with complex or continuing health care needs at home, parents should have access to a Registered Children's Nurse 24 hours per day to provide advice, support and care in their home
- CCN service should be subjected to regular audit including:
  — Surveying of the views of users of the service, to include parents, children and health care professionals
  — Risk assessment exercises, monitoring and seeking to minimise the possibility of adverse events or outcomes arising from the work of the CCN service
  — Evaluation and measurement (long-term and short-term) against pre-set criteria in order to identify possible positive clinical outcomes for children in receipt of the service
  — Evaluation of the impact of the service upon activity within hospital in-patient, out-patient and A&E departments as well as in primary health care
- Each child should be allocated a named nurse who is qualified both as a Registered Children's Nurse and a Community Children's Nurse
- When children are admitted to hospital and referral to the CCN team is anticipated, hospital and community based nursing staff should maintain effective on-going communication throughout the period of care in hospital and at the point of discharge
- When children are referred to the CCN service, the child and family should be advised of the referral in advance, and, where appropriate, the family should participate in the referral decision
- Each family should be provided with written information giving details of how to make contact with the CCN as and when necessary
- Each child should have a written plan of care which has been negotiated, agreed and signed by the nurse, parent and (where appropriate) the child
- General practitioners, health visitors and school nurses should be notified either by telephone or in writing of a referral to a CCN service within three working days of the child's first visit. Telephone notifications should be followed up in writing within five working days
- When children are cared for in the community, arrangements for the provision of any necessary equipment should be made at the earliest opportunity. All professionals should be clear about their individual responsibilities in ensuring continuity of supply

Appendix

National Service Framework for children, young people and maternity services (DoH 2004)

PART I – Core Standards

Standard 1: Promoting Health and Well-being, Identifying Needs and Intervening Early

The health and well-being of all children and young people is promoted and delivered through a co-ordinated programme of action, including prevention and early intervention wherever possible, to ensure long-term gain, led by the NHS in partnership with local authorities.

Standard 2: Supporting parents or carers

Parents or carers are enabled to receive the information, services and support which will help them to care for their children and equip them with the skills they need to ensure that their children have optimum life chances and are healthy and safe.

Standard 3: Child, Young Person and Family-Centred Services

Children and young people and families receive high quality services which are coordinated around their individual and family needs and take account of their views.

Standard 4: Growing Up into Adulthood

All young people have access to age-appropriate services which are responsive to their specific needs as they grow into adulthood.

Standard 5: Safeguarding and Promoting the Welfare of Children and Young People

All agencies work to prevent children suffering harm and to promote their welfare, provide them with the services they require to address their identified needs and safeguard children who are being or who are likely to be harmed.

PART II

Standard 6: Children and Young People who are Ill

All children and young people who are ill, or thought to be ill, or injured will have timely access to appropriate advice and to effective services which address their health, social, educational and emotional needs throughout the period of their illness.

Standard 7: Children in Hospital

Children and young people receive high quality, evidence-based hospital care, developed through clinical governance and delivered in appropriate settings.

Standard 8: Disabled Children and Young People and Those with Complex Health Needs

Children and young people who are disabled or who have complex health needs receive co-ordinated, high quality child- and family-centred services which are based on assessed needs, which promote social inclusion and, where possible, which enable them and their families to live ordinary lives.

Standard 9: The Mental Health and Psychological Well-being of Children and Young People

All children and young people, from birth to their eighteenth birthday, who have mental health problems and disorders have access to timely, integrated, high quality multidisciplinary mental health services to ensure effective assessment, treatment and support, for them, and their families.

Standard 10: Medicines Management for Children

Children, young people, their parents or carers, and health care professionals in all settings make decisions about medicines based on sound information about risk and benefit. They have access to safe and effective medicines that are prescribed on the basis of the best available evidence.

PART III

Standard 11: Maternity Services

Women have easy access to supportive, high quality maternity services, designed around their individual needs and those of their babies.

References

Amarnath, R.P., Fleming, C.R. & Perrault, J. (1987) Home parenteral nutrition in chronic intestinal disease: its effects on growth and development. *Journal of Pediatric Gastroenterology and Nutrition*, **6**, 89–95.

Atwell, J., Burn, J.M.B., Dewar, A.K. & Freeman, N.V. (1973) Paediatric day-case surgery. *The Lancet.* October 20th, 895–897.

Atwell, J. & Gow, M. (1985) Paediatric trained district nurse in the community: expensive luxury or economic necessity? *British Medical Journal*, **291**, 227–229.

Audit Commission (1993) *Children First: a study of hospital services*. HMSO, London.

Beardsmore, S. & Alder, S. (1994) Terminal care at home: the practical issues. In: *Caring for dying children and their families*, Hill L. (ed). Chapman Hall, London.

Bergman, A.B., Shrand, H. & Oppe, T. (1965) A pediatric home care programme in London: ten years experience. *Pediatrics*, **36**(3), 314–321.

Bosanquet, N., Connoly, M., Hart, D. & Dzapasi, L. (1994) *Paediatric nursing service – North Middlesex Hospital: integrating the A&E department service for children with the paeditric home care nursing service*. Health Policy Unit, Department of General Practice, Lisson Grove Health Centre, London.

Bowlby, J. (1951) *Maternal care and mental health*. Monograph series number 2, World Health Organization, Geneva.

British Paediatric Association (1992) *Outcome measurements for child health* (2nd edn). BPA, London.

British Paediatric Association (1993) *Flexible options for paediatric care: a discussion document*. BPA, London.

Brooten, D., Kumar, S., Brown, L.P., Butts, P., Finkler, S.A., Barkwell-Sachs, S., Gibbons, A. & Delivoria-Papadopoulos, M. (1986) A randomised clinical trial of early hospital discharge and home care, follow-up of very-low-birth-weight infants. *The New England Journal of Medicine*, **315**, 934–939.

Burr, B.H., Guyer, B., Todres, I.P., Abrahma, B. & Chiodo, T. (1983) Home care for children on respirators. *New England Journal of Medicine*, **309**(21), 1319–1323.

Casey, A. (1995) Partnership nursing: influences on involvement of informal carers. *Journal of Advanced Nursing*, **22**, 1058–1062.

Cash, K., Compston, H., Grant, J., Livesley, J., McAndrew, P. & Williams, G. (1994) *The preparation of sick children's nurses to work in the community (P2000) evaluation*. English National Board, London.

Clayton, M. (1997) Traction at home: the Doncaster approach. *Paediatric Nursing*, **9**(2), 21–23.

Couriel, J.M. & Davies, P. (1988) Costs and benefits of a community special care baby service. *British Medical Journal*, **296**, 1043–1046.

Department of Health and Social Security (1976) *Fit for the future. The report of the Committee on child health services*. HMSO, London.

Department of Health (1989a) *Working for Patients*. HMSO, London.

Department of Health (1989b) *Caring for People: Community Care in the Next Decade and Beyond*. HMSO, London.

Department of Health (1991) *The Welfare of Children and Young People in Hospital*. HMSO, London.

Department of Health (1993) *Making London Better*. HMSO, London.

Department of Health (1997a) *The New NHS: Modern, Dependable*. The Stationery Office, London.

Department of Health (1997b) *Government response to the Report of the Health Committee on Health Services for Children and Young People, session 1996–97*: 'The specific health needs of children and young people' (307–1); 'Health services for children in the community, home and school' (314–1); 'Hospital services for children and young people' (128–1); 'Child and adolescent mental health' (26–1). The Stationery Office, London.

Department of Health (1998) *A First Class Service: Quality in the New NHS*. DoH, London.

Department of Health (1999) *Making A Difference*. DoH, London.

Department of Health (2000a) *The NHS Plan: a Plan for Investment, a Plan for Reform*. The Stationery Office, London.

Department of Health (2000b) *The NHS Plan: an Action Guide for Nurses, Midwives and Health Visitors*. DoH, London.

Department of Health (2000c) *National Census Day* (DoH Press Release 2000/0317). DoH, London.

Department of Health (2000d) *Shaping the Future NHS: Long term Planning for Hospitals and Related Services. Consultation document on the findings of the National Beds Enquiry – supporting analysis*. DoH, London.

Department of Health (2002a) *Liberating the Talents: Helping Primary Care Trusts and Nurses to Deliver the NHS Plan*. DoH, London.

Department of Health (2002b) *Delivering the NHS Plan*. DoH, London.

Department of Health (2004a) *The Chief Nursing Officer's Review of the Nursing, Midwifery and Health Visiting Contribution to Vulnerable Children and Young People*. DoH, London.

Department of Health/Department for Education and Skills (2004a) *National Service Framework for Children, Young People and Maternity Services: Core Standards*. DoH, London.

Department of Health/Department for Education and Skills (2004b) *National Service Framework for Children, Young People and Maternity Services: Ill Child.* DoH, London.

Department of Health/Department for Education and Skills (2004c) *National Service Framework for Children, Young People and Maternity Services: Disabled Child.* DoH, London.

Department for Education and Skills (2003) *Every Child Matters.* The Stationery Office, London.

Department for Education and Skills (2004) *Every Child Matters: Next Steps.* The Stationery Office, London.

Dryden, S. (1994) The Nottingham paediatric community nursing service. *Cascade,* **13**, 8–9.

Edwards, N. (2000) Primary Care Trusts: Barrier Grief. *Health Service Journal,* **110**(5696), 28–29.

Farrell, M. & Allen, S. (1998) Hospice at home: our first year. *Paediatric Nursing,* **10**(7), 18–20.

Fradd, E. (1992) Working with the specialists. *Community Outlook,* **2**(6), 29–30.

Frates, R.C., Splaingard, M.L., Smith, E.O. & Harrison, G.M. (1985) Outcome of home mechanical ventilation in children. *Journal of Pediatrics,* **86**, 850–856.

Freeland, A.M. & Munro, K.M. (1995) All part of the service: an audit of follow-up care after day surgery. *Child Health,* **3**(4), 154–158.

Gillet, J.A. (1954) Children's nursing unit. *British Medical Journal,* **i**, 684–685.

Great Ormond Street Hospital for Children NHS Trust (1996) *Quality quest: standards 1995–1996.* Hospital for Children NHS Trust, London.

Green, A. (2000) *Audit data from the Barking, Havering and Brentwood Children's Home Care Team 1995–1999 (BHB).* Personal Communication.

Gould, C. (1996) Multiple partnerships in the community. *Paediatric Nursing,* **8**(8), 27–31.

Gow, M. & Campbell, C. (1996) Paediatric community nursing: doctor's views. *Professional Nurse,* **11**(6), 365–367.

Hill, A. (1989) Trends in paediatric medical admissions. *British Medical Journal,* **298**(6686), 1479–1481.

Hogg, C. (1996) *Health services for children and young people.* Action for Sick Children, London.

Hogg, C. (1997) *Emergency health services for children and young people.* Action for Sick Children, London.

Hogg, C. (1998) *Child friendly primary health care.* Action for Sick Children, London.

Holden, C.E., Puntis, J.W.L., Charlton, C.P.L. & Booth, I.W. (1991) Nasogastric feeding at home: acceptability and safety. *Archives of Disease in Childhood,* **66**, 148–151.

House of Commons Health Select Committee (1997) *Health Services for Children and Young People in the Community, Home and School (third report).* The Stationery Office, London.

Hughes, J. & Collins, P. (1998) Neonatal nursing in the community. *Paediatric Nursing,* **10**(1), 18–20.

Hunt, J. & Whiting, M. (1999) A re-examination of the history of children's community nursing. *Paediatric Nursing.* **11**(4), 33–36.

Jardine, E. & Wallis, C. (1998) Core guidelines for the discharge home of children on long term assisted ventilation in the United Kingdom. *Thorax,* **53**, 762–767.

Jefferson, H. & Gow, M.A. (1995) *Paediatric Community Nursing Standards*: Southampton. Southampton Community Health Services.

Jennings, P. (1994) Learning from experience: an evaluation of 'Hospital at Home'. *Journal of Advanced Nursing,* **19**, 905–911.

Joseph, K., MacKewan, G.D. & Boos, M.L. (1982) Home traction in the management of congenital dislocation of the hip. *Clinical Orthopaedics and Related Research,* **165**, 83–90.

Kahn, L. (1984) Ventilator-dependent children heading home. *Hospitals,* March 1st, 54–55.

Kelly, P.J., Taylor, C. & Tatman, M.A. (1994) Hospital outreach or community nursing. *Child Health,* **2**(4), 160–163.

Lauer, M.E. & Camitta, B.M. (1980) Home care for the dying child: a nursing model. *Journal of Pediatrics,* **97**(6), 1032–1035.

Lightwood, R. (1956) The home care of sick children. *Practitioner,* **177**, 10–14.

Marland, J. (1994) Back where they belong: caring for sick children at home. *Child Health,* **2**(1), 40–42.

May, C. (1984) Antibiotic therapy at home. *American Journal of Nursing,* March, 348–349.

McEvilly, A. (1991) Home management on diagnosis. *Paediatric Nursing,* **3**(5), 16–18.

Ministry of Health (1959) *The welfare of children in hospital: report of the Committee.* HMSO, London.

Moldow, D.G., Armstrong, G.D., Henry, W.F. & Martinson, I.M. (1982) The cost of home care for dying children. *Medical Care,* **20**(11), 1154–1160.

Mulhern, R.K., Lauer, M.E. & Hoffman, R.G. (1983) Death of a child in the hospital or at home: subsequent psychological adjustment of the family. *Pediatrics,* **71**(5), 743–747.

National Association for the Welfare of Children in Hospital (NAWCH) (1984) *Charter for Children in Hospital*. NAWCH, London.

National Association for the Welfare of Children in Hospital (1987) *Quality Checklist: caring for children in hospital*. NAWCH, London.

National Association for the Welfare of Children in Hospital (1989) *Setting Standards for Children in Health Care*. NAWCH, London.

National Health Service Executive (1996a) *The Patient's Charter: services for children and young people*. The Stationery Office, London.

National Health Service Executive (1996b) *Child Health in the Community: a guide to good practice*. The Stationery Office, London.

National Health Service Executive (1996c) *Primary Care: the future*. The Stationery Office, London.

National Health Service Executive (1998a) *Evaluation of the Pilot Project Programme for Children with Life Threatening Illness*. The Stationery Office, London.

National Health Service Executive (1998b) *National Service Frameworks*. The Stationery Office, London.

National Health Service Executive (1999) *Clinical Governance: in the New NHS*. The Stationery Office, London.

Neill, S. (2000a) Caring for the acutely ill child at home. In: *Textbook of Community Children's Nursing*. J. Muir & A. Sidey, Baillière Tindall, Edinburgh.

Neill, S. (2000b) Acute childhood illness at home: the parent's perspective. *Journal of Advanced Nursing*, **31**(4), 821–32.

Øvretveit, J. (1992) *Health Services Quality: an introduction to quality methods for health services*. Blackwell Science, Oxford.

Parker, G., Bhakta, P., Lovett, C.A., Paisley, S., Olsen, R., Turner, D. & Young, B. (2003) A systematic review of the costs and effectiveness of different models of paediatric home care. *Health Technology Assessment*, **6**, 35.

Proctor, S., Biott, C., Campbell, S., Edward, S., Redpath, N. & Moran, M. (1998) *Preparation for the Developing Role of the Community Children's Nurse*. English National Board, London.

Robertson, J. (1953) *A Two Year Old Goes to Hospital*. Tavistock, London.

Robertson, J. (1958) *Young Children in Hospital*. Tavistock, London.

Robottom, B. (1969) The contribution of the children's nurse to the home care of children. *British Journal of Medical Education*, **3**(4), 311–12.

Royal College of Nursing (1989) *Standards of Care: a framework for quality*. RCN, London.

Royal College of Nursing (1998) *Buying Children's Community Nursing*. RCN, London.

Royal College of Nursing Society of Paediatric Nursing (1990) *Standards of Care: paediatric nursing*. RCN, London.

Royal College of Nursing Society of Paediatric Nursing (1994) *Standards of Care: paediatric nursing*, 2nd edn. RCN, London.

Royal College of Nursing Paediatric Community Nurses Forum (1996) *Evidence submitted to the House of Commons Health Select Committee*. RCN, London.

Royal College of Nursing (2001) *Directory of Community Children's Nursing Services*, 15th edn. RCN, London.

Royal Hospital for Sick Children, Edinburgh (1987) *Standards of Paediatric Nursing*. Lothian Health Board, Edinburgh.

Sappa, M., Newton, J. & Morey, J. (1990) *Standards of care for the Paediatric Community Nursing Team*. Waltham Forest Health Authority, Unpublished.

Sappa, M. (1991) *There's no place like home: a report on a survey of users of the Waltham Forest Paediatric Community Nursing Team*. Waltham Forest Health Authority, Unpublished.

Sidey, A. (1998) CF and me. *Paediatric Nursing*, **10**(7), 21–2.

Sleath, K. (1989) Breath of life. *Nursing Times*, **85**(44), 31–3.

South West Thames Regional Health Authority (1990) *Paediatric Standards of Care*. SWTRHA, London.

Smellie, J.M. (1956) Domiciliary nursing service for infants and children. *British Medical Journal*, **i**, 256.

Smith, J., Hughes, A. & Wiles, R. (1996) *Loddon NHS Community Trust paediatric community nursing team – service evaluation*. College of Health, London.

Tatman, M.A., Woodroffe, C., Kelly, P.J. & Harris, R.J. (1992) Paediatric home care in Tower Hamlets: a partnership with parents. *Quality in Health Care*, **1**, 98–103.

Tatman, M.A. & Woodroffe, C. (1993) Paediatric home care in the UK. *Archives of Disease in Childhood*, **69**, 677–80.

Taylor, J. (2000) Partnership in the community and hospital: a comparison. *Paediatric Nursing*, **12**(5), 28–30.

The Children Act 2004. TSO, London.

The Hospital for Sick Children (1880) *The 28th Report of the Hospital for Sick Children, Great Ormond Street*. Folkard & Sons, Bloomsbury.

Torr, G. & Peter, S. (1996) Paediatric hospital at home: the first year. *Paediatric Nursing*, **8**(5), 20–23.

United Kingdom Central Council for Nursing, Midwifery and Health Visiting (1999) *Professional self-regulation and clinical governance*. UKCC, London.

Walker, A. (2000) *Audit data from the St George's Children's Community Nursing Service (StG)*. Personal Communication.

While, A.E. (1991) An evaluation of a paediatric home care team. *Journal of Advanced Nursing*, **16**, 1413–1421.

While, A.E. (1992) Consumer views of health care: a comparison of hospital and home care. *Child Care Health and Development*, **18**, 107–116.

While, A.E., Citrone, C. & Cornish, J. (1996) *A study of the needs and provisions for families caring for children with life limiting incurable disorders*. King's College, London.

Whiting, M. (1988) *Community paediatric nursing in England in 1988*. Unpublished MSc Thesis, University of London.

Whiting, M. (1991) Caring for children with asthma using Orem's self-care model. In: (ed) *Caring for children: towards partnership with families*, A.E. While. Edward Arnold, Kent.

Whiting, M. (1995) Nursing children in the community. In: *Whaley and Wong's Children's Nursing*, S. Campbell & E.A. Glasper. Mosby, London.

Whiting, M. (1999) Communty children's nursing. In: (ed) *Current issues in community nursing (2): Specialist practice in primary health care*, J. Littlewood. Churchill Livingstone, Edinburgh.

Whiting, M. (2000) 1888–1988: 100 Years of community children's nursing. In: *Community children's nursing*, J. Muir & A. Sidey (eds). Bailliere Tindall, Edinburgh.

Whyte, D.A., Barton, M.E., Lamb, A., Magennis, C., Mallinsong, A., Marshall, L. *et al.* (1998) Clinical effectiveness in community children's nursing. *Clinical Effectiveness in Nursing*, **2**(3), 139–144.

Chapter 12 **School Nursing**

Val Thurtle and Anne Akamo

School nursing is one of the longest established groups within the family of community nursing, working with a defined population that is important both now and for the future. Despite their significance, school nurses have been invisible for much of their history and not afforded the same status as their community health nursing colleagues. This chapter seeks to examine some of the functions of the school nurse and review the position of school nursing in the 21st century. The government's renewed emphasis on public health, as well as the continued interest in children and young people, has provided all those who promote health in the school-aged population with the potential to raise their profile. This opportunity requires all those involved in this field of employment to clarify the effectiveness of their work and make their interventions far more widely known than is currently the case.

Children as the future

Throughout recent history children and young people have been recognised as important both for the present and more significantly for the future. Their education has been regarded as an area for investment for the workforce and the nation's security. Additionally, diseases of adulthood and emotional problems have increasingly been found to have their origins in early life (Blair *et al*. 2003; Townsend *et al*. 1992).

The development of the school health service in 1907 was seen as a way of promoting the positive health of the future population. This has continued with more recent initiatives such as *Health of the Young Nation* (DoH 1995) and the *Healthy School Standard* (DfEE 1999). The increasing interest and concern with the health and well-being of children throughout the twentieth century is not a concern specific to the UK. Whilst it is evidenced in the Children Act 1989 and the Children Act 2004, this theme is

also highlighted in the United Nations Convention on the Rights of the Child (1991).

Education high on agenda

The education of children and young people has been given prominence in recent government agendas and both health and education have been the remit of different government departments which, together with social services, are concerned with the welfare of children (Mayall & Storey 1998). The development of children's trusts (DfES 2003a) integrating education, social services and some health services, may take this further. From the educational perspective, the development of the national curriculum, standard attainment tasks (SATs) and changes in the inspection system have put the spotlight on the academic achievements of schools. Attention paid by parents and estate agents to these school scores and league tables has led to the fear that there is an over-emphasis on 'academic' attainment. This had placed extra stress on teaching staff and pupils influencing their current and future mental health. Recent changes include interest in the 'value added' input of the school to the child's attainment, the move to more creativity in the curriculum (DfES 2003b), partnership beyond the classroom (DfES 2002a), and concern with children's emotional well-being. This requires all professionals concerned with children and young people to take a holistic approach to promoting their health.

Health and education are linked. Education influences a person's position in the work place, which influences his or her health outcomes (DoH 1998a). The Department of Education (1997) White Paper *Excellence in Schools* referred to 'good education as a lifeline for children on the wrong side of the health divide' (p. 63). On the opposite side of the coin, the child who is wrestling with health difficulties and marked inequalities is unlikely to make the best use of educational opportunities.

Emphasis on public health for school health

Public health is not a new idea; it came to the fore in the nineteenth century and contributed to the development of the school health service. The end of the twentieth century saw its re-emergence in a different form, with an emphasis on a population approach, active involvement of communities and addressing of inequalities. Further development of this and its outworking on government policy is discussed in Chapter 2.

Saving Lives: Our Healthier Nation (DoH 1999b) highlighted the public health role of the school nurse. Kuss *et al.* (1997) argue that public health nursing involves community empowerment, working with communities, families and individuals to achieve prevention of illness, promotion and protection of health and a developing concern with the environmental conditions surrounding a population. This involves working in partnership with children and young people and their families. The practical implications of this require school nurses to go beyond working with individual children and specific schools, and to work collaboratively with community groups and organisations. The coming of primary care trusts strengthened the opportunity to do this, allowing health care services to be delivered by a variety of health workers who are involved with children and young people. Such an approach requires that health needs be assessed, both on an individual and group basis, and steps be taken to meet them through inter-agency working (DoH 2003; Dooris 2004). Families, teachers and other staff should be involved in this process, but the school nurse for whom health is a priority will often be the team leader and 'driver' in ensuring that health needs are identified and responded to.

Examples of such a co-ordinated approach can be seen in the Healthy Schools programme announced in partnership with *Our Healthier Nation* (DoH 1998c) the *National Healthy School Standard* (DfEE 1999) and the *Healthy Living*

Blueprint for Schools (DfES 2004a). In particular schools or geographical areas, action might be realised through the design and implementation of programmes that encourage physical activity, promote a positive diet and seek to reduce the incidence of smoking or stress. The school nurse might also consider risk reducing activities in the health skills programme as well as incorporating citizenship and personal and social education, and in so doing integrate health related issues into the national curriculum.

The focus of *Saving Lives* (DoH 1999b) encouraged all schools to become 'healthy' schools, characterising the principle that 'good health and social behaviour underpin effective learning and academic achievement which in turn promote long term health gain' (p. 46). The accent that *Saving Lives* placed on the promotion of the concept of community highlighted the school nurse's role within the wider neighbourhood, which also makes up a significant component of the young person's life. Public sector legislation since 1997 has promoted the concept of 'joined up thinking', through the development of partnerships between health-related agencies and government departments. Education and health staff need to liaise and develop a corporate agenda, which many are already doing at both school and strategic level. This is reflected in the *Healthy Schools Standard* (DfEE 1999) and in the links with government targets to reduce heart disease and stroke, accidents, cancer, mental ill health and child ill health (DoH 1998c, 1999c, 2000a, 2003).

Other roles government departments take in relation to public health include issues such as the control of drugs and alcohol, fluoridation of water, road safety, improved housing and leisure facilities. To strengthen the public health approach, ongoing development of skills is required as outlined in *Skills for Health* (2004).

The development and implementation of the public health role of the school nurse has been much discussed. It was pointed out in *Making a Difference* (DoH 1999a) that school nurses play 'a vital role in equipping young people with the knowledge to make healthy lifestyle choices' (p. 13). This highlighted the proactive nature of their work rather than merely responding to ill health and developmental difficulties. The document advised that school nurses, taking a public health role and leading teams of nurses and community and education workers were expected to:

- Assess the health needs of children and school communities, agree individual and school health plans and deliver these through multi-disciplinary partnerships
- Play a key role in immunisation and vaccination programmes
- Contribute to personal and health and social education and to citizenship training
- Work with parents to promote positive parenting
- Offer support and counselling, promoting positive mental health in young people
- Advise and co-ordinate health care to children with medical needs

Building on this, *Saving Lives* (DoH 1999b) highlighted that school nurses are public health practitioners with a specific role in the healthy school programme, tackling teenage pregnancy and working with families. It suggested that school nurses could provide advice and help regarding personal relationships and stress management. They could also advise on risk taking behaviours thereby providing a safety net for all, especially the most disadvantaged who had not received a comprehensive child health service before school entry. The school-nursing role was seen as needing further development to enable them to lead teams and assess the health needs of individuals and school communities. The resultant findings would be used to develop and agree health plans and to develop multi-disciplinary partnerships with a variety of professionals including teachers, general practitioners, health visitors and young peoples' mental health practitioners, in order to implement health care strategies. The adoption of these functions would enable the school nursing team to engage in a range of health improvement activities as indicated in Box 12.1. Much of this has been in evidence.

The practice development pack for school nurses (DoH 2001a) (see Figure 12.1) shows how

a continuum of public health, with concern for individuals through to communities, could be implemented.

Many would argue that school nurses with a focus on groups of children in schools have always had public health at the fore while others call for more activity with individual children with specific health needs or disabilities. School nursing within the public health agenda (DeBell & Jackson 2000), a shared document published by the three key professional organisations, outlined school nurses' responsibilities in promoting healthy lifestyles and healthy schools. It also drew attention to the school nurses' role in promoting health in childhood and adolescence and managing chronic and complex health care needs in children and young people. The school nurse, as a specialist practitioner nurse in the UK setting, has the multiple roles of clinician, health

---

Box 12.1 School nursing teams' health improvement activities

School nursing teams' health improvement activities to include:

- Immunisation and vaccination
- Support and advice to school staff on a range of child health issues
- Support to children with medical needs
- Support and counselling to promote positive mental health in young people
- Personal health and social education programme and citizenship training
- Identification of social care needs, including the need of protection from abuse
- Advice on relationships and sex education building on clinical experience and pastoral role
- Liaison between schools, primary care groups and special services in meeting the health and social care needs of children
- Contribution to the identification of children's special educational needs
- Work with parents and young people alongside health visitors to promote parenting

Saving Lives: Our Healthier Nation,
p. 134–135 (DoH 1999b)

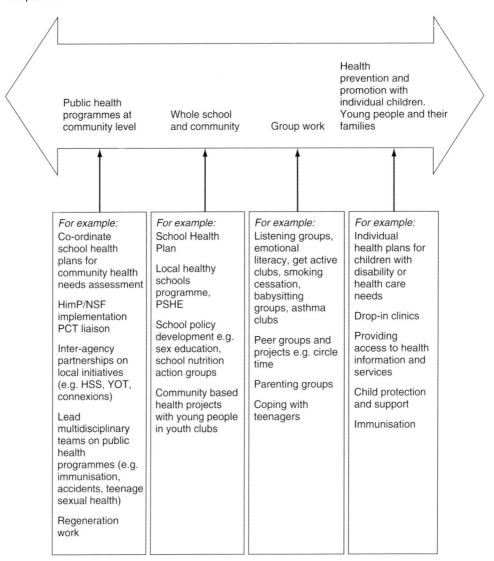

For example:
Co-ordinate
school health
plans for
community health
needs assessment

HimP/NSF
implementation
PCT liaison

Inter-agency
partnerships on
local initiatives
(e.g. HSS, YOT,
connexions)

Lead
multidisciplinary
teams on public
health
programmes (e.g.
immunisation,
accidents, teenage
sexual health)

Regeneration
work

For example:
School Health
Plan

Local healthy
schools
programme,
PSHE

School policy
development e.g.
sex education,
school nutrition
action groups

Community based
health projects
with young people
in youth clubs

For example:
Listening groups,
emotional
literacy, get active
clubs, smoking
cessation,
babysitting
groups, asthma
clubs

Peer groups and
projects e.g. circle
time

Parenting groups

Coping with
teenagers

For example:
Individual
health plans for
children with
disability or
health care
needs

Drop-in clinics

Providing
access to health
information and
services

Child protection
and support

Immunisation

Public health
programmes at
community level

Whole school
and community

Group work

Health
prevention and
promotion with
individual children.
Young people and their
families

Figure 12.1   A continuum for public health practice in school nursing. (Source: DoH 2001)

education provider, consultant, researcher and manager.

These ongoing discussions were strengthened by government documents putting the emphasis on public health (DoH 1999b, 2001a). The setting up of the third part of the Nursing and Midwifery Council (NMC) register for specialist community public health nurses, to which all school nurses with a recordable specialist practitioner qualification will move, formalises their role as public health practitioners.

The recent past and contemporary situation

Despite the renewed focus on public health and the recognition of the part school nurses can play in promoting this agenda, there is limited evidence that the service is being developed to meet this need. In 1986, Harrison and Gretton dubbed the school nursing service the 'invisible service'. While concerned with the all round health of children, school nurses are different from most other community health workers, in that they seek out health needs in a population that meets for the purpose of education rather than health care.

Establishing the number of school nurses involved in school health is difficult. The Health Committee of the House of Commons (1997) noted that school nurse/child ratios were not available centrally. The Chief Nursing Officer's review suggests there are around 2500 school nurses (DoH 2004b), but it is unclear from where this figure originates or what qualifications the practitioners hold. Bagnall and Dilloway (1996a) reported vast differences in the school nurse/child ratios in their 1995 survey of NHS trusts. Ten years later this information cannot be found and anecdotal reporting indicates big differences in the number of children or schools covered and the numbers and types of staff involved in school health activities. Numbers alone do not indicate the needs and demands of the caseload which are influenced by the type of schools that make up the workload. The socio-economic status of the area and the availability of other health workers in these schools will influence the demand.

Cotton *et al.* (2000) concluded that the allocation of resources between districts was not equitable and argued that the use of school nurse time was out of step with current evidence of need and effectiveness. In subsequent years changes have occurred but the extent to which improvements have been achieved must be considered. Mayall and Storey (1998) also suspected there was duplication with general practice based services. Primary care has been largely focused on co-ordinated services in general practice. Bagnall and Dilloway (1996a) argued that increasing liaison with general practices was a way forward for the school health service. Work by Baptiste and Drennen (1999) in an inner city area indicated that primary care professionals were not fully aware of the role of the school nurse. The general practitioners (GPs) in particular saw them concerned with problem-solving rather than health promotion. GPs and practice nurses saw little need for collaboration or joint working with school nurses and while they wished to increase their awareness of the school nursing service they felt the onus was on the school nurses to liaise with them. Furthermore, Richardson-Todd (2002) found that GPs had a poor understanding of the school nurse role and did not know how to contact the service. In many areas it would seem as though school health and general practice services are running in parallel, with limited partnership working.

In the 1990s the image of the school nurse seemed of low status. As there was a small or unknown number of them and their role was not well known, they were vulnerable as efficiency savings were sought (CPHVA 1998a; Cowley & Houston 1999). Then, as now, some had chosen school nursing for the convenience of the hours and school holidays that fitted with their child-care commitments but they still believed it was a worthwhile and satisfying role, staying in post when their domestic commitments were no longer paramount (Thurtle 1996). The age profile of school nurses, like many nurses, is tilted, with a significant proportion approaching retirement age (NMC 2002). In addition, their status in comparison to health visitors and district nurses is often viewed as lower, with many school nurses being paid at an F or even E Grade. Formal educational training for school nursing came later and was at first of lower status in terms of length and academic value compared to health visitors and district nurses. These factors have combined to encourage school nurses, and others with whom they work, to see themselves as less valued than other community health care nurses. The coming of the Specialist Community Public Health Nurses register (NMC 2004) with those who undertake traditionally health visiting or school nursing public health work having the same registration may make some impact.

Education and training

Compared with other community nurses at the end of the twentieth century, school nurses are at a disadvantage. Unlike health visiting there is no mandatory specialist qualification. An HVA study (1996) found that only 55% of the respondents held the school nurse certificate based merely on a twelve-week course. DeBell and Everett (1997) found school nurses felt ill-prepared to respond to the range of needs they encountered. In particular they felt insufficiently trained as regards counselling skills for 'children in need'. While not mandatory, the delivery of the school nurse specialist practice award at degree level (UKCC 1994) moved the professional group forward, though limited provision by higher education institutions meant it was not available to all who wished to do it (DeBell 2000). Studying alongside other community nurses and health visitors has broadened their horizons. Having a comparable educational base and the experience of team leadership, school nurses now have the confidence to move on to acquire senior management positions. The future of school nursing or public health with school-aged children depends, as *Making a Difference* (DoH 1999a) highlighted, on the proportion of leaders who are able to influence the development of this specialist branch of nursing.

New future

School nursing may be one of the longest established groups of community nurses but it cannot afford to rest on its laurels. Recognition of their work in public health by inclusion in the Specialist Community Public Health Nursing (SCPHN) part of the NMC register, and an educational preparation comparable to other community practitioners, is to be celebrated, but the future remains unsettled. Those involved in school health need to ensure that the services provided are beneficial to the population of children and young people. Some would suggest that health visitors and school nurses have come closer together in becoming specialist public health nurses, and may be moving to a combined role, something akin to what has happened in Scotland. However, school nurses may want to sustain their identity, not out of nursing tribalism, but to ensure that skills and experience related to the school aged children and young people are not lost or enveloped in a wider pool.

The employment structures in which school nurses operate may help or hinder their work. The majority of school nurses in England are employed in primary care trusts (PCTs) where

they are a small group but are in a position to make their voices heard through contact with school nurses in neighbouring trusts or by working with health visitors and others. Some are employed in acute trusts where they run the risk of health promotion activities being swamped by the focus on the acutely ill child. The outcomes of *Agenda for Change* (DoH 2004a) may raise school nurses' status or impact negatively on their self-esteem.

While there may be those that fear the role of the school nurse is being lost, others see great opportunities. School nurses are increasingly taking on new roles such as specialist nurses for looked after or excluded children, teenage pregnancy co-ordinators or nurse consultants. Practitioners in school health are researching and publishing work allied to their area of practice in which the evidence base has often been lacking. Some in school health have hit the headlines, having been involved with nurse prescribing particularly in relation to emergency contraception through PCT based group directions. School nurses transferring onto the SCPHN part of the NMC register with health visitors who can prescribe from a limited formulary, raises further questions at to whether prescribing is an area that might be developed.

In the last decades of the twentieth century, school nursing appeared fragmented and disjointed. The national service framework for children brings the concerns of school nurses to the fore, heightening opportunities for them and allowing them to metamorphose from the 'chrysalis' state of the recent past into public health butterflies (Kiddy & Thurtle 2002).

The outworking of the public health nurse in school health

Standards of proficiency to become a specialist community public health nurse, which underpin the ten principles of public health, are cited by the NMC (2004) and these are grouped into four domains:

- Search for health needs
- Stimulation of awareness of health needs
- Influence on policy affecting health
- Facilitation of health enhancing activities

These four domains were originally identified as the principles of health visiting (CETHV 1977) and have been adapted to develop the principles of school nursing (CPHVA 1998b). They provide a useful framework to consider the work of school nurses.

Search for health needs

Screening children's hearing, vision, height and weight, is, in part, the search for health needs. The Hall report (Hall & Elliman 2003) led to a questioning of the effectiveness of universal screening of school children. Taking a population approach necessitates the identification of local priorities and the specific needs of a school community so that the service provided is needs led. Health needs assessment (discussed elsewhere in this volume) should be central to the work of school health. Bagnall and Dilloway (1996b) comment that profiles provide a comprehensive record of the health and social needs of a school population and can reveal clear differences between schools even if they are located in similar areas. The data can inform the commissioning process, be used to negotiate service led agreements, and inform school and wider policy. Profiling helps define where most effort should be focused, in accordance with national and local priorities and with those identified by primary care trusts. In turn, the data will be used to define new concerns and assist in evaluating and resetting goals and targets. Establishing local priorities has reduced routine screening, and indicated the need to focus on health promotion and illness prevention. There is much discussion about profiling but in some areas it is little more than an annual paper exercise that makes little impact on practice. Staff need to accept its relevance and utilise the views of service users, children and young people.

Stimulation of awareness of health needs

Making individuals aware of actual and potential health needs may have limited impact. Graham *et al.* (2002) considered the improvement of teenagers' knowledge of emergency contraception through a teacher led intervention. The teaching sessions led to young people knowing more about emergency contraception but did not change the pupils' sexual activity or use of emergency contraception. No doubt the same would hold in terms of healthy eating, taking more exercise and even valuing self and each other. Raising awareness of health needs requires collaboration with individuals, schools and the wider community. It may be, for example, working with an individual to encourage them to participate in physical activity, or with school staff, parents and governors to improve facilities for drinking water, or with the local community to work towards safer roads and more play spaces. The school nurse should be influencing policies affecting health in the local school and beyond.

School nurses are few in number and are therefore limited in their capacity to raise awareness of health needs. Current thinking on empowerment and partnership supports the idea that the 'community' should have a central role in deciding upon its own health needs. School nurses may be catalysts in this process, co-ordinators or just members of a group.

Influence on policies affecting health

School nursing teams may interact with the teaching and governing bodies to ensure that workable and realistic policies on personal and social education, nutrition and physical activity are designed and implemented. The day to day operation of the school is included in this perspective on health promotion, for example, considering the provision of special events including health weeks, influencing what is put in a packed lunch, what is sold in the tuck shop and the condition of the school toilets.

Multi-agency working is seen to be most effective in changing knowledge, attitudes and risk behaviours at school and community level. It is also important in identifying and addressing the wider determinants of health such as poverty, poor educational attainment, social exclusion, poor housing and environmental factors (DoH 1999a, 2004b; SEU 1999) in which school nurses should also be involved.

Advocacy for individuals and groups of children will underpin much of school nurses' activities representing parents and young people on issues such as after school activities, play space and sexual health facilities.

Facilitation of health enhancing activities

Schools remain an important setting for offering an efficient and effective way to reach children and through them, families and the wider community (DfEE 1999; ENHPS 2000; WHO 2001). Inequalities often start in childhood but all stages of childhood offer scope for improving health and preventing health risk behaviour among children, adolescents and young adults. Hence a healthy school setting can help children and adolescents attain full educational and health potential now and for the future.

Traditional childhood diseases may have diminished but new health problems have emerged which have a negative effect on child and adolescent development. These include an increase in chronic health conditions such as asthma, allergies and diabetes as well as drug and alcohol abuse, teenage pregnancies and sexually transmitted diseases, suicides, accidents, injuries or deaths from child abuse.

The intensity of school health promotion (in its widest sense) varies from one school to another and between PCTs. School nurses have a clear role to ensure that they are developing local healthy schools and have a prominent role in their management (DoH 2002).

Increased consumption of fruits and vegetables has been advocated as a preventative strategy (DoH 2000a). Around two-thirds of the UK population are overweight and if the present pattern is not curbed the greatest cause of early death for the present generation of children will be obesity (House of Commons Health Committee 2004). Not surprisingly the Children's National Service Framework (NSF) (DoH 2003) linked childhood obesity with the need to promote a healthy diet and increase physical activity.

School nurses promote healthy eating through direct teaching via the PSHE curriculum, school health days, and working in partnership with parents to discuss healthy options including provision of healthy lunch boxes. Many children consume too little fruit and vegetables and school nurses support the schools in the government introduction of the National School Fruit Scheme, which allows every 4–6 year old to receive a piece of fruit daily (DoH 1999d).

School nurses work with schools in drawing up and supporting school policies (linking back to policies influencing health) that present informed messages about healthy eating. Encouraging schools to provide healthy options in vending machines, tuck shops and school meals is all part of this.

Children and young people's sedentary lifestyle is another issue of concern to school nurses. The National Diet and Nutrition survey (DoH 2000b) found 40% of boys and 60% of girls surveyed in Britain were failing to exercise adequately. Encouraging physical activity is an important focus for health promotion, helping to reduce excessive weight gain and chronic illnesses, and improving psychological well being. School nurses working alongside community health project co-ordinators are being involved in the assessment and referral of children and young people who are overweight.

Health promotion activities may be discharged in different ways, and include 'opportunistic drop in sessions' or open access clinics with young people. The latter have been implemented in many school settings and received positive evaluation (Osborne 2000). The school nursing service provides opportunities to maintain good health, to identify health problems, to offer appropriate advice or make referrals and generally to promote health of young people, parents and at times the teaching staff.

Another opportunity for school nurses to facilitate their health-enhancing role exists within the *Extended Schools Initiative* (DfES 2002a). The Education Act 2002 provided the legislative framework for schools to extend their facilities to pupils and the local community outside the normal school hours. Services run might include parenting groups, performing arts, social clubs; whatever is needed locally. School nurses can be available to families in setting up a range of health promotion and public health services on, for example, healthy eating, accident prevention, smoking cessation support, breakfast clubs, sexual health and contraception, or through organising a farmers' market in partnership with local businesses. The scope for health enhancing activities is vast with school nurse linking into national campaigns to promote the health of all children and young people.

The emphasis on health enhancing activities is not at the expense of those with specific health issues. Technology has led to more children who have complex health needs surviving through childhood and into adulthood (Hall & Elliman 2003). Excellence for all children (DfEE 1997) and the Special Educational Needs and Disability Act 2001 sets out rights for inclusion of children in mainstream education. If parents want a place for their child, the utmost should be done to facilitate this. This is fully supported in the *Special Educational Needs Code of Practice* (DfES 2002b). Not all children with special educational needs have a health problem and not all those with a diagnosed health difficulty need support with their education, but there is a strong overlap in the two groups. Croll and Moses (2000) set out teachers' descriptions of key stage 2 (7–11 year old) classes with special needs in a variety of classes and schools in 1998. Considering all the children in their classes, 26% were seen as having special educational needs. Not surprisingly, learning was the most mentioned area of difficulty with 23% of children being in this category, 5% having emotional and behavioural difficulties, and 4% having health, sensory and physical difficulties. Some children may experience one or more of these areas of need. With the reduction of places in special schools and the commitment to the concept of inclusion, there are more children with complex health and social needs in mainstream schools.

The range of chronic complex needs varies; the most prevalent include epilepsy, anaphylaxis, asthma, diabetes, sickle cell disease, hyperkinetic disorders, co-ordination difficulties, speech and language problems, enuresis, obesity, soiling or foot deformity (Meltzer *et al.* 2000). The majority

cope well, gaining full education and enriching the experience of their peers. The practical health care of these children may be delegated to teachers, secretaries, classroom assistants or community children's nurses (DfEE 1996). However, school nurses often assume a leadership role in developing a care plan in partnership with parents, teachers, support workers and the child. This ensures care is co-ordinated, information is shared as necessary, medication or equipment is available and intimate or invasive treatments can be given if necessary (DfEE 1996). Children needing invasive treatment remain the minority. Health in most schools for most children is concerned with promoting the best outcomes for all children, that affords them the opportunity to achieve their personal potential (DfES 2001a, 2002a). Leadership and organisation are key qualities for developing the school nursing service.

Leadership and organisation

Leadership has been highlighted as a priority in nursing generally (DoH 1999b, 2001b) and school nursing in particular (DeBell 2000). As all health staff work in a changing context and school health is being modified or developing itself, there is a need for those who can be leaders and change agents.

There is much discussion about styles of leadership and transformational leadership as described by Burns (1978). Leaders and staff encourage each other and the approach is mobilising, inspiring, exalting and uplifting. Rosener (1990) claims that transformational leadership is essentially a woman leader's style. As school nursing remains predominately female the use of charisma, interpersonal skills as well as hard work are very appropriate. In practical terms, being a leader in school health means building alliances within and outside the team and ensuring the vision is rooted in research-based evidence, which in school nursing has been limited, but is growing. Creativity in outlook is vital requiring the readiness to take risks and, being prepared to tell others what has been achieved, through publications and websites and by talking at meetings and conferences.

Thinking creatively about the role of the school nursing service involves a division of labour. Different ways of working should involve a genuine skill mix, which will vary depending upon the needs of the local population. School nurses with different interests and expertise, perhaps in mental health, sexual health, behavioural or learning difficulties, could make up the school health team. These staff should work with those without nursing qualifications but with skills and interests in children and young people, health promotion, group work, interviewing and counselling. Leadership of such teams will raise the status of school nursing and provide the individuals involved with renewed professional confidence. Nurses generally are in short supply, and school nursing needs to attract those who are committed to it. This in itself may necessitate the evolution of teams with a variety of nursing and non-nursing skills and abilities, which in turn will promote richness and diversity.

Such challenges lead to changes in the way that neighbourhoods and schools are allocated to the school nurses' workload. Information from the profiling can be used to allocate schools or areas, not merely by numbers but by current priorities. Many would argue that it is imperative to ensure that all children, in both private and maintained schools, are offered a core, evidence-based service through which they can access further services. Commitment to school health needs to be at all levels, supplemented by a mix of staff who are adequately prepared and deployed to meet the health related needs of children and young people.

Working in different ways will involve school nurses working in a variety of settings other than educational establishments. By meeting them in places which provide youth activities such as children's clubs, young people may be accessed with a readiness to take up the issue for themselves rather than because it is part of the school day or curriculum. Despite the fact that educational settings are likely to remain dominant, a chance for school nurses to do some evening work and all year round activity, will inevitably occur in the future. Whilst this will have financial and personal implications for the nurses, such changes in working patterns will change the base and improve the effectiveness of health care activity with school aged children.

The concerns of the school health service have changed over time. At one point their focus might have been infection and infestation later shifting to screening and surveillance. There is breadth in the school nurses' responsibilities (Madge & Franklin 2003) and public health is now key with the focus of concern changing, as health needs are identified.

Mental health – a specific issue

Good mental health of school age children is of crucial significance as it contributes to maintaining a good level of personal and social functioning, and influences future health behaviour. The Mental Health Foundation (1999) states that mental health means being able to grow and develop emotionally, intellectually and spiritually in a way appropriate for the child's age. Having low self-esteem, and being unfulfilled and stressed can result in mental distress, which is also a risk factor for physical health problems. This consequently has an impact on self-esteem as well as on health choices such as engaging in physical activity, healthy nutritional intake, liking own image, substance misuse and risky sexual behaviour (Ramrakha *et al.* 2000).

Political commitment to put mental health at the forefront of health policy was reiterated in *Saving Lives: Our Healthier Nation*, (DoH 1999b) and the *National Service Framework for Mental Health* (DoH 1999c). This was followed by *National Suicide Prevention Strategy* (DoH 2002) and supported in the *National Service Framework for Children* (DoH 2003). The focus of these documents is that mental health is a major cause of ill health and suicide is reported to be the leading cause of death amongst 15–24 year olds (DoH 1999c). Targets set on a national basis to reduce the incidence of mental illness and suicide strive for a reduction by one fifth by 2010, thereby saving up to 50 000 lives (DoH 1999c). Current data from the Office of National Statistics (ONS 2004) reports that 1 in 10 children and young people aged 5–15 years living in England have a clinically recognisable mental disorder (11% of boys and 8% of girls).

Young Minds, a children's mental health charity, estimated that in any secondary school where there are 1000 pupils, there is a likelihood of 50 pupils being seriously depressed, 100 suffering serious distress, between 10 and 20 pupils having a compulsive disorder and between 5 and 10 girls having an eating disorder (Young Minds 2002). The incidence of poor mental health is noted to be prevalent amongst vulnerable children, particularly those looked after by the local authority, those leaving care, those who are homeless, and young offenders (ONS 2004; SEU 2004). Other risk factors include being in one-parent families, educational underachievement, parental mental illness, domestic violence, low family income and children with neurological problems such as epilepsy and co-ordination difficulties.

Mental illness has been identified as a barrier to learning and strategies to promote mental health need to begin in early childhood (DfES 2001b). Since the 1990s most areas have run children and adolescent mental health services (CAMHS) leading to a more comparable service in different areas (Fawcett *et al.* 2004). *Every Child Matters* (DfES 2003a) and other government documents have advocated an expansion of this service. The coming of CAMHS led to a four-tier model of service approach. First level staff, which would include school nurses, identifies health problems, offers advice treatment in less severe cases and promotes good mental health. Clear routes need to be available for school nurses and others to refer young people to more specialised help in the other tiers and clinical supervision needs to be available for the practitioner.

School nurses recognise that positive mental health is essential for academic success and that services that support prevention, early identification and treatment of mental illness are necessary to support pupils' achievement (DeBell & Jackson 2000). They can provide mental health promotion activities within the school community to address developing self-esteem, positive coping skills and stress management. The profile of mental health promotion could be further raised through the national healthy schools standards.

Mental health services that are easy to access and which provide comprehensive co-ordinated services are needed to reduce the incidence of mental health problems in school children (DfES 2001b). School nurses are in a position to recognise the potential impact mental ill health can have on pupils' development and can act as strong advocates for child mental health in the political and public arenas, including campaigning for early intervention for the pre-school population (Espeland 1998).

School nurses may feel wary and unskilled in this area but have much to offer in Circle Time, a programme that is being utilised both within primary and secondary school settings to promote mental health and improve self-esteem. 'Drop in' sessions provide direct access for the students to the school nurse within the school environment.

Offering parenting groups and support to parents with school age children, selective reception health interviews with new entrants and parents, response to individuals via referral system, either self/teacher, all contributes. Working with other professionals and agencies on anti-bullying strategies, friendship clubs and young person's clinics, takes the issue forward.

School nurses can be the liaison between child and adolescence mental health services, the family and school staff. By joining forces with other health professionals to promote a whole school approach to mental health their profile in this area can be expanded. At present school nurses work with educational psychologists, clinical psychologists, educational social workers, special educational needs co-ordinators, counsellors, social workers, learning mentors and other support staff to plan and implement mental health services.

The challenges for school nurses and other health professionals contributing to mental health promotion within the school setting are to eliminate stigma and discrimination, to reduce fragmentation of services and work towards achieving a comprehensive wider community model that includes partnership, prevention, early identification and intervention.

The need for marketing

Adopting a marketing perspective is a strategy for survival (Edwards 1992). More positively, to take advantage of the new opportunities in public health there is a need for the development of a concerted marketing strategy by school nurses. Polnay (1998) noted there had been a 'conspicuous lack of marketing about school health, with many people, parents, children, teachers, health purchasers and providers not having correct knowledge about the service and indeed being cluttered with misinformation' (p. 98). A few years later Teachernet (2004), the DfES web site for teachers stated,

> 'To many, the image of the school nurse is that of a stern or matronly nit checker. Sweeping changes in health education in schools have meant that the role of the school nurse in both primary and secondary schools is now impressively wide-ranging'.

Teachers, perhaps school nurses' closest allies, appreciate the changes, yet some school nurses themselves are still relying on outdated views of their function. For the school nursing service to develop, its value must be recognised by children and their parents and beyond, with school nurses advertising their role and the need for it in every available arena. With local trusts seeking to match services to their local communities, school nurses need to be working with them in locally and medically based practice groupings, rather than being marginalised and potentially competing with others concerned with the welfare of children and young people. Instead of working separately from practice nurses, outreach workers, sexual health nurses and others, it is essential that school nurses explain their role and function to them clearly and with conviction, and even more importantly, they should identify what could be achieved in partnership with others, within the context of realistic resource allocation.

Conclusion

The past ten years have seen a huge development in the practice and confidence of school nurses. They are concerned with the search for health needs, of individuals and schools as well as communities. Having identified them, they are competent to stimulate an awareness of health needs and to facilitate health-enhancing activities, though influencing health policies needs may need further development in some areas. Working in these four domains is not revolutionary to school nurses, they have developed such practice over the past decade. School nurses' inclusion in the specialist community public health nurses register is a consolidation and celebration of their role and will hopefully enable them to fulfil this role, for which there is a great need, more effectively than ever before.

References

Bagnall, P. & Dilloway, M. (1996a) *In search of a blueprint: A survey of school health services*. Department of Health and Queen's Nursing Institute, London.

Bagnall, P. & Dilloway, M. (1996b). *In a different light: school nurses and their role in meeting the health needs of school age children*. Department of Health and Queen's Nursing Institute, London.

Baptiste, L. & Drennan, V. (1999) Communication between school nurses and primary care teams. *British Journal of Community Nursing*, **4**(1), 13–18.

Blair, M., Stewart-Brown, S., Waterson, T. & Crowther, R. (2003) *Child public health*. Oxford University Press, Oxford.

Burns, J. (1978) *Leadership*. Harper and Row, New York.

Council for the Education and Training of Health Visitors (1977) *An Investigation into the Principles of Health Visiting*. Council for the Education and Training of Health Visitors, London.

Community Practitioners' and Health Visitors' Association (1998a) *The Cambridge Experiment*. CPHVA, London.

Community Practitioners' and Health Visitors' Association (1998b) *The Principles of School Nursing: Foundations for good practice*. CPHVA, London.

Cotton, L., Brazier, J., Hall, D., Lindsay, G., Marsh, P., Polnay, L. & Williams, T. (2000) School nursing: costs and potential benefits. *Journal of Advanced Nursing*, **31**(5), 1063–1071.

Cowley, S. & Houston, A. (1999) *Health Visiting and School Nursing: The Croydon Story*. King's College/Croydon Community Health Council, London.

Croll, P. & Moses, D. (2000) *Special needs in the primary school. One in five?* Cassell, London.

DeBell, D. (2000) *Translating School Nursing Research into Practice. An assessment of change in the management and delivery of school nursing.* Report to the Department of Health.

DeBell, D. & Everett, G. (1997) *In a Class Apart: A Study of School Nursing.* The Research Centre City College, Norwich.

DeBell, D. & Jackson, P. (2000) *School Nursing within the Public Health Agenda: A strategy for practice.* CPHVA/Queen's Institute/RCN, London.

Department for Education and Employment (1996) *Supporting Pupils with Medical Needs.* Stationery Office, London.

Department for Education and Employment (1997) *Excellence in Schools.* Stationery Office, London.

Department for Education and Employment (1999) *National Healthy School Standard Guidance.* DfEE, Nottingham.

Department for Education and Skills (2001a) The Special Educational Needs and Disability Act. www.dfes.gov.uk

Department for Education and Skills (2001b) *Guidance: Promoting Children's Mental Health within Early Years and School settings.* DfEE 0121/200, Nottingham.

Department for Education and Skills (2002a) *Extended Schools: Providing Opportunities and Services for all.* DfES, Nottingham.

Department for Education and Skills (2002b) *Special Educational Needs Codes of Practice.* DfES, Nottingham.

Department for Education and Skills (2003a) *Every Child Matters.* DfES, Nottingham.

Department of Education and Skills (2003b) *Excellence and Enjoyment: A Strategy for Primary Schools.* DfES, Nottingham.

Department for Education and Skills (2003c) Excellence in Cities: An evaluation of an Education Policy in Disadvantaged Areas, www.dfes.gov.uk/ excellenceincities

Department for Education and Skills (2004a) *Teachernet. School Nurses.* http://www.teachernet. gov.uk/teachingandlearning/library/schoolnurses

Department for Education and Skills (2004b) *Health living blueprint for schools.* DfES, Nottingham.

Department of Health (1995) The *Health of the Young Nation.* HMSO, London.

Department of Health (1997) *The New NHS: Modern, Dependable.* DoH, London.

Department of Health (1998a) *Independent Inquiry into Inequalities in Health.* (Acheson Report): DoH, London.

Department of Health (1998b) *A First Class Service: Quality in the new NHS.* Department of Health, Leeds.

Department of Health (1998c) *Our Healthier Nation.* DoH, London.

Department of Health (1999a) *Making a Difference: Strengthening the nursing, midwifery, and health visiting contribution to health and health care.* DoH, London.

Department of Health (1999b) *Saving Lives: Our Healthier Nation.* DoH, London.

Department of Health (1999c) *National Service Framework for Mental Health.* DoH, London.

Department of Health (1999d) *The School Fruit Scheme.* Healthy Schools, London.

Department of Health (2000a) *National Service Framework for Coronary Heart Disease: Modern Standards and Service Models.* Department of Health, London.

Department of Health (2000b) *National Diet and Nutrition Survey: Young People aged 4–18 years. Volume 1: Report of the Diet and Nutrition Survey.* DoH, London.

Department of Health (2001a) *Liberating the Talents.* DoH, London.

Department of Health (2001b) *School Nurse Development Resource Pack,* The Stationery Office, London.

Department of Health (2001c) *Shifting the Balance of Power within the NHS – Securing Delivery.* Department of Health, London.

Department of Health (2002) *National Suicide Prevention Strategy for England. Great Britain.* The Stationery Office, London.

Department of Health (2003) *Getting the Right Start: The National Service Framework for Children, Young People and Maternity Services Emerging Findings.* Consultation document, Department of Health, London.

Department of Health (2004a) *Agenda for Change Proposed Agreement* (September 2004), Final draft. Department of Health, London.

Department of Health (2004b) *The Chief Nursing Officer's review of the midwifery and health visiting contribution to vulnerable children and young people.* Department of Health, London.

Dooris, M. (2004) Joining up Settings for health: a valuable investment for strategic partnerships? *Critical Public Health,* **14**, 49–61.

Edwards, J. (1992) Market in practice. *Health Visitor,* **65**(10), 352–353.

Espeland, K. (1998) Promoting mental wellness in children and adolescents through positive coping mechanisms, *Journal of School Nursing.* **14**, 22–25.

European Network of Health Promoting Schools (ENHPS) (2000) http://www.euro.int/eprise/main/ who/progs/ENHPS/home

NORTHBROOK COLLEGE LIBRARY

Fawcett, B., Featherstone, B. & Goddard, J. (2004) *Contemporary Child Care Policy and practice*. Palgrave, Basingstoke.

Graham, A., Moor, L., Sharpe, D. & Diamond, I. (2002) Improving teenagers' knowledge of emergency contraception: cluster randomised controlled trial of a teacher led intervention. *BMJ* **324**, 1179–1185.

Hall, D.M.B & Elliman, D. (2003) *Health for All Children*. 4th edn, Oxford University Press, Oxford.

Harrison, A. & Gretton, J. (eds.) (1986) *Health Care UK: An economic, social and policy audit*. Hermitage, Berkshire.

Health Visitor Association (1996) *School Nursing: Here Today for Tomorrow*. HVA, London.

House of Commons (1997) *Health Committee. Third Report Health Services for Children and Young People in the Community Home and School*. The Stationery Office, London.

House of Commons (2004) *Health Committee Obesity*. The Stationery Office, London. www.parliament. the-stationery-office.co.uk/pa/cm200304/cmselect/ cmhealth/23/23.pdf

Kiddy, M. & Thurtle, V. (2002). From chrysalis to butterfly – the school nurse role. *Community Practitioner*, **75**(8), 295–298.

Kuss, T., Proulx-Girouard, L., Lovitt, S., Katz, C.B. Kennelly, P. (1997) A Public Health Nursing Model. *Public Health Nursing*, **14**(2), 81–91.

Madge, N. & Franklin, A. (2003) *Change Challenge and School Nursing*. National Children's Bureau, London.

Mayall, B. & Storey S. (1998) A School Health Service for Children. *Children and Society*. **12**(2), 86–97.

Meltzer, H., Gatward, R., Goodman, R. & Ford, T. (2000) *Mental Health of Children and Adolescents in Britain: A survey carried out in 1999 by the social survey division of the ONS*. The Stationery Office, London.

Mental Health Foundation (1999) *Bright Futures*. Mental Health Foundation, London.

Nursing and Midwifery Council (2002) *Statistical analysis of the register 1 April 2001 to 31 March 2002*. NMC, London.

Nursing and Midwifery Council (2004) *Standards of proficiency for specialist community public health nurses*. NMC, London.

Office for National Statistics (2004) *The Health of Young People*. www.statistics.gov.uk/.children

Osborne, N. (2000) Children's Voices: Evaluation of School Drop-in Health Clinic. *Community Practitioner*, **73**(3), 516–518.

Polnay, L. (1998) A School Health Service for Children: A Commentary. *Children and Society*. **12**(2), 98–100.

Ramrakha, S., Caspi, A., Dickinson, N., Moffit, T.E. & Paul, C. (2000) Psychiatric disorders and risky sex in young adulthood: a cross sectional study in a birth cohort. *BMJ*, **321**, 263–266.

Richardson-Todd, B. (2002) GPs: Do they know what school nurses do? *Primary Health Care*, **12**(8), 38–41.

Rosener, J. (1990) Ways women lead. *Harvard Business Review*. Nov–Dec. 119–125.

Skills for Health (2004) *National occupational standards for the practice of public health guide*. Skills for Health, Bristol.

Social Exclusion Unit (SEU) (1999) *Teenage Pregnancy*. Social Exclusion Unit, London.

Social Exclusion Unit Report (2004) *Mental Health and Social Exclusion*. Office of the Deputy Prime Minister, Yorkshire.

Teachernet (2004) www.teachernet.gov.uk/ teachingandlearning/library/schoolnurses/

Thurtle, V. (1996) Why Nurses Choose to Enter School Nursing. *Health Visitor*, **69**(6), 231–233.

Townsend, P., Davidson, N. & Whitehead, W. (1992) *Inequalities in Health*. Penguin, London.

UKCC (1994) *The future of professional practice, the council's standards for education and practice following registration*. UKCC, London.

United Nation Convention on the Rights of the Child (1991) HMSO, London

World Health Organization (2001) *The World Health Report*. http://www.who.int/whr2001/2001/archives/ 1998/exsum98e.htm

Young Minds (2002) *Mental health services for adolescents and young adults*. Young Minds, London.

Chapter 13 **Occupational Health Nursing**

Anne Harriss

Occupational health nurses (OHNs) provide specialised nursing care in a specific primary health care setting – the workplace. The International Labour Organisation (ILO) and the World Health Organization (WHO) are two international institutions that regularly comment on both health and health and safety at work and both have defined the aims and objectives of an occupational health (OH) service. One of the ILO's recommendations (recommendation 112) states that the aim of an OH service is to protect workers against health hazards arising out of their work or their working environment and adapting work processes so that optimum physical and mental health of the worker can be achieved. (ILO 1959). The WHO in their technical report 535 take a similar stance but also comment on the identification and control of all 'chemical, physical, mechanical, biological and psychosocial agents that are known to be or expected to be very hazardous' (WHO 1973).

Occupational health nurses as specialist practitioners

This chapter provides an overview of the role of the OHN as a specialist practitioner. In order to give the reader an understanding of contemporary OH nursing, a historical perspective and the influencing factors and the domains of OHN practice are explored.

OHNs work with a predominantly well client group and are aware that inequalities in health arise as a result of the complex interplay between employment, socioeconomic status, housing and education. It is not an easy task for most nurses to be able to influence many of these factors but OHNs have the opportunity to influence the health of a workforce that may consist of a 'crunchy social mix' of people of differing cultures, ethnicity and social backgrounds. They

are well placed to offer advice to employers on preventing, or at least reducing, the incidence of workplace accidents and work related ill-health in order to meet the aims proposed by the ILO and WHO referred to above. They practise as part of a distinct specialty within the family of nursing and employ a distinct body of knowledge. Their practice is multi-faceted and involves utilising a unique range of general and specialised nursing skills. These skills include:

- Undertaking health needs assessments for their client group – people at work
- Identifying health inequalities and devising strategies that can be utilised in the workplace with the aim of reducing these
- Planning, implementing and evaluating programmes designed to protect and promote health in the workplace
- Working collaboratively with other practitioners and employers to identify and address health needs

The Royal College of Nursing (RCN) defines an OHN as a nurse who holds a recordable qualification in occupational health nursing (RCN 2003), that is, one which is eligible to be recorded on the register maintained by the Nursing and Midwifery Council. There is currently no mandatory requirement for nurses to hold a specialist qualification in occupational health nursing and many nurses work in the specialty without one. However the author proposes that holding a specialist qualification is essential in this very specialist area of nursing practice that encompasses independent functioning, autonomous decision-making, and employee health management (Rogers 1994, p. 34). It is the role of the OHN specialist practitioner that will be explored in this chapter.

OHNs practice nursing in a unique way. Although their role is diverse and complex, it is primarily concerned with promoting general health status and preventing work related ill health and accidents. Experienced OHNs play an important part in organisational health policy development, risk and health assessment and they are able to contribute to attendance management and rehabilitative interventions. These interventions will be explored later in this chapter.

An effective OH service has the potential to add value to the organisation that employs them as there are clearly benefits to both employee and employer by improving the quality of working life as well as having a positive impact on business productivity. Employer commitment to employee health improvements therefore not only contributes to the long-term health status of the community but also benefits the organisation through an improvement in worker retention, a reduction in sickness absence and accident rates, and an increase in productivity. As the Health and Safety Executive assert 'good health means good business' (HSE 1995).

The effect of work on health

It can be argued that there is a paradoxical relationship between work and health; work is usually a financial necessity and often socially rewarding but it must be acknowledged that it results in significant adverse health effects. Some work areas such as construction sites have obvious dangers including working at heights, in adverse climatic conditions and with dangerous machinery. Furthermore this industry has a predominantly itinerant workforce. Although construction industry workers are highly skilled the majority are semi- or unskilled employees and many of these people speak English as a second or subsequent language and a number may not speak any English at all. The combination of these factors results in an increased risk of accidents. Indeed construction sites are probably the most dangerous work areas in the UK today. The HSE recognise the dangers associated with construction work and note that between 1999–2004 almost 300 people died in that industry as a result of accidents including falls during work carried out at height, accidents involving the movement of vehicles and machinery and accidents occurring during lifting operations involving heavy loads. This accounts for over 70% of all fatal injuries in that industry and this has been the focus of a nationwide HSE campaign that aims to reduce such accidents.

Not only are construction workers more likely to be involved in serious accidents than people employed in less dangerous work areas but their work is also associated with a range of occupational illnesses. Working with noisy, vibrating tools can result in them developing occupational deafness and circulatory disorders such as hand arm vibration syndrome. Their exposure to materials such as oils and cement predispose them to developing occupational dermatitis and chemical burns. There are now a growing number of OHNs who choose to work in the construction industry as a result of the diversity of the hazards associated with such employment.

Many less hazardous occupations also have illnesses associated with them. For example, work related upper limb disorders are associated with repetitive tasks such as poorly designed work involving extensive keyboard use. Occupational asthma is a work related condition associated with a number of work processes including exposure to flour in food production; exposure to isocyanates in the paint spraying of motor vehicles; and exposure to dander and body fluids from working with animals. Noise-induced hearing loss is not confined to the construction industry and is also associated with a number of occupations including factory work and amongst professional musicians. Unsurprisingly a number of high profile rock musicians are reputed to have developed noise induced hearing loss. These performers are particularly at risk due to both their ongoing exposure to noise and their probable reluctance to wearing hearing protection.

Members of other performing arts such as actors, singers and dancers are also predisposed to developing occupationally related conditions. Dancers are prone to joint and other musculo-skeletal injuries whilst singers and actors may develop problems with their voice. There is a small group of OHNs working specifically in this highly specialised field of OH practice. Their client group is interesting and unusual as it includes every age-range from child (including babies) to older age actors.

An appreciation of the effect of work on health is not new. Indeed more than 300 years ago, Ramazzini, a professor of medicine at Padua, Italy, acknowledged that work impacts on health. Ramazzini is widely considered to be the father of occupational medicine and his practice involved looking after the health needs of artisans and labourers. He stressed the importance of asking patients a particularly important question 'What is your occupation?' (Lee 1994). This question is often forgotten by many medical (and nursing) practitioners of today but is not forgotten by nurses working in occupational health as they appreciate the possible adverse effects of work on health and health on work performance.

Historical perspective

OH nursing has a long history in the UK. The first nurse working in the industrial setting is reputed to be Phillipa Flowerday who was employed in the late nineteenth century in the Coleman's mustard factory in Norwich. Her role was innovative at that time and encompassed a public health dimension as she offered a treatment service in the factory during the morning then spent the rest of her working day working with sick employees and their families in their own homes. Contemporary OHN practice has evolved from such a treatment-based approach to one that is both evidence-based, pro-active and has a preventative focus.

OH nursing education also has a rich history in the UK. The first course in what was then known as industrial nursing was offered to qualified nurses by the Royal College of Nursing in the early 1930s. Over the years that course has evolved to meet the needs of OHNs and has kept pace with contemporary OHN practice. The early certificate in industrial nursing then became the occupational health nursing certificate which in turn evolved into a course offered at diploma level and finally into a BSc (Hons) degree conferring specialist practitioner status initially validated by the English National Board for Nursing Midwifery and Health Visiting (on behalf of the United Kingdom Central Council for Nursing Midwifery and Health Visiting) and more recently by the Nursing and Midwifery Council (NMC). The BSc (Hons) Occupational Health Nursing transferred from the RCN to London South Bank University in 2000.

OH services of the 21st century are directly involved in employee health management and they work towards reducing employee exposure to health risks and preventing illnesses associated with occupation. This is congruent with the ILO/WHO's stated aim of occupational health as being:

> 'the promotion and maintenance of the highest degree of physical, mental and social well-being of workers in all occupations by preventing departures from health, controlling risks and the adaptation of work to people, and people to their jobs'.

In order to accomplish this aim OHNs must have an understanding of the factors impacting on the health of workers and be innovative in their approach to the client care offered by them to all strata within the organisation. They have an understanding of how organisations function and an appreciation of the social influences on health status. The Acheson report (DoH 1998) indicates that poverty continues to exert a negative effect on health with the gap between the social classes widening. OHNs are able to work with employees at all levels and within all social groups. Consequently, they contribute to the improvement of the health of all strata of the workforce and are able to focus on particularly vulnerable groups. One such group are people, often low paid unskilled workers, employed to operate hazardous processes which may involve the use of chemicals or work that requires them to use vibrating tools or dangerous machinery. These people are already disadvantaged and such exposure to workplace hazards has the potential to further contribute to the health divide between the social classes.

Provision of occupational health services in the UK

Unfortunately there is currently no legal requirement in the UK for employers to provide an

OH service for their employees. Large organisations, or those with exposure to workplace hazards such as dangerous chemicals, often do provide one. The provision of such a service is not mandatory and is therefore an option for businesses rather than an obligation. The decision whether to provide an OH service is usually a financial one. A consequence of the provision of OH services not being obligatory is that OH provision in the UK is patchy, in short there is no 'National Occupational Health Service'. Harling (1999) suggests that OH as a specialty has been slow to progress owing to its exclusion from the National Health Service at its inception in 1948. This omission was probably due to financial reasons resulting from concerns regarding the cost of developing a new National Health Service. The Government's stance that employers are responsible for OH provision has resulted in this inconsistent approach and, until recently, there was little collaborative working evident between the NHS and the workplace. NHS Plus, which is discussed later in this chapter is helping to bridge this gap.

The changing nature of UK workplaces

The nature of UK workplaces is changing and the role of the OHN is developing to meet the challenges these changes present. Their role can be as diverse as the workplaces in which they are employed. There is now a decline in the number of large manufacturing industries in the UK and work is increasingly undertaken within a multi-cultural context. Non-discriminatory governmental policy has resulted in employers being required to make arrangements to facilitate the employment of people with a range of physical and mental disabilities. Employers must also offer equality of opportunity for both men and women; women of all ages now form a much larger proportion of the workforce, particularly so in what had previously been occupations dominated by male workers. This raises particular health and safety issues in respect of those who are pregnant or those who have recently returned to work following maternity leave. Pregnant women and new and nursing mothers

are at risk from some work processes including exposure to some chemicals or the moving and handling of loads.

The rapid growth of information technology has had a significant influence on work practices. This development has led to a growth of 'call centres' in which people are employed to undertake work that depends on the use of both telephones and computers. On the face of it this would appear to be a safe place of work. However, on closer inspection there are a number of health problems associated with work of this nature. One of the most significant is voice strain; it is arguable that there is also the potential for some degree of hearing loss associated with loud noise from a poorly adjusted volume control on telephone headsets. Other health problems are not specific to workers in call centres but are common to other occupations requiring work with computers such as work related upper limb disorders. Doke (2004) outlines recent research undertaken in the UK and Sweden that suggests that working in a call centre is generally more stressful than other occupations. Careful work planning and equipment design can alleviate some of this stress and an OHN can advise on such issues.

OHN practice requires an appreciation of the biopsychosocial sciences and recognises that employment is an integral part of adult life and health should not be harmed as a result of it. The ability to participate productively in workplace activities can, and should, contribute to ongoing physical and psychological well being. However, not all work is free from risk. Workers of lower social status experience more injuries and work related ill health than those from the middle classes. The financial circumstances of those living in socially deprived areas, single parents or those without skills or qualifications may be forced into hazardous, low paid occupations. Cognisance of this situation enables OHNs to focus workplace health promotion activities on this group of workers – people who may not access such information from other sources.

Semi-skilled and unskilled workers frequently undertake tasks on poorly designed production lines pre-disposing these people to musculo-skeletal disorders. An example of a successful initiative put in place by one company is the protection of people working on a poultry processing production line. Their work tasks had hitherto included lifting plucked, semi-processed turkeys from a production conveyor belt located behind them and at waist height. The birds were then lifted onto a hook positioned in front of and at the shoulder height of the operatives. Many of these workers subsequently developed a range of work related musculo-skeletal disorders including neck, shoulder and back pain. The design of both the equipment with which they worked and their work tasks pre-disposed them to such pain as they resulted in repetitive twisting actions of the trunk, lifting a load (the turkeys) away from the body and re-positioning and anchoring it at shoulder height. The high-risk operations they were required to undertake included twisting, reaching and handling a heavy load held at a distance from the body. The OH service took a pro-active involvement in the redesign of both the work process and work equipment. Risk assessment proformas were developed in order to identify any future problems associated with the process. The OHNs were able to refer clients with musculo-skeletal problems into a fast track, in-house, physiotherapy service. These initiatives resulted in a dramatic reduction in musculo-skeletal disorders with reduced costs relating to labour relations and turnover, sickness absence and possible future litigation. These employees were fortunate to have access to such a pro-active occupational health service that was funded by their employer. This was possible due to the size and financial turnover of their company. Employees in many other workplaces in similar factories are not so fortunate.

Changing work patterns

It must be acknowledged that the world of work is rapidly changing with fewer large industries and a higher proportion of small and medium sized business enterprises. Employment does not always take place in a conventional workplace even in large organisations. Paton (2004) comments that more than a million people are now estimated to regularly work from home. Such working has been facilitated by developments in information technology. Paton goes on to discuss the benefits and challenges of using the home as a workplace. Reduced travel costs with fewer distractions are appealing, however, isolation, the potential for longer working hours and higher levels of stress may result in workers employed in this way experiencing more emotional difficulties than their colleagues employed in a conventional office environment. Home working brings challenges to the OHNs who provide a service for people who work in this way

Employers have a duty of care under legislation including the Health and Safety at Work etc. Act 1974. They must ensure the health, safety and welfare of their staff no matter where they work. It is also in the employer's financial interest to reduce absences resulting from work-related ill health. OHNs are suitably positioned and experienced to work collaboratively with workers, their representatives, management and other health and health and safety practitioners to improve worker health. Changing work patterns, work requirements and improved control strategies have resulted in a reduction of health deficits linked to exposure to hazardous chemicals. However, there has been an increase in work related upper limb disorders associated with the use of computers. Likewise, workplace stress seems to be a topical subject of much debate. Work should not lead to mental ill-health. Indeed Payne (1999) suggests that most research indicates poorer mental health amongst those who are unemployed compared to those in employment. Some studies also indicate higher rates of suicide and para-suicide amongst the unemployed. Managers have a moral and legal responsibility to ensure that workers do not suffer from mental health as a result of their work and the OHN is well positioned to advise on promoting both mental and physical health at work.

Workplace practices

An important aspect of the role of the OHN requires cognisance of the organisational, sociological and psychological factors that affect workplace practices and can adversely impact worker health status. They are able to advise and work with management, employees and their representatives towards ensuring a safe and a health-promoting workplace. OHNs are well placed to influence the health of the community as the workplace provides a captive audience for strategies to further promote health amongst a group of well adults who are often otherwise difficult to access. As the Department of Health states, the workplace offers potential for improving the health status of the population because of:

- 'Access to a large number of people many of whom are at risk for adverse health effects
- A potentially low level of attrition as the population is relatively stable
- Cohesion of the working community which can offer benefits such as positive peer pressure and peer support
- Established channels of communication which can be used to publicise programmes, encourage participation, provide feedback and assist in the process of change' (Department of Health 2003)

Although some OH services offer a very limited service with an emphasis on pre-employment screening and attendance management as highlighted by Pickvance (1993), other services have a much more pro-active and holistic approach more closely aligned to the broader public health agenda. Such pro-active services provide very much a preventative role integrating the skills of risk and health assessment. Many OHNs are highly experienced in formulating return to work recovery programmes for employees who have been absent from work as the result of accidents or following serious ill-health.

The discussion so far has indicated that OHNs are specialist practitioners aware of the effect of work on health and health on work and able to work with both individuals and groups to improve health. Their advice to all concerned aims to minimise any adverse effects of work on health and assist in reducing accidents (Harriss 2004). Most OHNs undertake health and risk management to achieve this aim whilst experienced and more senior OHNs also contribute to policy formation and professional leadership in the organisations in which they work.

The domains of occupational health nursing practice

OHNs face challenges and practice in a way that differs from that undertaken by nurses employed in other community or hospital settings. Although their practice has a different emphasis OHNs bring with them the values and beliefs developed as a result of having initially qualified as general or mental health nurses. Much, but not all, of what OHNs undertake as part of their practice would be unrecognisable to many other nurses as 'nursing skills' and their role will now be explored.

Having discussed some of the influences on, and elements of, OH nursing practice the specific aspects of that practice will now be highlighted. The role of the OHN incorporates a number of domains including professional, managerial, environmental and educational spheres. How these are applied depends on their area of practice and the needs of their employing organisation but there are certain commonalities.

The professional domain

The professional domain is very broad and encompasses the 'nitty-gritty' of practice as nurses in the workplace setting. They must be able to work within the requirements of both legislation and the NMC professional code of conduct. This is often challenging as many of the people with whom OHNs work, including managers and human resources professionals do not fully appreciate the implications of their professional code of conduct particularly in relation to client confidentiality.

OHNs have the potential to undertake an important role in research and epidemiology – identifying work related health issues. They use their nursing skills in the assessment of health in a range of activities including pre-employment health assessments to ensure that prospective employees are fit to take on the requirements of their proposed job. They are involved in providing ongoing health surveillance for workers exposed to workplace hazards such as work involving exposure to a vast array of hazardous chemicals including iso-cyanates, chrome, lead and solvents. Chemicals used in the workplace can have numerous patho-physiological effects of which the

OHN should be aware. They have the potential to impact on a number of organs and body systems including the skin, liver, kidneys and the respiratory, reproductive, haematopoetic and central nervous systems. Health surveillance provides an opportunity to identify early changes linked to such exposure in order to identify people at risk.

Increasingly OHNs are undertaking a role in attendance management as the costs of sickness absence is a significant drain on the profitability of many organisations and is consistently estimated to cost the UK economy more than £11 billion each year. The OHNs' knowledge of health and work requirements means that they can make a valuable contribution to an attendance management strategy (Harriss 2001). However, it is essential that they clarify their role to ensure that there is no conflict between maintaining an impartial role as employee advocate and acting as an advisor to management. Part of their contribution to attendance management strategies put in place by organisations is the undertaking of health assessments for employees following periods of repeated short-term or one episode of long-term absence prior to their return to work. This offers an ideal opportunity to identify whether a health problem is caused or exacerbated by their job requirements. They are then able to devise return to work recovery programmes facilitating a successful and productive return to work, a benefit to all concerned.

It is appropriate that the OHN is asked for an opinion on the health of employees with a tendency to repeated short-term absences as well as those who have had a long-term absence whether or not these are work related. An automatic OH review is advisable following a period of long-term sickness absence, of say three weeks duration, or following a reportable workplace accident as this offers the opportunity to decide whether the person is now fit enough to carry out the full requirements of their job or whether a phased return to work programme should be negotiated with both the client and their manager.

A competent assessment of a worker's fitness to return to work involves consideration of the extent of fitness or any degree of impairment and current health status in the light of their job demands. A skilled and competent assessment requires consideration of aspects of the individual, their job, the hazards to which they may be exposed at work considered in the light of a range of legal requirements. These requirements are incorporated into the Murugiah *et al.* health assessment model: Fitness to Work (Figure 13.1). This model, developed by three practicing occupational health nurse educators, is designed specifically for use in the occupational health setting and assists in the decision making process regarding whether a worker who had previously experienced a significant health deficit is fit to return to work. Their return to work may, in the short term, be on restricted duties (Murugiah *et al.* 2002).

There are occasions when a return to work following serious illness or injury would be difficult without modifications being made to the work-process and/or the equipment used at work. The Disability Discrimination Act 1995 requires employers to make such reasonable adjustments for people who are disabled, as defined by the Act. In order to do so they need access to competent and professional advice. The specialist OHN is well placed to do this as they have knowledge of health and illness, the requirements of the worker's job coupled with an understanding of both employment and health and safety legislation. They are able to integrate clinical and problem solving skills with other expertise such as the skills of risk assessment, problem solving and multidisciplinary team working.

In order to facilitate a successful return to work programme it may be necessary for the OHN to make effective links with a range of practitioners including medical practitioners and those who work in the allied health professions such as occupational and physiotherapists and disability advisers. This facilitates them giving the best possible advice to both worker and manager. Although an employee may be fit to undertake work of some type, a multitude of factors, not least continuing health problems may preclude them from returning to their previous post. Unfortunately under such circumstances redeployment may be the only option in order to keep that person at work. Occasionally even redeployment is not an option owing to the nature,

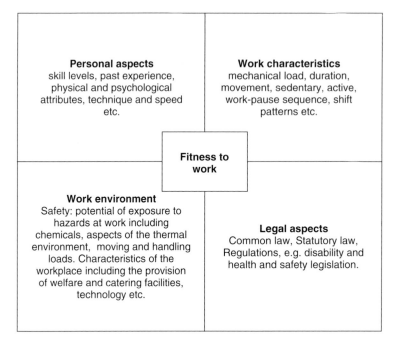

Personal aspects
skill levels, past experience, physical and psychological attributes, technique and speed etc.

Work characteristics
mechanical load, duration, movement, sedentary, active, work-pause sequence, shift patterns etc.

Fitness to work

Work environment
Safety: potential of exposure to hazards at work including chemicals, aspects of the thermal environment, moving and handling loads. Characteristics of the workplace including the provision of welfare and catering facilities, technology etc.

Legal aspects
Common law, Statutory law, Regulations, e.g. disability and health and safety legislation.

Figure 13.1 The fitness to work framework of assessment. (Source: Murugiah *et al.* 2002. Reproduced with permission)

severity or circumstances or of their health status and the person chooses to retire from work on the grounds of ill health seeing this as a positive step and the OHN can give valuable advice and support at this time.

The managerial domain of OHN practice incorporates policy development. The range of health related policies an organisation may need to formulate is very broad and reflects the type of work they undertake. Some of these include those covering home working, work with computers, moving and handling of loads, food hygiene, waste management, and working with chemical and microbiological hazards. OHNs also contribute to the formulation of policies focused on human resources including attendance management policies and strategies as already discussed. Senior OHNs manage and lead multi-disciplinary teams, a role previously only assigned to a physician.

Increasingly many OH services outsource their services; this is particularly the case since the advent of NHS Plus which has facilitated services initially set up for NHS establishments offering their services to businesses leading to valuable

income generation. This process must be well managed if it is to be successful. There are commonalities with managing any OH service as both require significant leadership and business acumen. Outsourcing involves the setting and negotiation of service level agreements, effective budgeting and procurement of human and other resources. The final part of the process is the effective management of both these contracts and the staff required to service them.

The environmental domain
The environmental domain is perhaps the aspect that is least recognisable to a 'generalist' as 'nursing care'. This can be the most challenging owing to the range of skills required in order to perform it with any degree of competence and an in-depth understanding of health and safety and employment legislation is therefore required. Particularly pertinent is an appreciation of the requirements of the myriad of regulations covering both health and safety and disability, much of which results from the UK being part of the European Union. In 1992 six regulations under

the Health and Safety at Work Act 1974 became law. These regulations are generally known as the 'six-pack'. A recurring theme within these regulations is the need for both risk and health assessments. All employers are required to undertake a general risk assessment supplemented with health surveillance for people exposed to hazards that have an identifiable adverse effect on their health such as exposure to respiratory or skin sensitising agents. In addition to the need for a general risk assessment, further risk assessments are included within the 'six-pack' for workers who use computers or who manually handle loads or patients. OHNs are skilled and considered competent to undertake, or teach others to undertake, such risk assessments. They are able to evaluate control measures such as local exhaust ventilation extracting chemicals in work areas such as laboratories or car spraying booths.

Many people work in industries that are intrinsically noisy. OHNs who practise in such industries are well placed to undertake a risk assessment to identify if employees are at risk, measure noise levels, comment on current exposure and suggest ways of reducing exposure by putting in place engineering or other controls. They are also able to comment on the suitability of personal protective equipment such as ear defenders including in-ear devices and ear muffs. They can interpret legislation covering noise in the workplace and decide which employees could be at risk of developing noise induced hearing loss. Under such circumstances they undertake audiometry in order to detect its very early signs enabling protective strategies to be instigated as a matter of urgency.

The educational domain of practice

The educational domain interlinks with the environmental domain previously discussed. It involves the OHN in teaching managers and workers on a range of issues as part of workplace health promotion. This is complementary to, but often different from, the health promotion interventions undertaken by nurses outside the occupational health setting. An example of such an activity is raising awareness of workplace hazards from managers to 'shop floor' staff and

being involved in developing strategies and policies to prevent exposure. This may, for example, involve developing and presenting a health education package teaching people who work with hazardous chemicals how they can protect themselves from exposure. This may include highlighting safe and unsafe working practices during the storage, use and disposal of hazardous material, protective mechanisms including local exhaust ventilation and finally advising on the suitability of personal protective equipment. This is a health promotion activity but not as most nurses would recognise it.

Public health strategies

OHNs are well placed to influence the health of the community and as such they are public health nurses. Having discussed the domains of their practice the contribution they are able to make to the Government's public health strategy will now be briefly explored. The end of the 20th and start of the 21st century has seen the publication of a number of public health documents including *Saving Lives: Our Healthier Nation* (DoH 1999); *Revitalising Health and Safety* (Department of the Environment, Transport and the Regions 2000); and the Occupational Health Advisory Committee report on improving access to occupational health support (Health and Safety Commission 2000). These publications acknowledge the extent and costs of work-related ill health and recognise the potential for the workplace to become a platform to achieve the Government's overall aim of reducing accidents and improving the health of the population. They have influenced the practice of OHNs by engaging them in public health agendas and are essential if they are to meet the aims of the ILO and WHO already highlighted earlier in this chapter. The Department of Health in association with the RCN and Association of Occupational Health Nurse Practitioners have underlined the contribution of OHNs to public health in their document *Taking a Public Health Approach in the Workplace* (DoH 2003). This guide states, 'Occupational health nurses are a key part of the public health workforce. Changing health needs, increasing public expectations and new Government policies make this role more important than ever before.' It acknowledges the contribution that OHNs may make in reducing health inequalities and improving physical and mental health of the community through workplace interventions. Interestingly Thornbory (2004) refers to the Health and Safety Commission's strategy for improving health and safety in Great Britain to 2010 and beyond whereby 'occupational health is acknowledged as a rising challenge now that "causes of safety failure" have been brought under some sort of control' (HSC 2004).

Specialist community public health nursing – Part 3 of the register maintained by the Nursing and Midwifery Council

So what will the future hold for OH nursing? The year 2004 saw the Nursing and Midwifery Council (NMC) opening a new three-part register which incorporates the 15-part register previously maintained by the United Kingdom Central Council for Nursing, Midwifery and Health visiting (UKCC). The third part, which does not allow for direct access for those not already registered with the NMC, is for specialist community public health nurses (SCPHN) and this includes health visitors and occupational health nurses. The NMC have demonstrated their commitment to the public health agenda by supporting a new qualification for qualified nurses that will lead to additional registration on this new part of the register. The NMC had debated whether the SPCHN qualification should be of a generic nature covering all aspects of specialist community public health nursing. This concept was rejected as it was quite rightly decided that it would be very difficult to ensure that graduates from such a programme would be 'fit for practice' across the whole field of public health nursing.

Validating a qualification that leads to registration on a separate part of the nursing register is a significant move. Previously qualifications in OH nursing were recordable but in contrast to the position with health visitors such a qualification did not lead to registration of the holders on a special part of the register. The establishment of a new third part of the register for public

health nurses which includes OHNs recognises their contribution to the public health agenda. It will undoubtedly benefit those who have specialist practitioner status. In the view of many practitioners a registerable qualification for OHNs is essential to ensure public protection. There may be implications for nurses who are practising in the OH setting without such a specialist practitioner qualification.

The NMC is responsible for setting standards for the length and key learning outcomes of courses conferring SCPHN status and these will include general competencies. Practitioners already having a recordable qualification conferring specialist practitioner status were automatically registered on the third part of the register from its inception as the content of these courses were congruent with the NMC requirements for registration as a public health nurse. (The NMC requirements for entry to the third part of the register mapped against the UKCC requirements for courses preparing specialist practitioner occupational health nurses are included as an appendix to this chapter.)

In future, practitioners who have completed an approved course offered at first or Masters' degree level completed in a minimum of 52 weeks and incorporating evidence-based, practice-centred learning will be eligible to register. One of the principles underpinning the design of these courses is the integration of theory with practice and an emphasis on inter-professional working.

In conclusion, this chapter has presented to the reader an overview of the aim of OH services and the role of the OHN as a specialist practitioner within them. The context of their practice and historical perspective has been explored with particular reference to their contribution to public health initiatives. The OHN can directly influence the health, health and safety, and productivity of the workforce and indirectly the health of the nation as a whole. It is an excellent career choice for nurses who enjoy a high degree of autonomy working with a predominantly well population.

Appendix

In 2004 radical changes were made to the register held by the Nursing and Midwifery Council (NMC). A complex register consisting of 15 parts

Table 13.1 NMC requirements for entry to the third part of the register mapped against the UK requirements preparing specialist practitioner occupational health nurses.

		NMC requirements for entry to the third part of the register			
		Search for health needs	Stimulation of awareness of health needs	Influences on policies affecting health	Facilitation of health enhancing activities including developing services and programmes
UKCC requirements for courses preparing specialist practitioner qualified occupational health nurses	Assess, plan, implement and evaluate occupational health nursing care	X	X	X	X
	Assess, manage and provide care in clinical and other emergencies including environmental incidents ensuring care and safety	X	X	X	X
	Promote effective use of OH services in the workplace	X	X	X	X
	Search out the health and health-related learning needs of the workforce & identify and initiate steps for health promotion, health maintenance, effective care for individuals and groups within organisations	X	X	X	X
	Build health alliances with other agencies for health gain	X	X	X	X
	Interpret and apply health and safety legislation and approved codes of practice with regard for the environment, the well being and protection of those who work, and the wider community	X	X	X	X

was simplified to a register consisting of a total of three; one part each for registered nurses and midwives and a third part for specialist community public health nurses. There is no direct entry to the third part of the register as it is dependent on prior NMC registration and on holding a recognised qualification in an area of public health nursing. The framework includes four broad principles including:

- Identifying health needs
- Strategic leadership to promote and protect health
- Policy and research development
- Service development

Each of these principles is underpinned by a number of public health domains with identified skills and associated competencies.

After consultation with a range of stakeholders including practitioners and educators it was decided by the NMC that on the inception of that new part of the register occupational health nursing practitioners holding an NMC recognised specialist practitioner qualification were eligible for third part registration. This decision was made as the NMC recognised specialist qualifications are focused on public health principles and cover four key areas of clinical nursing practice, care and programme management, practice development and practice leadership. The match between the NMC requirements for entry to the third part of the register mapped against the UKCC requirements for courses preparing specialist practitioner occupational health nurses are illustrated in Table 13.1.

References

Department of the Environment, Transport and the Regions (2000) *Revitalising Health and Safety: strategy statement*. The Stationery Office, London.

Department of Health (1998) *Report of the Independent Inquiry into the Inequalities in Health*. DoH, London.

Department of Health (1999) *Saving Lives: Our Healthier Nation*. Department of Health, London.

Department of Health (2003) *Taking a public health approach in the workplace*. Department of Health, London.

Doke, D.D. (2004) Happy talking. *Occupational Health*, **56**(4), 14–16.

Harling, K. (1999) In: *Perspectives in Public Health*, S. Griffiths & D. Hunter (eds). Radcliffe Medical Press.

Harriss, A. (2001) Attending to sickness absence. The experience of OH nursing degree students. *Occupational Health Review*, **92**, 24–27.

Harriss, A. (2004) Erring on the side of danger. *Occupational Health*, **56**(4), 24–27.

Health and Safety Commission (2000) *Occupational health advisory committee: report and recommendation on improving access to occupational health support*.

Health and Safety Commission (2004) *A strategy for workplace health and safety in Great Britain to 2010 and beyond*. HMSO21, London. HSC, London.

Health and Safety Executive (1995) *Good Health is Good Business: An Introduction to Managing Health risks at Work*. HSE, London.

International Labour Organisation (1959) *International Labour Organisation Occupational Services Recommendation no. 112*. International Labour Organisation, Geneva.

Lee, W.R. (1994) In: *Hunters Diseases of Occupations*, 8th edn. P.A.B. Raffle, P.H. Adams, P.J. Baxter & W.R. Lee (eds). Edward Arnold, London.

Murugiah, S., Thornbory, G. & Harriss, S. (2002) Assessment of fitness. *Occupational Health*, **54**(4), 26–29.

Paton (2004) Putting OH centre stage. *Occupational Health*, **56**(4), 10–11.

Payne, S. (1999) In: *Health and Work Critical Perspectives*. N. Daykin & L. Doyal (eds). Macmillan Press Ltd., London.

Pickvance, S. (1993) In: *Health and Work Critical Perspectives*. Daykin & Doyal (eds). Macmillan Press Ltd., London.

Rogers, B. (1994) *Occupational Health Nursing Concepts and Practice*. W.B. Saunders, London.

Royal College of Nursing (2003) *Nurses Employed Outside the NHS Recommended Pay, Terms and Conditions*. Royal College of Nursing, London.

Thornbory, G. (2004) In with the new. *Occupational Health*, **56**(6), 20–21.

World Health Organization (1973) *Environmental and health monitoring in occupational health*. Report of a WHO expert committee. Technical report series 535. World Health Organization, Geneva.

Chapter 14 **Community Mental Health Nursing**

Ann Long

Introduction

Community mental health nurses (CMHNs) may be located in health clinics, outreach centres, GP practices, voluntary organisations and accident and emergency departments. They practise a wide variety of therapies ranging from behavioural psychotherapy, family interventions and grief counselling to psychodynamic psychotherapy, relaxation and visualisation. Their raison d'etre is to represent people with mental health needs and to provide high quality therapeutic care founded on a code of professional practice (NMC 2002). Being accountable to that code gives nurses licence to enhance and own a personal practice methodology which is unique to each individual nurse's style and personhood.

Five defining characteristics underpin the professional practice of community mental health nursing:

- A guiding paradigm
- Therapeutic presence
- The therapeutic encounter
- The National Service Framework
- The principles of community mental health nursing

The fundamental portrait of the CMHN as a reflective practitioner (Schön 1983) is succinctly interwoven into each of the *distinct characteristics*. Moreover, these essential aspects are not displayed in order of priority. They are operationalised continuously and simultaneously. It is their dynamic combination in practice that illustrates the distinctive nature of community mental health nursing.

A guiding paradigm

The axioms underpinning community mental health nursing are to respect, value and facilitate the self-propelling and self-generating growth

unique within each individual (Rogers 1990). For CMHNs the adoption of a person-valuing paradigm can serve as a means of utilising systematically the powerful healing forces both within and between individuals, families, groups and nations. A person-valuing paradigm necessitates the use of a co-participative, person-centred perspective of a nurse *being* with and for the individual who is in need of mental health care as advocated by Long (1997a).

Being as a therapeutic experience

At an individual level, *being with* and *caring for* the person is both a valuable and therapeutic experience (Benner 1984; Leininger 1978; Long 1997a; Travelbee 1971; Watson 1985). It emphasises the role of the nurse as caring for the person with an illness. The person-valuing paradigm demands that community mental health nurses facilitate people to understand and make sense of their 'self' through listening, exploration, clarification and interpretation rather than by observing and explaining illnesses and behaviours. The person-valuing paradigm suggested here has its foundations in, and was developed from, a synthesis of Parse's theory of human becoming (Parse 1992), Rogers' human science perspective of a unitary human being (Rogers 1980) and existential phenomenology (Heidegger 1987; Merleau-Ponty 1974; Satre 1969).

Therapeutic ambience

Therapeutic activities should be conducted within a therapeutic ambience marked by a high degree of emotional nourishment and containment for feelings (conscious and unconscious), acceptance, genuine concern for, and openness to, sharing. The person-valuing paradigm paradoxically implies that mental health and well-being are embroiled in the process of 'becoming' (Rogers 1990). Mental health and well-being are embedded into each individual's chosen way of living, their cherished ideals, and into the way in which he or she works to become an autonomous person (Mills 1986). At the *same time*, it means believing oneself to be part of and concerned for the general community and a wider universe of people (Long 1997a). Mental health is profoundly featured in each person's own experience of both valuing and living in their internal and external world; and this can be made known to the nurse only by their personal description. Herein lies the complexity, quality and richness of the process of community mental health nursing.

It is imperative that CMHNs master the ability to show their clients that they value, and convey accurate empathy with, the latters' communicated expressions of felt helplessness and experiences of distress. Coupled with this, CMHNs must demonstrate the ability and confidence to listen authentically, explore, clarify and interpret the immediate experience that occurs during each therapeutic encounter (Long 1999; Rogers 1977). This is an empowering process. The use of a person-valuing paradigm as a basis on which to build practice methodology demands that nurses actually believe that every person is a unique being within the social context of each experience as it is lived (Heidegger 1992). Hence, mental health providers and professionals might benefit from recognising that everyone in distress is an individual and has different needs, preferences and potential ways of coping; thus support for their ways of coping must be provided through their inclusion in the decision making processes involved in 'the planning and delivery of care' (*The National Service Framework*, DoH 1999c, p. 4) and in case/care reviews (Mental Health Foundation, *Strategies for Living* 2000).

Becoming a mirror image for the person

To achieve a successful outcome and recovery the client must observe descriptions of lived experiences and personal histories of need and distress being validated in the eyes of a non-judgemental nurse who demonstrates empathy with, mutuality, genuineness and concern for the other person, namely that client. Community mental health nursing begins from, and within, the essence of the person/client's own perception of their needs. Moreover, as catalysts for healing and change, nurses must rely upon the client for the direction, pace and movement of the healing process (Long 1999; Rogers 1961).

Providing a new focus of care: shifting the power base

Shifting to a new person-valuing paradigm as a guide to practice means more than adding to or replacing wide and unacceptable variations in provision (DoH 1999c, p. 5). It presents a formula for helping to raise standards, tackle inequalities and meet the special needs of women, men and different ethnic groups (DoH 1999c).

A person-valuing paradigm, because of its integral, unifying, community and global aspects, is an ideal foundation on which to build the practice methodology of community mental health nursing. The *Code of Professional Conduct* (NMC 2002) allows nurses to develop a unique, individualised style of practice based on the person-valuing paradigm. This gives CMHNs the freedom to work in co-participation with clients and the community and demands that the clients direct the clinical decision making process.

Self-monitoring

In view of these humanistic, esoteric and essential health-giving and life-nurturing dimensions, CMHNs must come to believe that they, too, possess essential life-affirming and health-giving inner strengths and resources including the human quality to care. They too need to continue to develop and grow as persons and as professionals. Because of this, they should be facilitated to believe that they are self-actualising people with a need to further enhance this human capacity to care (Brykczynska 1999; Heidegger 1992). In addition, they must be endowed with skills and provided with opportunities to become open and genuine, self-monitoring, self-reflective and self-receptive people. This goal may be achieved through the belief in, and adoption of, structured, sensitive, clinical supervision (Hawkins & Stohet 1992).

Therapeutic presence

Community mental health nursing in its uniqueness attributes precedence to the interpersonal, dynamic process of enabling individuals, families and nations to restore equilibrium between their internal and external worlds (Long & Chambers 1993). Through the therapeutic use of self the nurse embraces the concept of self to influence all therapeutic approaches to care (DHSS NI 1993, 1995, 1999). Implicit in this concept is the belief that a nurse's therapeutic presence has a complex role to play in the promotion of healing and in the recovery process – in liberating self-propelling growth and recovery in clients. The unique attributes of the CMHN, coupled with the salience of what he or she says, feels, thinks and believes, when accepted and introjected, can lead to clients internalising a positive experience of self. *Being with* and *for* clients is the quintessential health-giving way in which CMHNs can meet the psychotherapeutic needs of clients (Slevin 1999).

Community mental health nursing is an interactive process and as such its primary purpose is to restore clients' dignity and worth as healthy, unique human beings. Both the CMHN and the client are human beings first. Both possess given, individual variances: all the characteristics and attributes of being human. In this very real sense, both the client and the nurse are equal, yet each is unique in individual expression of these characteristics. This has implications for the interactions that occur in the nurse–client relationship and also for the pace and direction of the healing work.

A central tenet of the nurse–client relationship is *therapeutic* communication. It is a two-way process. Communication embraces the notions of giving and receiving, opening up, reflecting and responding (Hargie & Dickson 1997). Working within a therapeutic encounter, communication also involves *empathic being* and having an ability to invite, 'stay with', contain and interpret a client's painful thoughts and emotions, thus help the person to work through distressing experiences. Keltner *et al.* (1991) believe that:

> 'Therapeutic communication relies on client disclosure of personal and sometimes painful feelings, with the professional at an emotional distance, near enough to be involved but objective enough to be helpful.'

> 'Nurses' unresolved conflicts about authority, sex, assertiveness and independence will tend to create, rather than solve problems.'

Unexamined life histories, coupled with unexplored and unresolved feelings *in nurses*, may render them unable to stay with and contain clients' painful thoughts and feelings. When this happens, a nurse's presence is no longer that of a catalyst for healing and recovery rather she/he becomes instead atherapeutic. Therefore, CMHNs require an understanding and awareness of their own *therapeutic presence* in order that they may be able to stay with and contain their clients' innermost thoughts, feelings and emotions. Otherwise, they may find it impossible to integrate their therapeutic presence into the nurse–client relationship. Rogers (cited in Baldwin 1987) has written:

> 'Recently I find that when I am closest to my inner intuitive self whatever I do seems to be full of healing, simply my presence is releasing and helpful.'

The therapeutic encounter

Being and working with another human being is quintessential for the development and maintenance of a therapeutic relationship, which is the crux of community mental health nursing. Keltner *et al.* (1991) have said that:

> 'The therapeutic relationship can be described in terms of three stages of development, namely, orientation, working and termination.'

The essence of the therapeutic relationship is referred to by Buber (1937, 1987), as the *interhuman*. The interhuman is not owned by either the nurse or the client, it exists between them. Community mental health nursing is, therefore, located within the interhuman. The central tenet in Buber's philosophy is that to be human is to relate (Buber 1988; Buber & Rogers 1965; Slevin 1999). In community mental health nursing, then, the nurse–client relationship *takes centre stage as* a therapeutic channel for healing and growth and as such it is an end in itself. Each therapeutic encounter should therefore become a lived experienced for both the nurse and the client on the basis of co-participation.

Community mental health nursing also aims to help clients to gain an awareness of the meaning of life and the purpose of living (Long 1997a). In co-participation with clients, intentions are identified for achieving that aspiration by designing specific goals and plans (DoH 1999c). Thus, the promotion of such decision making and decision taking contributes greatly to empower-ment and to the holistic healing process (DoH 1999c; Long 1999; Mental Health Foundation 2000).

The National Service Framework

The National Service Framework for mental health was designed to drive up quality by setting national standards and defining service models for promotiong mental health and treating mental illness. It emphasises the need to ensure that programmes of care can be deliverd locally. In addition, it established milestones and a specific group of high-level performance indi-cators against which progress within agreed timescales could be measured. To ensure this framework starts and remains up-to-date a national group has been set up to oversee both implementation and future development. The standards have been set out in seven areas, which are:

- Standard one: mental health promotion
- Standards two and three: primary care and access to services
- Standards four and five: effective services for people with severe mental illness
- Standard six: caring about carers
- Standard seven: preventing suicide

The standards are realistic, challenging and measurable, and are based on the best available evidence. Interestingly, all of these standards had already been interwoven within the principles of community mental health nursing, which were designed prior to the framework. They will now be integrated into the following discussion.

The principles of community mental health nursing

In its uniqueness, community mental health nursing recognises the diversity and breadth of the role of CMHNs. They aim to offer a proactive outreach service which embraces a professional responsibility to seek out, challenge and influence public policy related to mental health. Govern-ment, health education and health promotion agencies have been asked to support and promote positive images of people living with mental health problems (Mental Health Foundation 2000). Hence, the overall objective of CMHNs is to work in co-participation with clients, their carers and communities to maximise overall mental health potential.

In this section the four principles of health visiting, as recommended by the CETHV (1977), and the standards and service models prioritised in the *National Service Framework* (DoH 1999c) are incorporated and reformulated into five principles of community mental health nursing. These five principles were recommended in a policy document to all community nurses, mid-wives and health visitors in Northern Ireland as their guide to practice (DHSS 1996):

- The search for recognised and unrecognised mental health needs
- The prevention of a disequilibrium in mental health
- The facilitation of mental-health-enhancing activities
- therapeutic approaches to mental health care
- influences on policies affecting mental health

These principles draw on the notion that 'principles state a relationship between two facts that may be used to explain, guide and predict action' (Chater 1975).

The first principle: the search for recognised and unrecognised needs

The search for and identification of recognised and unrecognised mental health needs is integral to the concept of a facilitative and empowering partnership with clients and communities. In order to practice this principle, CMHNs are required to research, analyse and audit detailed health and social profiles of the specific recog-nised and unrecognised needs they identify within the population they serve. A systematic health and social needs-based model is suggested here, which is based on four key factors:

- Health and social needs profiling
- Prioritising mental health care
- Primary care and access to services
- Specification of mental health targets and the identification of measurable mental health outcomes

Health and social needs profiling

Mental health cannot be divorced from the socio-economic and cultural context in which it is experienced (Anderson 1984; Cowley 1991; DoH 1999c; Long 1997b). Consequently, many unre-solved mental health needs have continued to be unaddressed. Health and social profiling is one way of endeavouring to redress this situation as it is a specific attempt to identify the level and distribution of poverty and poverty-related health and social needs (current and potential) in a defined population (Blackburn 1992). A health and social profile is essentially a contextualising profile. It assigns identified health information about recognised and unrecognised mental health needs into a social context. It offers CMHNs an overview of poverty and an awareness of how people's experience of poverty shapes their lives and affects their mental health.

Further, a health and social profile acts as a baseline and information source for prioritising, planning, implementing and evaluating practice (DoH 1999c; Rowe *et al.* 1997; Twinn *et al.* 1990). In addition, it generates objective and comparable information and data that can be used by practi-tioners and addresses a major deficit in the information base that exists regarding mental illness in the communities and GP practices within which CMHNs work (DoH 1999c). At a wider level, the development and updating of com-munity mental health and social profiles provides evidence for the evaluation of the effectiveness of mental health services by using approaches that are tailormade to meeting clients' needs and perceptions rather than simply recording the

activities and skills of each individual practitioner (DoH 1999c; Rowe & Mackeith 1991).

Prioritising

Practitioners will require the support of managers skilled in their area of professional practice if they are to draw up priorities and develop their work to the highest standard and effectively and efficiently deliver community mental health nursing care. Standards two and three of the *National Service Framework* (DoH 1999c) indicate that primary care and access to services are fundamental to the effective delivery of mental health services. This seems justifiable as mental health indicators range on a continuum from suicide, severe depression and phobia through to the whole range of identity, sexual, marital and human relationship problems for which it is both humane and realistic to offer high-quality nursing care (Long & Chambers 1993).

Primary care and access to services

A primary care led NHS is a fundamental health service priority that is built on the proposition that primary care professionals are best placed to assess, plan, deliver and evaluate services that are based as near to service users as possible (DoH 1999c; NHSME 1996). Further strengthening of clinical effectiveness initiatives and extending the role of primary health care through primary care trusts that emphasise health care quality are currently features of the Government's evolving health service strategies (DoH 1997). Such features include reductions in the number of people admitted to psychiatric hospitals and in the onset of mental illnesses in addition to support for carers and cost-effectiveness.

Clearly, services must be developed to ensure that all members of the community have equal access to health services (DoH 1999c). Evidence reveals that 25% of of routine GP consultations are for people with a mental health need (Goldberg & Bridges 1987) and around 95% of mental health care is provided solely by primary care teams (Goldberg & Huxley 1992). Further, it is essential to ensure that most of the guidance provided by all team members is honest and consistent. In terms of first-level guidance, members of the primary care team must work with other agencies and the voluntary sector organisations, for example, the Samaritans and Saneline, to ensure that access is available 24 hours daily. Whatever the point of contact the principles of The new NHS Direct (DoH 1998a) should apply. In addition, a duty doctor, section 12 approved, and an approved social worker must be available around the clock, every day of the year (DoH 1999c).

However, it must be acknowledged that not all members of the primary care team are educated and trained in contemporary evidence-informed interventions. Consequently, community mental health nurses often act as consultants to other team members on mental health issues. The importance of carrying out on-going accurate needs assessment is stressed.

Specification of targets and the identification of measureable outcomes

The ways in which mental health services are commissioned need further development to ensure that resources and priorities reflect a planned approach and an overall strategy for promoting mental health, preventing mental ill health and ensuring the therapeutic care of people who are mentally ill and their carers (DoH 1999c). Indeed, CMHNs should use the commissioning process (Roy 1990) to improve, change and expand services to meet the needs and preferences of users, carers and communities. *The Health of the Nation* (DoH 1991) set out a comprehensive strategy for health which has been adopted by the World Health Organization as a model for other countries to follow (Yeo 1993).

Moreover, mental health outcomes/objectives must be identified and evaluated yearly to measure how effectively the objectives have been met. Contracts can be informed by the *needs profile* which will need annual updating (Rowe *et al.* 1997).

The second principle: the prevention of disequilibrium in mental health

This principle reflects standard one, mental health promotion, of the National Service Framework (DoH 1999c). The Caplan (1961) model of primary,

secondary and tertiary prevention can be used as a practical guide to focus on this principle. Primary preventative measures are carried out by CMHNs through designing mental health promotion programmes and health education packages, for example, the promotion and maintenance of healthy relationships (Duck 1992; Kelley *et al.* 1988); preconceptual mental health care; promoting healthy bonding (Bee 1994; Sluckin *et al.* 1992); facilitating emotional health and well-being; healthy, non-shaming and non-punitive communication patterns (Dwindell & Middleton-Moz 1986); human sexuality and education for love (Iven 1994); and death, dying and letting go as natural experiences in living (Gunzberg & Stewart 1994; Sherman 1988; Worden 1982). CMHNs are in a key position to initiate, develop, implement and research such health-promoting and life-enriching programmes. Such mental health activities challenge nurses to redirect their focus and promote positive mental health at a wider level.

Secondary prevention

Secondary preventative measures are conducted by CMHNs who offer individuals, families, groups and communities a diversity of health promoting strengths and strategies for coping with identified disequilibrium in mental health. Some examples of such health-giving activities are anxiety and stress management (Gaylin 1989); dealing with rational fear (Beck 1979); resolving anger, resentment and shame (Bradshaw 1992); screening and identifying 'at risk' indicators for self-destructive and self-abusive behaviours (Beck *et al.* 1974, 1979); and planning screening programmes for the early identification and remediation of addictive behaviours (Long & Mullen 1994). Examples of service models and of good practice include the provision of 24 hour crisis response teams, assertive outreach teams, one-stop clinics, the CALM programme (campaign against living miserably), local mental health helplines and self-harm intervention services (DoH 1999c, p. 34–39).

To put any of these programmes into action requires an advanced level of planning, educative, therapeutic and management skills (Cowley 1991).

Tertiary prevention

Tertiary prevention embraces standards four and five, effective services for people with severe mental illnesses, of the National Service Framework (DoH 1999c). Tertiary prevention involves planning current mental health care and preventing further deterioration in people who endure chronic mental ill health. To be successful in carrying out this role, CMHNs must be competent in advanced skills, which include monitoring clients' and carers' satisfaction. In addition, they must be competent to assess, monitor and evaluate the therapeutic modalities provided including their own health care skills. This principle also embraces the notion that CMHNs are proficient in assessing, monitoring and evaluating the uses, benefits and positive and negative side effects of drugs and other chemicals used in psychiatry (Healy 1993) as well as in the field of addictions (Long & Mullen 1994). For further information on service models and examples of good practice please see the National Service Framework (DoH 1999c, p. 52). However, it must be cautioned that many of the models cited in this framework have not yet been empirically investigated.

The third principle: the facilitation of mental-health-enhancing activities

Long and Chambers (1993) defined mental health as:

'A process of equilibrium both within and between the inner and outer Self, the social environment and the natural world in which people live. Within individuals it is manifest by self-awareness; self-acceptance; the ability to cope with changing life circumstances; a personal recognition and acceptance of inner strengths and resources; and a desire to aim for continuous personal potential and self-development throughout life. Positive mental health leads to a true value of all people as unique individuals and, therefore, the awareness of the existence of one humanity in an evolving world.'

The facilitation of mental-health-enhancing activities can be promoted by designing health and self-awareness programmes. Such educative experiences should be designed and implemented in ways that empower people to come to *believe in* themselves as unique individuals; enable them to come to know, understand and accept both self and others; improve relationships; increase their understanding of life's meaning and purpose; and realise their creative potential. One of the key findings in the *Strategies for Living* report (Mental Health Foundation 2000) demonstrated that the 71 interviewees with mental distress included in this study highlighted the need for professionals to acquire 'people valuing' strategies. People strategies were categorised into: ongoing survival strategies, crisis or life saving strategies, medication, physical exercise, religious and spiritual beliefs, money and other activities, such as hobbies, receiving information and the need for creative expression.

At community level, to protect the individual's autonomy within defined limits, society imposes norms of behaviour on its members (Prior 1993). In the most permissive range, compliance brings personal acceptance and the enhancement of social esteem, social status and material rewards. Alternatively it is difficult, if not impossible, for others to sustain and maintain mental health and retain their dignity in a climate where poverty and unemployment are paramount; where there is gross inequality and social injustice; where the young, the homeless, and those who are socially disadvantaged, including those who belong to minority groups are undervalued and deprived of equitable opportunities and equal civil liberties for personal, social, educative and futuristic self-growth and development (Long 1997b; DoH 1999c).

The fourth principle: therapeutic approaches to mental health care

The role of the CMHN has undergone significant reclarification as community mental health care services have continued to expand and develop. The search for a more specialised role for CPNs has evolved as service responses become more sophisticated. This will demand an holistic approach to care based on the principle tenet that CMHN's should be able to utilise a range of therapeutic interventions. Carr *et al.* (1980) were early in calling upon CPNs to develop a range of skills which would enable them to be recognised as clinical consultants, a term which has now been discussed at length by the Mental Health Nursing Review (DoH 1994) and the DHSS (NI) (1999).

Others counter-argued that specialisation was nothing more than a form of professional escapism. Barker (1997); Barker *et al.* (1998); Skidmore and Friend (1984); White (1993) indicated that specialisation did little to improve the quality of nursing care offered by CPNs. These authors cautioned against this developing trend. They contended that the needs of certain clients would be overlooked if particular clients and their needs did not match the appropriate specialty, hence they challenged the benefits of specialisation on client-care outcomes.

In the present era, however, CMHNs care for a wide variety of clients in the community. Hence, it is argued here that all CMHNs are specialist practitioners in that they are concerned with the totality of mental health care at individual, family, community, society and global levels. It is imperative, therefore, that they have a solid, eclectic and integrated theoretical grounding on a wide range of contemporary psychotherapeutic approaches to mental health care. Meanwhile, in order to function holistically, they must become purists in community mental health care nursing and consultants in the provision of high quality mental health care. Consequently, they must be exposed to the whole gamut of current psychotherapeutic modalities. The extent of the clients' needs for specialist mental health nursing intervention, however, requires further research.

Community mental health nurses: using therapeutic modalities to facilitate change

Examination of the differering approaches to care demonstrates that mental health nurses are continuing to advance new, culturally-sensitive approaches to nursing and a new epistemology of change for clients, carers and communities. As their role has evolved a number of levels of change have been witnessed:

Change at *level one* refers to a change in a specific behaviour such as smoking, which can be brought about by the provision of a behaviour modification technique.

Change at *level two* refers to a change in a set of behaviours that are controlled by a belief or a construct regarding how to operate in the world. Change is brought about by insight and this can be achieved by the use of cognitive therapy (Beck *et al.* 1985) or rational emotive therapy (Ellis 1984) or the 'gentle art of reframing' (Watzlawick 1974).

Change at *level three* refers to a change in a set of beliefs that are held within a world view or paradigm. An example of such a change might take place when individuals reach retirement. Their sense of meaning in life and their identities which might have been established through their work are lost. Most 'depth' therapies, such as psychoanalytic or psychodynamic operate at this level.

Change at *level four* refers to a change in a set of paradigms or world views. Level four is related to not being identified in any world view but rather being truly oneself. Work at this level does not involve therapy as such but spiritual discipline such as meditation or yoga.

Change at *family/carer level* research has demonstrated that people experiencing severe psychotic symptoms are very sensitive to their environments (Hatfield & Lefley 1987; Gournay 1995a,b). Since families provide the essential psychosocial environment for patients, working with families must be a necessary part of caring for peole with severe and enduring mental ill health. The evidence of the efficacy of practical family interventions in schizophrenia is well documented and has been the focus of a systematic review by the Cochrane Collaboration (Mari & Steiner 1996). Psychosocial interventions have the potential to engage with families and carers in a meaningful way and contribute significantly to psychosocial adjustment and change of clients within their families and the local community. Programmes have already received national recognition as they are part of the prestigious Thorn Initiative (Gamble 1995). Much of the theoretical base of these programmes has been derived from work around high expressed emotion (EE) in families of people living with schizophrenia (Brooker 1990). Other units in the course include 'training in principles and practices of case management and in the psychological management of psychoses' (Hannigan 1998).

Change at European and global levels

Mental health and social inclusion have been chosen as key priorities for care at the global network of WHO Collaborating Centres for Nursing and Midwifery (1999). Six priority areas were highlighted to advance and strengthen cross-national cooperation, invigorate new activity and redefine priorities in the field of mental health care. This European innovation provides a platform for listening to the voices and recognising the expertise of users of mental health services, as well as nurses, and all those involved in mental health care. All have a role in shaping and influencing the care and service delivery of the future. Priorities are:

- Enhancement of the value and visibility of mental health
- Development of mental health indicators
- Promotion of mental health of children and young people
- Promotion of mental health in old age
- Working life, employment policy and promotion of mental health

Examination of these levels and styles of change, in combination with Long's (1998) work on the stages of healing, demonstrates that some people might wish to change only their behaviours. Others might wish to change a particular belief without wishing to change their world view. Appreciating the different levels of change can enable community mental health nurses to assess both at what level clients want to change and at what level they want to remain the same. Therapeutic approaches to care would be enhanced if they could be matched accordingly.

Listening to the voice of users and their carers

This section embraces standard six of the National Service Framework (DoH 1999c). People who are ill and their carers have a right to expect considerate and competent care. To achieve this practitioners must feel supported to take ownership of their practice. To make decisions based on clinical judgement CMHNs must accept responsibility for the maintenance and advancement of standards of care and for the protection of clients. In so doing CMHNs should ensure that practice is founded on the belief that each individual is capable of achieving his or her full potential and is respected as the primary player in the care-transaction process.

As new care pathways develop in mental health the quest for evidence-informed approaches to interventions has been promoted. Unfortunately, the voice of users has not been integrated within the evidence base. All too often mental health service users and their carers have been the subject of research – providing details of their lives – to be used by others. However, rarely has their expertise and experience actually been used to influence service development and treatment response. In this regard pressure groups and consumer organisations add an important dimension to the debate.

Carers play a vital role in helping to look after service users, particularly those with severe mental illness. The Government has shown the importance it assigns to ensuring that all carers get the services and support they need in its strategy for carers (DoH 1999d). The approach is built around three fundamental issues; information, support and care. Carers of service users, including young carers, should be involved in their own assessment of their caring and their physical and mental health needs and this should be carried out on an annual basis (DoH 1999c). In addition to this, they should be given their written care plans, which are designed and implemented in partnership with them.

Further, the emphasis on collaboration and cooperation, with the plurality of statutory, voluntary and private providers, stimulates a need for quality assurance and clincial governance, which hopefully will increase the choices available to individuals and their carers (DoH 1998a; NHSME 1992).

The fifth principle: influencing policies affecting mental health

Mental health is political. It cannot be divorced from the decisions made by local councils or from policies created and legislated at government level. As such, CMHNs should be politically aware and assume positive action roles on behalf of their clients. This could be achieved through the creation and utilisation of local networks with the aim of influencing the political agenda and promoting positive mental health for all members of the population.

Managed care

The concept of *managed care* is a recent variant of the terms care management and case management (Cochrane 2001). Managed care has been established largely against a backdrop of the dialogue on best practice versus best value. Essentially, it involves designing planned programmes that specify what will be provided, the range of interventions, diagnostic tests and the protocols to be followed in providing the services. Care provision, therefore, is determined by guidelines, which are broad in that they state the general range of provision and some guidelines on delivery. In addition, managed care involves the formation of *integrated care pathways*, which state the activities that will take place at each stage in the course of the care provided to users.

Designing integrated care pathways involves cooperation and collaboration among health and social services providers to meet the holistic needs of people with mental health problems and their carers. This includes all those people who will be, or have been, discharged from mental hospitals and other institutions.

The National Service Framework (DoH 1999c) operates at the level of providing broad guidelines; however, they operate largely within a managed care philosophy, which is increasingly commonplace within UK health services. Managed care could be used for people considered to present a risk of harm, either to self or others, along with the use of the supervision register (DoH 1995). Supporting this guidance are legislative powers enshrined in the Mental Health Act 1983 and the Mental Health: Care in the Community Act

1995, which introduced the concept of supervised discharge. Combined, they provide a set of principles to frame managed care and service co-ordination. In practice, however, implementation is fragmented.

The approach demands the allocation of a key worker who appropriately reflects the needs of individual clients and their carers and also ensures that different professional skills are utilised to best effect. CMHNs are in the ideal position to act as key workers.

Supervised discharge planning

The notion of developing a concept of *supervised discharge*, and the action taken to ensure that CMHNs play a central role in the planning and implementation of managed care is crucial for the advancement of community mental health services and a locally based approach to care. It is fundamental that managed care with its integrated care pathways approach provides effective, safe and appropriate intervention strategies and proactive support systems for all patients generally and for ensuring the safe and therapeutic preparation for and transition of patients from hospital to the community setting (Mental Health Nursing Review, DoH 1994; MIND publication, *Discharged from Mental Hospital* (Bean & Mounser 1993).

Further, primary care trusts were implemented against a background of growing public and media concern, consequently greater emphasis is currently placed on ensuring the provision of effective support systems and continuing holistic, psychotherapeutic care for people with serious and enduring mental illness. The most prominent response to the reporting of high profie incidents where risk has been poorly managed has been the call for greater powers to ensure compliance with medication in the community setting. These powers have featured in the latest review of mental health legislation in the form of a community treatment order (CTO) (DoH 1999a).

Overall, nurses and other mental health professionals, for example, could set about designing strategies to meet the current government's five challenges set out in the National Service

Framework for Mental Health (DoH 1999c). They are:

- Tackling the causes of inequalities
- Ensuring fast and easy access to a range of therapeutic interventions
- Keeping patients fully informed at all stages of their illness and the recovery process
- Involving patients in their own care by working in partnership with them and planning their care with them
- Designing actions to improve both the clinical performance and the productivity of the NHS
- Promoting flexibility in education and training and also in working practices and removing fudged professional boundaries to ensure that the NHS has the right skills, organised in the right way, to deliver modern, flexible and patient centred services

Ultimately, mental health care means supporting individuals and communities to make choices, to explore and test out their options and to learn from their experiences in life. It does not ignore the need to protect individuals and others from potential harm but it strives for a better balance between professional enforcement and patient choice, which needs to take place in a therapeutic and nurturing environment.

Risk assessment

There is no doubt that the benefits to be achieved by real community care, and concomitant increased normalisation for people who are mentally ill and their carers, far outreach the deficits. This may be especially true for our future generations. However, there are real concerns about the dangers that a minority of people with serious mental illness may pose to the community. These concerns have been focused on a small, but tragic, number of high profile incidents of violence and suicide, prompting an internal review by the government on the care of vulnerable people with mental health problems who might slip through the net of services. There is an urgent need to review current practice and to define ways which help identify and protect individuals 'at risk', and also safeguard the

community. The implementation of the managed care approach, involving the concept of a 'named' key worker, will require mental health nurses to offer more formal specifications of their risk assessment methods, including the criteria underpinning clinical judgements. *Assessing and Managing Risk* has been published as a training package that could be used nationally to establish some systematic multidisciplinary approaches to this complex issue (Morgan 1999).

Risk management falls into three distinct categories; before, during and after an incident or event. Prevention is the key as neither practitioners nor patients wish to be on the giving or receiving end of serious harm. The content of the care plan will also help to prevent risk. Risk assessment can be carried out through the channel of continuous assessment and reassessment of holistic needs together with an open policy on information sharing and exploration of the thoughts and feelings of patients and carers and an openness to mutual learning. Risk management should be an implicit or explicit goal for interventions. The most appropriate activity for risk minimisation is initiating and maintaining a safe and therapeutic relationship with the services that can be achieved for example through assertive outreach (Allen 1998; Morgan 1999). The provision of evidence-based psycho-social interventions together with collaborative approaches to medication management further enhances risk minimisation. Paradoxically, risk-taking is also an important part of risk assessment and management. Positive risk-taking means supporting patients to make and take decisions about their lives, to explore and test out their choices and to learn from the experience of 'failure' as this is what living is about. This suggests that CMHNs take positive risks in the carrying out of their role.

Advocacy

The CMHNs advocacy role is primarily to safeguard and represent the rights of their clients and to assist, enable and empower clients to ensure that their needs are expressed and met. The possession of rights enhances the dignity of the rights held and so exemplifies the idea of respect for persons (Campbell 1988). People with a mental health problem have the right to liberty, equity of services with other citizens, acknowledgement of their mental illness, and access to survivor groups. They also have the right to refuse an assessment or treatment, and carers have the right to refuse to care (BMA 1992). Parallel to this, both clients and carers have the right to complain about the services provided, including that of the 'named' CMHN (NHSME 1992).

Thus, CMHNs have a duty to educate and empower clients and carers in the social and life skills necessary to enable them to make complaints and seek health and social justice. In this way clients are empowered to take decisions and so take control of their lives. Moreover, this enhances their self-advocacy skills. Advocacy, therefore, is an essential component of mental health nursing. CMHNs are required to protect and defend the rights of their clients to ensure that their strengths and needs and not just their diagnoses are recognised.

Homeless and 'rootless' people
It is also true to say that little attention has been given to the bulk of mentally ill individuals who generally have no home and few relatives (Bean & Mounser 1993). Nevertheless, it is fair to say that some progress has been made in this area. CMHNs have a key role in working alongside people who are homeless and motivating them to experiment with ideas and learn social and life skills. They may even encourage people who are homeless to share their real experience of what it means to be a homeless person in a wealthy society (Dewdney *et al.* 1994; Long 1997b).

The prevention of suicide
Standard seven of the National Service Framework (DoH 1999c) relates to preventing suicide. Statistics on suicide are a real cause for concern. Suicide is an avoidable form of mortality, yet it accounts for over 4000 deaths from suicide in England each year (DoH 1999c). The number of people dying from suicide is on a par with those dying from road traffic accidents (Long & Reid 1996). The likelihood of a person committing suicide depends on several factors including both physical and mental illness (Charlton *et al.* 1994), social deprivation and unemployment (Acheson 1998), and self-harm (Hawton & Fagg 1988). In addition, individuals in prison are at an especially high risk of suicide (Towl 1999). Suicidal ideations produce features of both a private depression and a public failure where there is a need to come to terms with the split between sentimental and unrealistic ideals and the reality, and pain, of living. Hence, the act of suicide can be defined as a short-cut to dying (Long *et al.* 1998). More work is required in this area. Clearly, suicide prevention must be targeted at individual, family, community and global levels. An example of an impressive suicide prevention strategy is one designed by the United States Air Force. This programme was designed to cultivate a community competent to deal with suicidal soldiers. One of its aims was to transform the soldiers' belief that 'seeking help is a sign of weakness' to the belief that 'it is a sign of strength'.

Therapist–client matching and multicultural community mental health care
The important challenge of meeting the needs of an increasingly diverse society remains controversial. Nonetheless, the *special needs* of people who belong to ethnic groups and of women who are mentally ill must be identified and met under the principle of influence.

Since many people who are mentally ill are female and from ethnic minorities and many CMHNs remain both white and male, it is imperative that CMHNs receive multicultural education and training. CMHNs working with different ethnic groups should be encouraged to examine their own values in relation to the needs of clients. Multicultural approaches require the avoidance of stereotyping and the encouragement of clients to explore their full potential, while realistically acknowledging social barriers to their aspirations.

A voice for women
Similarly, there is a need to critique and recast assumptions about the mental health of women in a way that elevates women's experiences.

Women frequently find their views being under-valued or discounted. CMHNs provide a voice for women who are mentally ill. They can also be instrumental in highlighting the real concerns of women's issues.

Gilligan (1977) and Benjamin (1984) suggest that important to women, including health professionals, is finding a balance between the extremes of self-definition: between autonomy (consideration of oneself) and connection (consideration of others). Mental health problems such as excessive dependency, anxiety and anger are subsequently explored as the consequences of narrow social and self definitions. The multi-factorial dimensions of mental health services for women are explored and debated by Belle (1982), Brodsky and Hare-Mussin (1980), Carmen *et al.* (1981), Kaplan (1983), Walker (1984), and the Mental Health Nursing Review (DoH 1994).

Moreover, CMHNs should be taught to identify and respect gender differences. They must hear and value women's perceptions about where their concerns and problems are coming from. Subsequently, it is the role of the CMHN to represent females and help influence policies affecting the mental health of all women.

A forum for children

The care of children and young people in addition to the promotion of their health and well-being is fundamental to enable them to reach their full potential. However, a deficit exists in the care of children with mental health needs and in the care of children who are living with parents who have a mental illness (McGreevey & Long 2000).

The effectiveness with which children's needs are assessed is the key to the effectiveness of subsequent interventions, the provision of services and ultimately to the health, growth and development of children. The duty to protect children from the emotional challenge of mental illness and the stress of living with parents with mental health problems demands knowledge, under-standing, guidance and multidisciplinary working. Determining who is in need, what those needs are and providing services to safeguard and care for these children requires urgent attention. All professionals must strive to ensure that children

grow up in circumstances consistent with the provision of safe and effective care.

Conclusion

Community mental health nursing services should be organised in a way that will help to accomplish the vision expressed about 'mental health for all' in the National Service Framework for Mental Health (DoH 1999c) and throughout this chapter. CMHNs engage in and strive to enhance the full spectrum of nursing care throughout the lifespan. This generic way of working enables the creative potential of professional practice to be fulfilled. Six key features are essential for the delivery and evaluation of high quality community mental health care:

- The primacy of mental health promotion and prevention at individual, family, group, community and global levels must be upheld
- The interface between primary care providers and specialist secondary mental health care providers needs to be strengthened
- The expertise of CMHNs and their unique and dynamic combination of therapeutic skills and psychotherapeutic approaches to care must be used to maximum effect at micro, median and macro levels
- Services must be proactive and responsive to recognised and unrecognised mental health needs
- Cooperative, collaborative and flexible approaches to practice must be adopted
- The views and perceptions of service users, their advocates and their families/carers must be paramount (UKCC 2000)

These aspects have long been recognised as the crucial factors in providing community mental health nursing services. Indeed, they were highlighted as important reasons for introducing both the NHS and Community Care Act 1990 and The Health Act 1999. However, the ways in which these Acts proposed to achieve these same health goals are markedly different from the ways put forward here. The key features addressed in this chapter emphasise the *empowerment* of clients, families, carers and communities and also of all practitioners who work in the field of mental health care. Implementation of the Act has created fundamental changes that need to be taken into account when considering the best way to plan community mental health nursing services. Primary care trusts will continue to develop their own philosophy or mission statement to guide the provision of the services they offer.

The fundamental principles of mental health for all, universal services for all and openness and availability for all remain unchanged. It is crucial therefore that all doctors, nurses and others who practise in the community work collaboratively and collectively to compile essential health and social data in order to promote the overall health of the community they serve. Finally, partnership between service users, government, local authorities, the voluntary and statutory services and community groups, both at national and local levels, is vital to improve the nation's mental health.

References

Acheson, D. (1998) *Independent inquiry into inequalities in health report*. DoH, London.

Allen, D. (1998) *Mental Health and Nursing*. Sage, London.

Anderson, D. (1984) Health Promotion – An Overview. *European Monographs in Health Education Research*, **6**(4), 4–19.

Baldwin, M. (1987) The Use of Self in Therapy: An Introduction. *Journal of Psychology and the Family*, Spring edition, **3**(1), 66–73.

Barker, P.J. (1997) *Assessment in psychiatric and mental health nursing: in search of the whole person*. Stanley Thornes, Cheltenham.

Barker, P.J., Keady, J., Croom, S., Stevenson, C., Adams, T. & Reynolds, B. (1998) The concept of serious mental illness: modern myths and grim realities. *Journal of Psychiatric and Mental Health Nursing*, **5**(4), 247–254.

Bean, P. & Mounser, P. (1993) *Discharged From Mental Hospital*. Macmillan Press, London.

Beck, A.T. (1979) *Cognitive Therapy and Emotional Disorders*. New American Library, New York.

Beck, A.T., Weissman, A., Lester, D. & Trexler, L. (1974) A measurement of pessimism: the hopelessness scale. *Journal of Consulting and Clinical Psychology*, **42**, 861–865.

Beck, A.T., Kovacs, M. & Weissman, A. (1979) Assessment of Suicidal Intention. The Scale for Suicidal Ideation. *Journal of Consulting and Clinical Psychology*, **47**, 343–352.

Beck, A.T., Emery, G. & Greenburg R.L. (1985) *Cognitive therapy of depression*. Guildford, New York.

Bee, H. (1994) *Tke Developing Child*. Harper Collins College Publishers, New York.

Belle, D. (1982) *Lives in Stress: Women and Depression*. Sage Publications, Beverly Hills, California.

Benjamin, L.S. (1984) Principles of Prediction Using Structural Analysis of Social Behaviour (SASB) In: *Personality and the Prediction of Behaviour* (eds R.A. Zucker, J. Aronoff & A.J. Rabin). Academic Press, New York.

Benner, P. (1984) *From Novice to Expert*. Addison-Wesley, Reading, Masachusetts.

Blackburn, C. (1992) *Poverty Profiling*. Health Visitors Association, London.

BMA (1992) *National Targets on Community Care: Targets for Service Provision* BMA, London.

Bradshaw, J. (1992) *Healing the Shame That Binds You*. Health Communications Inc, Florida.

Brodsky, A.M. & Hare-Mussin, R. (eds) (1980) *Women and Psychotherapy*. Guildford Press, New York.

Brooker, C. (1990) *Community Psychiatric Nursing. A Research Perspective*. Chapman and Hall, London.

Brykczynska, G. (1999) *Caring: The Compassion and Wisdom and Nursing*. Arnold, London.

Buber, M. (1937) *I and Thou*. T & T Clark, Edinburgh.

Buber, M. (1987) *I and Thou*. Translated by Walter Kaufmann. Scribners, New York.

Buber, M. (1988) *Knowledge of Man: Selected Essays*. Atlantic Highlands, Humanities Press, New York.

Buber, M. & Rogers, C. (1965) *Transcriptions of dialogue held 18 April 1965*. Ann Arbor, Michigan. Unpublished manuscript.

Campbell, T. (1988) *Justice*. Macmillan, London.

Caplan, G. (1961) *An Approach to Community Mental Health*. Tavistock Publications, London.

Carmen, E.H., Russo, N.F. & Miller, J.B. (1981) Inequality and Women's Mental Health. *American Journal of Psychiatry*, **138**, 1319–30.

Carr, P.J., Butterworth, C. & Hodges, B. (1980) *Community Psychiatric Nursing*. Churchill Livingstone, Edinburgh.

CETHV (1977) *An investigation into the principles of health visiting*. Council for the Education and Training of Health Visitors, London.

Charlton, J., Kelly, S., Dunnell, K., Evans, B. & Jenkins, R. (1994) *The Prevention of Suicide*. The Stationery Office, London.

Chater, S. (1975) *Understanding Research in Nursing.* WHO, Geneva.

Cochrane, D. (2001) *Managed care and modernization.* Open University Press, Buckingham.

Cowley, S. (1991) *A grounded theory of situation and process of health visiting.* PhD thesis, University of Brighton.

Dewdney, A., Gray, C., Minnion, A. & the residents of Rufford Street Hostel (1994). *Down But Not Out.* Trentham Books, Stoke-on-Trent.

DHSS NI (1993) *An Action Plan for Mental Health Nursing.* HMSO, Belfast.

DHSS NI (1995) *Community Nursing, Midwifery and Health Visiting in NI,* DHSS NI, Belfast.

DHSS NI (1996) *Valuing Diversity.* DHSS NI, Belfast.

DHSS NI (1999) *What Action? A Survey of Community Nurses, Midwives and Health Visitors Practice in NI,* DHSS NI, Belfast.

DoH (1991) *The Health of the Nation. A Consultative Document for Health in England.* Department of Health, London.

DoH (1993) *Secretary of State for Health announces ten point plan for developing successful and safe community care*: Press release. Department of Health, H/93/908.

DoH (1994) *Working in Partnership. A Collaborative Approach to Care.* Report of the Mental Health Nursing Review Team. Department of Health, London.

DoH (1995) *Building bridges: a guide to arrangements for interagency working for the care and protection of severly mentally ill people.* Department of Health, London.

DoH (1997) The New NHS: Modern, Dependable. Department of Health, London.

DoH (1998a) *Information for health: An information strategy for the modern NHS.* HSC (98) 168. Department of Health, London.

DoH (1998b) *A first class service: Quality in the new NHS Health Services,* circular 1998/113. Department of Health, London.

DoH (1999a) *The Patient's Charter: mental health services,* Department of Health, London.

DoH (1999b) *Review of the mental Health Act, 1983: draft outline proposals by the Scoping Study Committee.* Department of Health, London.

DoH (1999c) *National service framework for mental health: modern standards and service models.* Department of Health, London.

DoH (1999d) *Caring about carers: A national strategy for carers.* Department of Health, London.

Duck, S. (1992) *Human Relationships.* Sage Publications, London.

Dwinell, L. & Middleton-Moz, J. (1986) *After the Tears.* Health Communications, Pompano Beach, Florida.

Ellis, A. (1984) Rational emotive therapy. In: R. Corsini (ed) *Current psychotherapies.* Peacock, Itasca, IL.

Gamble, C. (1995) The Thorn nurse training initiative. *Nursing Standard,* **9**(15), 31–34.

Gaylin, W. (1989) Cited in: *Modelling awareness of feelings: a real tool in therapeutic communication workbox* (ed. L. Miller). *Perspectives in Psychiatric Care,* XX5(2).

Gilligan, C. (1977) In a different voice: women's conceptions of self and of mortality. *Harvard Educational Review,* **47**, 481–517.

Goldberg, D. & Bridges, K. (1987) Screening for mental illness in general practice: the general practitioners versus the screening questionnaire. *Journal of the Royal College of General Practitioners,* **37**, 15–18.

Goldberg, D. & Huxley, P. (1992) *Common mental disorders: A bio-social model.* Routledge, London.

Gournay, K. (1995a) Mental health nurses working purposefully with people with serious and enduring mental illness: an international perspective. *International Journal of Nursing Studies,* **32**(4), 341–52.

Gournay, K. (1995b) Future directions in community psychiatric nursing research. In: J. Carson, L. Fagin, & S. Ritter (eds) *Stress and coping in mental health nursing.* Chapman and Hall, London.

Gunzberg, J.C. & Stewart, W. (1994) *The Grief Counselling Casebook. A Student's Guide to Unresolved Grief.* Chapman and Hall, London.

Hannigan, B. (1998) Fragmentation or integration? *Mental Health Nursing,* **18**(2), 4–6.

Hargie, O.D.W. & Dickson, D. (1997) *The Psychology of Interpersonal Skills.* Croom Helm, London.

Hatfield, A.B. & Lefley, H.P. (1987) *Families of the mentally ill. Coping and adaptation.* Cassell, London.

Hawkins, P. & Stohet, R. (1992) *Supervision in the helping professions.* Open University Press, Milton Keynes.

Hawton, K. & Fagg, J. (1988) Suicide, and other causes of death, following attempted Suicide. *British Journal of Psychiatry,* **152**, 359–366.

Healy, D. (1993) *Psychiatric Drugs Explained.* Mosby Year Book, Europe.

Heidegger, M. (1987) *On Being and Acting: From Principles to Anarchy.* Translated by R. Shurrnann. Indiana University Press, Bloomington.

Heidegger, M. (1992) *The concept of time.* From the 1924 German Edition (translated by W. McNeil). Blackwell Publishers, Oxford.

Iven, H. (1994) Sex Education in Schools. In: *Teaching Today,* **8**. T. ASUW, London.

Kaplan, M. (1983) A Woman's View of DSM-III. *American Psychologist,* **38**, 78–92.

Kelley, H.H., Berscheid, E., Christensen, A., Harvey, J.H. & Houston, T.L. (1988) *Close Relationships*. W.H. Freeman, New York.

Keltner, I., Schroke, B. & Bostrom, M. (1991) *Psychiatric Nursing: A Psychotherapeutic Management Approach*. Mosby, London.

Leininger, M. (1978) *Transcultural Nursing*. Wiley, New York.

Long, A. (1997a) Nursing: a spiritual perspective. *International Journal of Nursing Ethics*, **4**(6), 496–510.

Long, A. (1997b) Avoiding abuse amongst vulnerable groups in the community: people with a mental illness, In: C. Mason (ed) *Achieving quality in community health care nursing*. Macmillan, London.

Long, A. (1998) The healing process, the road to recovery and positive mental health. *Journal of Psychiatric and Mental Health Nursing*, **5**, 1–9.

Long, A. (1999) *Interaction for Practice in Community Nursing*, Macmillan, London.

Long, A. & Chambers, M. (1993) Mental Health in Action. *Senior Nurse*, **13**(5), 7–9.

Long, A. & McGreevy, P. (1993) Advocating advocacy. *Community Psychiatric Nursing Journal*, October 1993, 11–14.

Long, A. & Mullen, B. (1994) An exploration of women's perceptions of the factors that contributed to their alcohol abuse. *Advanced Journal of Nursing*, **19**, 623–39.

Long, A. & Reid, W. (1996) An exploration of nurses' attitudes to the nursing care of suicidal patients in an acute psychiatric ward. *Journal of Psychiatric and Mental Health Nursing*, **3**(1), 29–37.

Long, A., Long, A. & Smyth, A. (1998) Suicide: A statement of suffering. *International Journal of Nursing Ethics*, (**5**)1, 3–15.

Mari, J.J. & Steiner, D. (1996) Family interventions for people with schizophrenia (Cochrane Review). In: *The Cochrane Library*. Issue 1. Oxford: Update Software.

McGreevey, C. & Long, A. (2000) *Children's perceptions of living with a parent who is mentally ill*. Unpublished MSc thesis, The University of Ulster, Northern Ireland.

Mental Health Foundation (2000) *Strategies for Living*. Mental Health Foundation, London.

Merleau-Ponty, M. (1974) *Phenomenology of Perception*. Humanities Press. New York.

Mills, J.S. (1986) *On Liberty*. Penguin, London.

Morgan, S. (1999) *Assessing and managing risk*. Pavilion: London.

NHS and Community Care Act 1990.

NHSME (1992) *Guidance on the Extension of the Hospital and Community Health Services Elements of GP Fundholding Scheme from 1 April 1993EL* 48 (92). NHS Management Executive, London.

NHSME (1994) *Introduction of supervision registers for mentally ill people*. HSG (94). NHS Management Executive, London.

NHSME (1996) *Annual Report 1995/96*. DoH, London.

Nursing & Midwifery Council (2002) *Code of Professional Conduct for the Nurse, Midwife and Health Visitor*, NMC, London.

Parse, R.R. (1992) Human Becoming: Parse's theory of nursing, *Nursing Science Quarterly*, **5**(35), 35–45.

Prior, L. (1993) *The social organisation of mental illness*. Sage, London.

Rogers, C.R. (1961) *On Becoming a Person*. Houghton-Mifflin, Boston, MA.

Rogers, C.R. (1977) *Carl Rogers on Personal Power*. Constable, London.

Rogers, C.R. (1990) *Client Centred Therapy*. Constable, London.

Rogers, M. (1980) Nursing: a science of unitary man. In: *Conceptual Model for Nursing Practice* (eds A. Reihl & C. Ray), 2nd edn. Appleton-Centur, Crofts, New York.

Rowe, A. & Mackeith, P. (1991) Is evaluation a dirty word? *Health Visitor*, **64**(9), 292–3.

Rowe, A., Mitchinson, S., Morgan, M. & Carey, L. (1997) *Health Profiling; all you need to know*. Liverpool John Moores University/Premier Health NHS Trust, Liverpool.

Roy, S. (1990) *Nursing in the Community. Report of a working group*, North West Thames Regional Health Authority, Sheila Roy (Chair). HMSO, London.

Satre, J.P. (1969) *Being and Nothingnesss*. Routledge, London.

Schön, D.A. (1983) *The Reflective Practitioner: How Professionals Think in Action*. Basic Books, New York.

Sherman, K.L. (1988) Grief is more than crying. In: *Reading in Psychosynthesis: Theory, Process and Practice* (eds J. Weiser & T. Yeomans). Department of Applied Psychology: Institute of Education, Toronto.

Skidmore, D. & Friend, W. (1984) Community psychiatric nursing. *Nursing Times, Community Outlook*, 10 October, 369–71.

Slevin, O. (1999) The nurse-patient relationship. In: *Interaction for practice in community nursing*. A. Long (ed) Macmillan, London.

Sluckin, W., Sluckin, A. & Herbert, M. (1992) *Maternal Bonding*. Blackwell, Oxford.

Towl, G. In: *Suicides in Prisons: research, policy and practice* (eds G. Towl, M. McHugh & D. Jones) Pavilion Publishing, Brighton.

Travelbee, J. (1971) *Interpersonal Aspects of Nursing*, 2nd edn. F.A. Davis, Philadelphia.

Twinn, S., Dancey, J. & Carnell, J. (1990) *The Process of Health Profiling.* Health Visitors Association, London.

UKCC (1988) *Project 2000: A New Preparation for Practice.* United Kingdom Central Council, London.

UKCC (1991) *Community Education and Practice Report.* United Kingdom Central Council, London.

UKCC (2000) *The nursing, midwifery and health visiting contribution to the continuing care of people with mental health problems: A review and UKCC action plan.* United Kingdom Central Council, London.

Walker, L.E. (1984) *Women and Mental Health Policy.* Sage Publications, Beverly Hills, California.

Watson, J. (1985) *Nursing: Human Science and Human Care.* Appleton-Century-Crofts, New York.

Watzlawick, P. (1974) *Change: the principle of problem formation and problem resolution.* W.W. Norton: New York.

White, E. (1993) *The 1990 National Quinquennial Community Psychiatric Nursing Survey.* Department of Nursing, University of Manchester, Manchester.

WHO Collaborating Centre for Research and Training for Nursing Development in Primary Health Care (1999) *Initiatives in European Mental Health.* WHO Collaborating Centre for Research and Training for Nursing Development in Primary Health Care, University of Manchester, Manchester.

Worden, J.M. (1982) *Grief Counselling and Grief Therapy. A Handbook for the Mental Health Practitioner.* Springer, New York.

Yeo, T. (1993) In: *Community Care and Mental Health: the Stanley Moore Memorial Lecture: Community Psychiatric Nursing Journal*, April, 1993 – Speech by the Health Minister. p. 223–225.

Chapter 15 **Community Learning Disability Nursing**

Owen Barr

Introduction

The chapter commences with an introduction to the definition of learning disabilities, an overview of the number of people with learning disabilities and their overall health status. This is followed by a review of the changing service principles within services for people with learning disabilities that have arisen as a result of the series of policy reviews that have been published since 2000 (SE 2000; DoH 2001; WO 2001). Following this, the growing evidence on the role of community nurses for people with learning disabilities and their families is presented. The key challenges presented in providing an effective community nursing service for people with learning disabilities are then explored before considering the future direction for community nursing in services for people with learning disabilities.

People with learning disabilities

The term 'learning disability' is used within the UK in the context of service planning and provision. The definitions used in the recent reviews in England and Scotland (SE 2000; DoH 2001) identified that learning disabilities is considered to have three components, namely;

- A significantly reduced ability to understand new or complex information, to learn new skills (impaired intelligence)
- A reduced ability to cope independently (impaired social functioning)
- Having started before adulthood (before the age of 18), with a lasting effect on development

Some clarification was provided within *Valuing People* (DoH 2001) that 'the presence of a low intelligence quotient, for example an IQ below 70, is not, of itself, a sufficient reason for deciding whether an individual should be provided with additional health and social care support' (p. 15). The guidance went on to state that in determining the level of need, an assessment of social functioning and communication skills should also be undertaken. Furthermore, it was clarified that the definition of learning disability is not the same as the term 'learning difficulty', which has been defined more broadly within the corresponding legislation relating to education.

The position of adults with autistic spectrum disorders in relation to the definition of learning disabilities is not always clear. Within the definition used in *Valuing People*, it was further stated that the definition covers adults with autism who also have learning disabilities, but not those with a higher level autistic spectrum disorder who may be of average or even above average intelligence – such as some people with Asperger's syndrome (p. 22). In contrast, within the policy review undertaken in Scotland (SE 2000) it was stated that the definition of learning disabilities was taken to include people with autistic spectrum disorders, for the purposes of that review (p. 116).

The above definitions provide an overview of the criteria that may be applied by service planners and providers in determining who has learning disabilities, and it is accepted that the term may be viewed from differing perspectives and the detail of the interpretation of the nature of learning disabilities alters to some degree depending on the perspective through which it is being viewed. However, it is generally agreed that if services for people with learning disabilities are to be effective they must be holistic in nature. The need for an effectively co-orientated interdisciplinary and interagency approach to working with people with learning disabilities is recognised as central to making a holistic approach to service a reality (DoH 1998).

The number of people who have learning disabilities

The current number of people in the UK who are considered to have learning disabilities is an estimate based on reported prevalence rates. These prevalence rates have been reported differently across different countries within the UK. Within England, a prevalence rate of 3–4 people per 1000 of the population for people with severe and profound learning disabilities and 20–25 people per 1000 of the population has been used to estimate the numbers of people with mild and moderate learning disabilities. On the basis of these figures it has been estimated there are about 210 000 people with profound and severe learning disabilities in England, of which approximately 65 000 are children and young people, with 120 000 adults of working age and 25 000 older people. In using the prevalence rate of 25 people per 1000 for people with mild and moderate learning disabilities it was estimated there were 1.2 million people with this condition in England (DoH 2001). A total figure of 120 000 has been given for the total estimated number of people with learning disabilities in Scotland, using a prevalence rate of 3–4 per 1000 for profound and severe learning disabilities and 20 people in every 1000 for people with mild/ moderate learning disabilities. Increasingly it was further estimated that only about a quarter of people with learning disabilities had regular contact with local authorities or the health service in Scotland.

A recent survey to calculate the prevalence of people with learning disabilities in Northern Ireland reported the overall prevalence rate for all levels of learning disability as 9.7 persons per 1000 people in the population. This calculates to a total population of 16 366 people with learning disabilities in Northern Ireland (McConkey *et al.* 2003). Within this total number it was reported that an estimated 14 000 people (85.5%) were living in community settings, either with family carers, in their own accommodation or in supported

housing. A further 1900 people (11.6%) were living in residential care and nursing homes, or supported living accommodation. The remaining 440–470 people (2.7–2.9%) were resident in long-stay hospitals.

The number of people with learning disabilities across the UK has been increasing since the 1960s with an estimated annual rate of increase of 1.2%. The life expectancy of people with learning disabilities has increased considerably in the past 50 years with many people living into their 60s, and although still lower, it is now approaching that of other members of the general population (Cooke 1997). At the other end of the age continuum, children with learning disabilities who may have died as children now more frequently live into adulthood owing to advances in and increased accessibility to treatment. At times, these children and young adults may have complex health needs which can lead to an increased need for physical care and support, such as specialist seating equipment, intensive physiotherapy, the availability of suction equipment and enteral feeding.

Given the increasing success of children with profound and severe learning disabilities surviving into adulthood and the increasing life expectancy of adults with learning disabilities, it is expected that the number of people with learning disabilities will continue to rise year on year over the next 10–15 years. It has been projected that the rate of increase will be approximately 1%; this will primarily be seen among younger people with profound and severe learning disabilities and the growth in the number of older people with learning disabilities (SE 2000; DoH 2001).

The majority of people with learning disabilities continue to live in community based settings with almost all people under 20 years of age living in their family home, as do about three quarters of adults with learning disabilities (McConkey *et al.* 2003). Increasingly, people with learning disabilities who move out of their family home seek accommodation in residential accommodation in the local community and a growing number are successfully living within supported living settings (Simons & Watson

1999). However, many adults with learning disabilities are living with older parents or other family carers who are often reluctant to see their son or daughter move into residential accommodation. Research findings in Scotland have reported that a quarter of people with learning disabilities live with a family carer over 65 years of age. Furthermore, 20% of people with learning disabilities have two carers aged 70 or over, and 11% have only one aged 70 or over (SE 2000).

Changing service principles

The past five years has seen the unprecedented level of revision in the policies that define how services for people with learning disabilities should be delivered. Policy reviews were published in Scotland under the title of *The Same as You?* (DoH 2000), and in England the first major review of learning disability policy in 30 years entitled *Valuing People* was published in 2001 (DoH 2001). The implementation of the recommendations of these reviews is ongoing and regular updates on progress are provided on their respective websites (www.scotland.gov.uk; www.valuingpeople. gov.uk). A new framework was presented in Wales during 2002 under the title of *Fulfilling the promises* (WO 2001: www.wales.gov.uk/ assemblydata) and a draft report of the review ongoing in Northern Ireland has been published under the title of *Equal Lives* (DHSSPS, 2004; see www.rmhldni.gov.uk) (see Boxes 15.1 and 15.2). Across these policy reviews, a consistent emphasis on the rights of people with learning disabilities to be included as valued citizens in the countries they live in can be seen in the principles identified to guide future services. The policy reviews within Scotland, England, Wales and Northern Ireland presented their future vision as a series of service principles.

These revised principles are intended to guide services for people with learning disabilities over the next 10–15 years, including community nursing services, representing a shift from the previous emphasis on normalisation. Inclusion emphasises the rights to people with learning disabilities as citizens of their respective countries and as citizens their entitlement to the same services as all other citizens. Citizenship refers to a respect for rights and freedoms and 'implies participation in and contribution to a community and to society in general…it also means that all members have equal opportunities to participate in and contribute to society' (http//:users.skynet.be/incluit/ 1999). Inclusion challenges the need for people with learning disabilities to meet extra conditions/criteria to use community facilities, make decisions about their lives or to receive the same services as other members of the local population.

The respect of citizenship means that community nurses will have to further develop their knowledge and skills in the establishment of anti-discriminatory practice. This is a major shift in emphasis in which the onus is on professionals, members of the public and local communities to make reasonable adjustments to accommodate people with learning disabilities, instead of the previous emphasis on people with learning disabilities having to 'fit in' to existing structures. The implementation of legislation such as the Disability Discrimination Act 1995 which covered access to areas such as goods, services and employment, together with the acceptance of the European Convention on Human Rights into UK law in 1997 are being used to further support the move towards development of inclusive services.

Another particular focus in policy reviews has been the to need deliver services in a person-centred manner and the need to promote choice for people with learning disabilities. This is consistent with the expectations of citizenship, inclusion and a holistic model to services. This will require a focus on the provision of information in a manner accessible to a person's individual abilities and needs. Attention will also need to be given to the criteria for informed consent in order to ensure that the procedures involved in providing information to people with learning disabilities and including them in overall decision making processes is consistent with these guidelines.

The need to improve the health of people with learning disabilities has also been identified as a major challenge to future services. There is a body of evidence that has accumulated since the

---

Box 15.1 Principles identified in policy reviews in Scotland, England and Northern Ireland since 2000

Scotland: Same as You? (SE 2000)

- People with learning disabilities should be valued. They should be asked and encouraged to contribute to the community they live in. They should not be picked on or treated differently from others
- People with learning disabilities are individual people
- People with learning disabilities should be asked about the services they need and be involved in making choices about what they want
- People with learning disabilities should be helped and supported to do everything they are able to
- People with learning disabilities should be able to use the same local services as everyone else, wherever possible
- People with learning disabilities should benefit from specialist social, health and educational services
- People with learning disabilities should have services which take account of their age, abilities and other needs

England: Valuing People (DoH 2001)

- *Legal and civil rights*: The Government is committed to enforceable civil rights for disabled people in order to eradicate discrimination in society. All services should treat people with learning disabilities as individuals with respect for their dignity, and challenge discrimination on all grounds including disability. People with learning disabilities will also receive the full protection of the law when necessary
- *Independence*: The starting presumption should be one of independence, rather than dependence, with public services providing the support needed to maximise this. Independence in this context does not mean doing everything unaided
- *Choice*: This includes people with severe and profound disabilities who, with the right help and support, can make important choices and express preferences about their day to day lives
- *Inclusion*: Inclusion means enabling people with learning disabilities to do those ordinary things, make use of mainstream services and be fully included in the local community

Northern Ireland: Equal Lives (DHSSPS 2004)

- *Citizenship*: People with learning disabilities are individuals first and foremost and each has a right to be treated as an equal citizen
- *Person-centred*: People with learning disabilities should be supported in ways that take account of their individual needs
- *Participation*: People with learning disabilities should be consulted about the services they want. They should be actively involved in making choices and decisions affecting their lives
- *Interdependence*: People with learning disabilities should be valued and encouraged to contribute to the life of the community
- *Equality*: People with learning disabilities should be able to use the same services and have the same entitlements as everyone else

---

mid 1990s which now conclusively shows that people with learning disabilities have a wide range of unmet health needs. Community nurses for people with learning disabilities have been identified as potentially having a significant role in promoting and maintaining the health of people with learning disabilities (DoH 2001).

The health of people with learning disabilities

In order to benefit from increased longevity, people with learning disabilities need to be able to maintain a high level of overall health. Physical and mental health is crucial if people are to have a satisfactory quality of life and be

---

Box 15.2   Principles that underpin the vision of future services for people with learning disabilities in Wales (WO 2001)

- Provide comprehensive and integrated services to achieve social inclusion
- Be person-centred
- Improve empowerment and independence
- Ensure effortless and effective movements between services and organisations at different times of life
- Be holistic in approach and delivery taking fully into account an individual's preferences, hopes and lifestyle
- Ensure that a range of appropriate advocacy services is available for people who wish to use them
- Be accessible – in terms of both service users and their carers and families having full information
- Have fully developed collaborative partnerships to deliver flexible services
- Services should be developed on evidence of their effectiveness and transparency about their costs
- Be delivered by a competent, well-informed, well-trained and effectively supported and supervised workforce
- The early completion of the National Assembly's resettlement programmes to enable all people with learning disabilities to return to live in the community

---

able to avail themselves of the developing opportunities for valued social inclusion. However, although the available evidence clearly shows an increasing life expectancy of people with learning disabilities, associated with this is the growing prevalence of physical and mental ill health. As for other members of the general population the physical and mental health of people with learning disabilities is impacted upon by broad factors such as their living and working conditions, their behaviour and way of life, and aspects within their wider environment including the degree of disadvantage or social exclusion they experience (DHSSPS 2002).

The influence of several of these factors may be stronger in the lives of people with learning disabilities, for instance, there may be a greater impact from disadvantage and social exclusion arising from higher rates of poverty, unemployment and low educational achievement (Emerson *et al.* 2001; Northway 2001). Limited opportunities for involvement in local community activities arising from a number of factors including lack of awareness of these opportunities, dependence on others for transport (often older carers) and the costs involved can result in people with learning disabilities leading a more sedentary lifestyle. Furthermore, poor nutrition and the long-term use of a large number of medications (polypharmacy) have been identified

as particular risk factors among people with learning disabilities (Beange 2002).

In addition to the above factors the health of people with learning disabilities may be further compromised by co-morbidity in which the presence of particular syndromes or conditions associated with their learning disabilities may increase their likelihood of having physical health problems (e.g. Down's syndrome, epilepsy, associated physical disabilities). The situation for people with learning disabilities may be further compounded by barriers in access to health care facilities and a resultant delay in the detection of their health needs and instigation of effective treatment (Thompson & Pickering 2002).

Physical health

It is clear that the pattern of morbidity and mortality among people with learning disabilities is altering to become similar to that of the general population, with the increasing longevity of people with learning disabilities considered to be a major contributing factor to these reported changes. There has been an increase in deaths arising from cardiovascular disease, stroke and cancers and at the same time there has been a reduction in the number of deaths arising from infections (Hatton *et al.* 2003).

Much debate has taken place in respect of whether the health of people with learning

Table 15.1 Overview of the findings of health screening projects within the other areas of the UK and internationally for people with learning disabilities in Northern Ireland. (Cassidy *et al.* 2002; Hatton *et al.* 2003; Horwitz *et al.* 2000; Hunt *et al.* 2001; Turner & Moss 1996)

Area of Health Screen	Examples of conditions detected
Optical/visual impairments	reduced vision, need for prescription glasses, cataracts, eye infections
Ear, nose and throat	hearing loss, ear wax
Dermatology	eczema, psoriasis, dry skin
Mobility problems	arthritis, obesity, foot problems
Dental health	problems with teeth, gums and mouth ulcers
Sexual health	menstrual problems, testicular and breast anomalies
Cardiovascular	obesity, hypertension
Endocrine	diabetes, thyroid problems
Gastrointestinal	pain & discomfort, reflux problems, peptic ulcers, constipation
Continence problems	reduced continence, urinary tract infections, pain & discomfort

disabilities is comparatively less healthy than that of the general population. Two main strategies have been used to answer this question; the first approach has involved the inclusion of control or comparison groups within research projects investigating the health of people with learning disabilities. In the main these studies have focused on hearing and visual impairments, conditions of the nervous system, skin disorders and obesity. These conditions are more 'visible' and data from observation and measurement can usually be collected to support the presence of these conditions without the need for most intrusive investigations that other conditions may need to confirm their presence. In undertaking a review of comparative studies on the health problems of people with learning disabilities Jansen *et al.* (2004) located eight studies undertaken since 1995 that they considered robust and included control groups. The evidence from these studies indicates that people with learning disabilities have increased prevalence rates for epilepsy, diseases of the skin, sensory loss and increased risk of fractures.

A second approach for conditions that require more intrusive investigation or have a lower frequency has been the comparison between the reported rates of particular conditions and illness among people with learning disabilities with national prevalence rates for that condition. The most comprehensive review in this area has been undertaken in relation to cancer among people with learning disabilities. The authors concluded that although the overall prevalence rates of cancer among people with learning disabilities are similar to that of the general population there is evidence of an increased prevalence of particular types of cancer among people with learning disabilities (Hogg *et al.* 2000). Cancers of the stomach and oesophagus, as well as testicular cancer have been reported at rates higher than those present in the general population. Conversely, people with learning disabilities appear to have lower rates for lung, breast, urinary tract and prostate cancers (Cooke 1997; Duff *et al.* 2001; Patja *et al.* 2001).

Irrespective of whether the overall rates for the above conditions are higher among people with learning disabilities, there is growing evidence of unmet health needs among people with learning disabilities in a number of areas (Table 15.1).

Mental health

A review of available studies reported prevalence rates of mental health problems (excluding challenging behaviour) among adults with learning disabilities ranging from 25–40% (Emerson *et al.* 2001). This compares with rates of 15–25% for adults without learning disabilities. A recently published population based study reported prevalence rates of mental health problems among children with learning disabilities as 39% compared to a rate of 8.1% for children who did not have learning disabilities (Emerson 2003).

A consistent finding across studies investigating the mental health of people with learning disabilities is that a wide range of mental health problems, similar to that found among the general population, can be present. In addition, on occasions, the presentation of the mental health problems among people with learning disabilities may be atypical owing to their level of verbal and cognitive abilities. Furthermore, some mental health problems may be over-prevalent among people with learning disabilities, including affective disorders, phobic states and dementia (Hassiotis *et al.* 2003). In children, similar rates have been reported for depressive disorders, eating disorders and psychosis, with higher rates reported for conduct disorders, anxiety disorders, hyperkinesis and pervasive developmental disorders (Emerson 2003). Whilst any attempt to provide definitive prevalence rates of mental illness among people with learning disabilities comes up against a number of difficulties it is clear that children and adults with learning disabilities do develop mental health problems and at a higher rate than members of the general population (FPLD 2002; Fraser & Kerr 2003).

Action to promote and maintain the health of people with learning disabilities is likely to become an increasing area of work for community nurses, both in relation to the direct care they provide and the need for more effective collaboration with staff in mainstream primary care, acute general hospitals and mental health services. Research on the role of community nurses demonstrates that they have already taken steps to improve the health status of people with learning disabilities, among a range of other roles they fulfil in present services.

The role of the community nurse for people with learning disabilities

The first research papers on the role of the community nurse learning disability (CNLD) appeared in the late 1980s (Mackay 1989) with several others published since that time. The findings emerging from these studies show that community nurses for people with learning disabilities report that they have a reasonably consistent range of reasons for visiting people with learning disabilities. These include support in responding to the presence of challenging behaviour, mental health problems, physical disability, epilepsy and sensory disability (Jenkins & Johnson 1991; Mackay 1989). More recently, the degree of community nurse support for issues relating to physical care needs, issues associated with people with learning disabilities growing older, and sexuality appear to becoming more prevalent (Parahoo & Barr 1996). It is also noted that although the majority of people with learning disabilities visited by community nurses are adults, community nurses are also actively involved with people with learning disabilities across a wide age range from young children through to people with learning disabilities who are over 60 years of age.

Mobbs *et al.* (2002) used postal questionnaires to managers of CNLD services across 170 NHS trusts in England and obtained responses from 136 NHS trusts (81%). The findings of this study showed that 99% of NHS trusts responding employed one or more CNLDs. However, it is clear from the information provided on clinical grades which range from A–I that this survey sought information on all nurses working in community learning disability services. It was reported that 44% of NHS trusts employed support staff at B grade, whilst staff at clinical grades D, E, F, G and H were employed by 12%, 57%, 30%, 97% and 43% of NHS trusts respectively, but no information was provided on the numbers of staff employed at each grade or grade mixture within individual services. Mobbs *et al.* (2002) outlined the increasing range of specific posts within community nursing services for people with learning disabilities and reported the presence of dedicated clinical posts in the following percentage of NHS trusts surveyed: challenging behaviour (27%), child health (25%), epilepsy (20%) and forensic (18%). However, despite these developments this study also reported that CNLDs were not employed to work with children less than 5 years of age, or between 6–19 years of age in 27% and 21% of

NHS trusts respectively. They also reported that 18% of NHS trusts provided an out of hours or on call service.

The top ten areas of clinical practice as identified by the managers on the basis of the time they felt allocated by nurses were:

- Assessment
- Advice and support
- Health monitoring (ongoing)
- Nursing care
- Counselling
- Health promotion
- Clinical procedures
- Health screening (assessment)
- Crisis intervention
- Client reviews

Whilst this study provides an overview from the perspective of managers, it does not provide information on the composition of services or the function of nurses within individual services. The authors also acknowledge that the views of managers may not reflect the views of individual community nurses in practice settings. It also appears that all nurses working with community services for people with learning disabilities have been considered as a homogeneous group, despite the range of specific posts identified which will impact on the activities the individual nurses will undertake.

In a qualitative study into the role of community nurses for people with learning disabilities, Boarder (2002) interviewed 20 experienced CNLDs (>5 years experience as a CNLD) in Wales about the key aims and features of their role. Participants reported caseloads of between 15 and 35 clients, three working with children and 17 with adults. In the analysis of the interview data a number of main themes were identified pertaining to the role of community nurses. Participants highlighted the increasing health focus on the community nurses and the continuing development of dedicated clinical posts, such as those reported by Mobbs *et al.* (2002).

They reported an emphasis on interdisciplinary teamwork and a wide range of tasks undertaken by community nurses was identified. These highlighted the role of community nurses in working with people with learning disabilities in relation to health maintenance and responding to specific physical and mental health difficulties they may experience. Community nurses also had key roles in respect of assessment, advocacy, assisting to maintain people with learning disabilities in a range of community settings, supporting people who present with challenging behaviour, skills development and personal relationships. Unfortunately the findings of this study may be confounded by the fact that two nurses were not RNMH qualified and four nurses (20% of sample) although working in the community did not work as part of the community learning disability nursing teams, but rather in two residential settings, one in a challenging behaviour service and one within a case management team (Boarder 2001).

The views that other professionals within community learning disability teams had of community nurses for people with learning disabilities was explored by Mansell and Harris (1998). They used postal questionnaires to collect information from a range of 96 professionals (including 32 nurses) working in community learning disability teams in South Wales and achieved a response rate of 83%. Respondents identified the top five skills of nurses to be:

- Client based interventions
- Co-ordination and planning of care
- Training
- Care management
- Health promotion

The authors reported that the majority of respondents (74 of the 96) indicated that if the registered learning disability nurse was not a team member, another professional could not undertake their role.

Powell *et al.* (2004) reported similar support of the role of community nurses by other health and social services staff community-based within residential services. In a questionnaire-based survey of 40 staff, the top five areas reported as part of the role of community nurses were consultancy, assessment, treatment, training and promoting access to services, care planning and health promotion. The need to improve

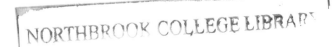
NORTHBROOK COLLEGE LIBRARY

communication with other services and take further action to promote the health of people with learning disabilities were identified as two areas that the services provided by community nurses could be further improved upon. Overall, the respondents rated the community nursing service as effective and valued the broad and varied role that community nurses undertook.

These developments in the role of community nurses are further evidenced in the published papers on individual service developments that provide detail of similar developments (Barr *et al*. 1999; Cassidy *et al*. 2002; Hunt *et al*. 2001; Martin 2003; Meehan *et al*. 1995). Overall, the emerging research knowledge on the role of community nurses and people with learning disabilities demonstrates a continued wide-ranging role of community nurses for people with learning disabilities but also the increasing focus on a health orientated approach and an increasing number of people appointed into dedicated clinical posts. These studies also provide a growing body of evidence as to the value attached to the role of community nurses by other health and social care professionals, in particular, the importance attached to the comprehensive knowledge and package of skills that community nurses have to work with people with learning disabilities across a wide range of tasks (Mansell & Harris 1998; Stewart & Todd 2001).

Whilst the above research findings do show considerable progress in the development of the role of community nurses for people with learning disabilities, they also identify three challenges that need to be considered in developing future services. First, there appears to have been a reduction in the number of community nurses who work with children with learning disabilities; it has been reported that up to a quarter of community nurses for people with learning disabilities in England do not work with children under 5 years of age and one fifth do not work with children under the age of 16 years old (Mobbs *et al*. 2002). Second, there continues to be a lack of recognition and understanding by staff in mainstream services as to the role of the community nurses for people with learning

disabilities and the need for greater role clarity within learning disability services. Third, there is a need to keep under review the impact that the development of dedicated clinical posts impacts on the access to these services for people with learning disabilities and the effect this has on the role of the domiciliary community nurse for people with learning disabilities.

The future role of community nursing services for people with learning disabilities

The direction of the future role of CNLD services appears clearly to be within a more health orientated framework than was previously the situation and developments within this area have been noted across the UK. The future CNLD role will be different in a number of ways from their previous role, namely:

- More work with people with complex physical and mental health needs
- A greater role in facilitating access to mainstream primary, secondary and tertiary care services
- A refocusing on the role and contribution of the 'nursing' component of the CNLD role and an increased 'throughput' in CNLD caseloads with more effective admission and discharge procedures

Existing services in many areas continue to be characterised by either perceived 'medical' or 'social' models of care. At times these models are unfortunately portrayed as having irreconcilable differences and that the medical model is less acceptable in developing services for people with learning disabilities. However, as Thomas and Woods (2003) have highlighted, both models have their strengths and limitations and it is important that a medical model is not mistaken for the provision with health care. Evidence has clearly shown the high level of unmet health needs among people with learning disabilities and action must be taken to address this. Future services will be required to become more holistic and accommodate a broader 'health' perspective. Health is holistic in nature as it encompasses physical, psychological and social aspects as well as primary, secondary and tertiary aspects. The emphasis should be on comprehensive holistic assessment of an individual's abilities and needs, whilst giving due recognition to their social circumstances. A holistic model of health such as that proposed by Seedhouse (1986) who defined health as 'the set of conditions which fulfil or enable a person to work to fulfil his or her realistic chosen and biological potentials' (p. 61) is consistent with services principles identified as guiding future services for people with learning disabilities and is in keeping with the need for increased interdisciplinary and interagency collaboration.

The assessment of health requires interdisciplinary collaboration in the completion of comprehensive assessments. The key rationale for a comprehensive assessment is bringing together the thoughts of the main people involved. Each professional inputs into their assessment either with a specific assessment instrument or in the process of joint assessments with other people. Nursing assessments can provide important information on which future decisions will be based and it is essential that nursing assessments are grounded in nursing models. Community nurses must be careful to match the assessment instrument/strategy they choose to the individual needs of the person with learning disabilities. Following the completion of a nursing assessment nurses will be able to contribute to a comprehensive assessment. Failure to complete a 'nursing' assessment and instead relying only on limited information obtained in some broader ranging but more superficial assessments considerably weakens the nursing contribution to a comprehensive assessment.

As more people with learning disabilities have their health needs met within primary care and other mainstream services, community nurses for people with learning disabilities will increasingly become a secondary specialist service working with people with more complex needs than can be met within mainstream services alone. This will involve the continued need for frequent visits to people with learning disabilities and their families together with close liaison with

other support services that are being provided. Community nurses will need to develop closer links with services such as community children's services, staff in dedicated clinical posts such as behaviour support, epilepsy services, mental health and child and adolescent psychiatry services, primary care, acute hospitals and at times palliative care services. Collaborative working in which some joint visits, as well as the exchange of knowledge and skills will need to be further developed to move beyond the separateness of some of these services, which now often work in comparative isolation from each other with differing priorities, aims and objectives.

Whilst this does not necessarily require community nurses to be physically based within primary and acute care services, at the very least it requires the development of more formal links between nurses and other professionals in learning disability and primary care services. For instance, community nurses for people with learning disabilities could attend local community nurse meetings within their trust and forge links with nursing colleagues or be nominally attached to general practitioner practices and develop effective liaison with local acute general hospitals. Actively promoting these links will increase the opportunities for CNLDs to make positive contributions, in collaboration with other community nursing services, to the lives of people with learning disabilities and their families. In relation to adults with learning disabilities such links will assist in overcoming barriers to accessing primary and acute care services for the increasing number of people with learning disabilities who need to access such services. In contrast, the continued 'isolation' of community nurses within separate learning disability and social work networks will do little to inform other nursing colleagues of their role and possible contributions.

Whilst it is important that more people become aware of the possible contribution of CNLD services, the admission of the people to caseloads should be more effectively managed and prioritised (Caffery & Todd 2002). Only on the completion of a nursing assessment and consideration by the CNLD of the contribution they can make in relation to specific nursing objectives should an individual be admitted to a CNLD caseload. This is not to argue against the need for person-centred planning approaches and it is strongly believed that nursing assessments should contribute to person-centred planning discussions. However, it is not acceptable professionally that nurses should become involved in nursing care that is not based on a nursing assessment. Nor is it acceptable to deliver nursing care to people and not record this intervention, for instance in the case of nurses who have direct involvement with people not on their nursing caseload. Whilst it is recognised that nurses may be asked for advice and support it is recommended that a note (not necessarily a complete file) be kept of this interaction. Such changes as outlined above are likely to require a revision of nursing assessments to ensure these reflect current approaches to nursing assessment and are suitable to CNLD services. More specific nursing assessment and determination of nursing needs will also go some way to removing the vagueness and uncertainties around the role of the CNLD (Boarder 2001).

When a nursing assessment identifies no nursing need (defined as a need identified within a structured nursing assessment undertaken by a registered nurse), then this should be communicated to the referring professional and alternative services can then be sought by them. It should not fall to the CNLD to fill the gap in existing services by responding to non-nursing needs; rather this should be identified as an unmet need and dealt with by the person making the referral through local arrangements for responding to such needs. A more focused approach to nursing assessment will contribute to smoother admission processes and to more effective discharge procedures. It follows that if an individual is admitted to a nursing caseload with specific identified objectives then once these objectives are achieved the person could be potentially discharged. However, in order for this to happen there is a need for comprehensive discharge policies that clearly provide procedures to staff as evidence exists that without such policies that address staff concerns they will not discharge clients (Caffery & Todd 2002;

Walker *et al.* 2003). CNLDs should start this process by reviewing the nursing needs of all people they have infrequent contact with (> once a month) and determine what the current nursing needs are that justify retaining these people on a CNLD caseload. If the need identified is primarily one of monitoring health (physical or mental) then steps should be taken to work collaboratively with primary care services towards a situation when they undertake this monitoring as they would for other members the community with ongoing health needs.

Conclusion

The role of community nurses for people with learning disabilities has altered considerably in the past few years and is becoming increasingly health focused. Community nurses continue to work with people who have a wide range of abilities and needs; however, there is some indication that a particular emphasis on their future role will be with people who have increasingly complex physical and mental health needs. The continued development of CNLD services requires the commitment of community nurses, their immediate managers and those managers within the services responsible for agreeing service structures and policies. Services planners need to consider how the comprehensive package of skills that a community nurse for people with learning disabilities brings to community services can be most effectively used within services that seek to take forward services for people with learning disabilities in line with revised principles that should underpin future services. Equally there is also a need for CNLDs to recognise that although the role they have performed for many years has been valued, it also will need to evolve further if it is to continue to be of value to people with learning disabilities and their families.

References

Barr, O., Gilgunn, J., Kane, T. & Moore, G. (1999) Health screening for people with learning disabilities by a community nursing service in Northern Ireland. *Journal of Advanced Nursing*, **29**, 1482–1491.

Beange, H. (2002) Epidemiological issues. In: *Physical health of adults with intellectual disabilities* V.P. Prasher

& M. Janicki (eds). Blackwell Publishing/IASSID, London.

Boarder, J.H. (2002) The perceptions of experienced community learning disability nurses of their roles and ways of working: an exploratory study. *Journal of Learning Disabilities*. **6**(3), 281–296.

Boarder, J. (2001) *Perceptions of experienced community learning disability nurses of their roles and ways of working: an exploratory study*. Report for Welsh National Board Training Research Fellowship.

Caffery, A. & Todd, M. (2002) Community Learning Disability teams: the need for objective methods of prioritisation and discharge planning. *Health Services Management Research*, **15**(4), 223–231.

Cassidy, G., Martin, D.M., Martin G.H.B. & Roy, A. (2002) Health checks for people with learning disabilities: community learning disability teams working with general practitioners and primary care teams. *Journal of Learning Disabilities*, **6**(2), 123–136.

Cooke, L.B. (1997) Cancer and learning disability. *Journal of Intellectual Disability Research*, **41**(4), 312–316.

Department of Health (1998) *Signpost for Success*. DoH, London.

Department of Health (2001) *Valuing People. A new strategy for learning disability for 21st century*, Department of Health, London.

Department of Health, Social Services and Public Safety (2002) *Investing in Health*, Department of Health, Social Services and Public Safety, Belfast.

Department of Health, Social Services and Public Safety (2004) *Equal Lives: Draft report of Learning Disability Committee*. Department of Health, Social Services and Public Safety, Belfast.

Duff, M., Hoghton, M., Scheepers, M., Cooper, M. & Baddeley, P. (2001). *Helicobacter pylori*: has the filler escaped from the institution? A possible cause of increased stomach cancer in a population with intellectual disability. *Journal of Intellectual Disability Research*, **45**(3), 219–225.

Emerson, E. (2003) Prevalence of psychiatric disorders in children and adolescents with and without intellectual disability. *Journal of Intellectual Disability Research*, **47**(1), 51–58.

Emerson, E., Hatton, C., Felce, D. & Murphy, G. (2001) *The Fundamental Facts*. London: Foundation for People with Learning Disabilities.

Foundation for People with Learning Disabilities (2002) *Count Us In: the report of the Committee of Inquiry into meeting the mental health needs of young people with learning disabilities*, Foundation for People with Learning Disabilities, London.

Fraser, W. & Kerr, M. (eds) (2003) *Seminars in the Psychiatry of Learning Disabilities*, 2nd edn. Gaskell Press, London.

Hassiotis, A., Tyrer, P. & Oliver, P. (2003) Psychiatric assertive outreach and learning disability services, *Advances in Psychiatric treatment*, **9**, 368–373.

Hatton, C., Elliot, J. & Emerson, E. (2003) *Key highlights of research evidence on the health of people with learning disabilities*. (available at http://www.doh.gov.uk/vpst/latestnews.htm#newdocs)

Hogg, J., Northfield, J. & Turnbull, J. (2000) *Cancer and people with learning disabilities*. British Institute of Learning Disabilities, Kidderminster.

Horwitz, S., Kerler, B.D., Owens, P. & Zigler, E. (2000) *The health status and needs of individuals with mental retardation*. Yale University, Connecticut.

Hunt, C., Wakefield, S. & Hunt, G. (2001) Community Nurse Learning Disabilities – a case study of the use of an evidence-based health screening tool to identify and meet health needs of people with learning disabilities. *Journal of Learning Disabilities*, **5**(1), 9–18.

Jansen, D., Krol, B., Groothoof, J. & Post, D. (2004) People with Intellectual disabilities and their health problems: a review of comparative studies. *Journal of Intellectual Disability Research*, **48**(2), 93–102.

Jenkins, J. & Johnson, B. (1991) Community nursing learning disability survey. In: *The community mental handicap nurse-specialist practitioner in the 1990s*. (ed P. Kelly) pp. 39–54. Mental Handicap Nurses Association, Penarth.

McConkey, R., Spollen, M. & Jamison, J. (2003) *Administrative Prevalence of Learning Disability in Northern Ireland. A Report to the Department of Health, Social Services and Public Safety*. DHSSPS, Belfast.

Mackay, T. (1989) A community nursing service analysis. *Nursing Standard*, **4**(2), 32–35.

Mansell, I. & Harris, P. (1998) Role of the Registered Nurse Learning Disability within community support teams for people with learning disabilities. *Journal of Learning Disabilities for Nursing, Health and Social Care*, **2**(4), 190–195.

Martin, G. (2003) Annual health reviews for patients with severe learning disabilities: five years of a combined GP/CLDN Clinic. *Journal of Learning Disabilities*, **7**(1), 9–22.

Meehan, S., Moore, G. & Barr, O. (1995) Specialist services for people with learning disabilities. *Nursing Times*, **91**(13), 33–35.

Mobbs, C., Hadley, S., Wittering, R. & Bailey, N.M. (2002) An exploration of the role of the community nurse, learning disability, in England. *British Journal of Learning Disabilities*, **30**, 13–18.

Northway, R. (2001) Poverty as a practice issue for learning disability nurses. *British Journal of Nursing.* **10**(18), 1186–92.

Patja, K., Eero, P. & Iivanainen, M. (2001) Cancer incidence among people with intellectual disabilities. *Journal of Intellectual Disability Research*, **45**(4), 300–307.

Parahoo, K. & Barr, O. (1996) Community mental handicap nursing services in Northern Ireland: a profile of clients and selected working practices. *Journal of Clinical Nursing*, **5**, 211–228.

Powell, H., Murray, G. & McKenzie, K. (2004) Staff perceptions of community learning disability nurses' role. *Nursing Times*, **100**(19), 40–42.

Scottish Executive (SE) (2000) *The same as you? A review of the services for people with learning disabilities.* Scottish Executive, Edinburgh.

Seedhouse, D. (1986) *Health: Foundations for Achievement.* Wiley, Bristol.

Simons, K. & Watson, D. (1999) *The view from Arthur's Seat: Review of services for people with learning disabilities – a literature review of housing and support options beyond Scotland.* Scottish Executive Central Research Unit, Edinburgh.

Stewart, D. & Todd, M. (2001) Role and contribution of nurses for people with learning disabilities: a local study in a county of the Oxford–Anglia region. *British Journal of Learning Disabilities*, **29**, 145–150.

Thomas, D. & Woods, H. (2003) *Working with people with learning disabilities: Theory and Practice.* Jessica Kingsley Publishers, London.

Thompson, J. & Pickering, S. (eds) (2002) *Meeting the needs of people with learning disabilities.* Bailliere Tindall, London.

Turner, S. & Moss, S. (1996). The health needs of adults with learning disabilities and the *Health of the Nation* strategy. *Journal of Intellectual Disability Research*, **40**, 438–450.

Walker, T., Stead, J. & Read, S.G. (2003) Caseload management in community learning disability teams; influences on decision-making. *Journal of Learning Disabilities*, **7**(4), 297–321.

Welsh Office (WO) (2001) *Fulfilling the Promises.* Welsh Assembly, Cardiff.

Chapter 16 Assessment of Competence to Practise and New NMC Teaching Standards

Anne Robotham

Introduction

The Nursing and Midwifery Council (NMC) succeeded the UKCC and four National Boards and came into being in 2002. Changes to registration rules, new rules for fees, midwifery and fitness to practice and standards of proficiency for specialist community public health nurses came into force in 2004. As has been mentioned elsewhere in this book, there are now three parts to the register, for nurses, midwives and specialist community public health nurses. This chapter explores the standards of proficiency and their meaning for assessment of education and practice. The major evolution in determining standards has been that competence and competency are no longer the standard measurement because Article 5(2)(a) of the order requires the NMC to:

'establish the standards of *proficiency* necessary to be admitted to the different parts of the register being the standards it considers necessary for safe and effective practice under that part of the register'.

The standards of proficiency were developed from previous competencies used for community health care nursing and health visiting and, following consultation, the framework has been expanded to include the ten standards for public health (NMC 2004b).

This chapter will now consider the implications of the third part of the register for specialist community public health nursing education and practice. It will consider the philosophy of the movement from competence to proficiency and explore ways in which practice might be assessed in order to reach standards of proficiency for entry to the register.

Entry to the register

How can public health nurses, health visitors, midwives, occupational health nurses and school nurses all aspire to the same standards of proficiency to enable them to be admitted to the third part of the register?

Earlier in this book, two chapters explore the work of specialist community public health nursing and specialist community public health nursing (health visiting). The similarities and differences in their actual and potential work lie, not so much with the way in which they proactively work towards ensuring the health and well-being of individuals and populations, but from the knowledge base and transfer of skills from one situation to another. These two groups of professionals are probably closest in practice philosophy than other professional groups, but the content of their education programmes differs in terms of breadth and depth of knowledge sources. For example, the health visitor course requires extensive understanding of human growth and development and social influences in order to be able to screen individuals for normal and abnormal development and behaviour. The public health nursing course requires extensive knowledge of disease patterns and social influences in order to screen groups and populations for illness and abnormal functioning.

The classic example given in Chapter 7 of the project on improvement in breastfeeding rates is a case in point. Health visitors (HV) and midwives work both antenatally and postnatally to encourage and prepare women to breastfeed their babies. The HV is concerned that the baby is given the best possible opportunity to develop immunity, nourishment, balanced feeding, bonding contact with enhanced communication with the mother, and so forth. The public health nurse is more concerned that in a deprived area breast-feeding is a cheaper option, the population benefits from well and correctly nourished infants, knows there is less likelihood of child neglect or abuse in infants and so forth. Ask each individual professional whether they are aware of the implications of breastfeeding that have been mentioned in this example, and they will probably both agree on a general knowledge base. However, this knowledge base comes from a different approach. The health visitor will use physio-psycho-sociological aspects of their knowledge, the public health nurse will use disease-data analysis-health promotion aspects of their knowledge. They aspire to satisfying the same principle and domain for specialist community public health programmes, but come from a different focus. It would seem therefore, that their proficiency lies in as accurate an assessment as is possible of their capabilities and knowledge following completion of their courses.

Standards of education for specialist community public health programmes

According to the Nursing and Midwifery Order, Article 15(1)(a) of the Order requires the NMC to establish *'the standards of education and training necessary* to achieve the standards of proficiency it has established under article 5(2)'.

Box 16.1 is a brief list of the standards for education as set out by the NMC (2004b).

It is standard 10 that this chapter is concerned with and initially academic assessment will be considered.

Levels of attainment in academia

In 1993/4 the first two education institutions offered a health visitor course at first degree level, and gradually the momentum gathered so that by 1997 it was a national requirement that all post-registered health visitor courses should be at degree level. As this was a top up degree

of one year, students needed to have completed a diploma standard of education to enable them to function at degree level. Academic assessment was mainly on the basis of at least one unseen examination paper as well as continuous assessment written assignments.

The basis of grading within academic levels was focused around the use of knowledge and reading sources to formulate arguments and analyses which became increasingly conceptually critical as the student moved through a course. Theoretical assessment for a good grade also required the student to be able to write coherently and with evidence of synthesis and balanced evaluative judgements and to be able to show clear relationships to experience derived from the practicum.

Having stated that lecturers were familiar with grading and levels of learning corresponding to the year of study, it must also be appreciated that academics were also cognisant of the fact that assessment of essay type continuous assessment was not an easy responsibility. Inevitably there are the assertions of subjectivity that show wide differences between the marking of very experienced examiners (Jarvis & Gibson 1985) and which may also show the problem of norm-referencing rather than criterion-referencing (Rowntree 1992). A further difficulty familiar to all examiners is that of overlap between descriptors of grades and levels. For example, the descriptors for a high grade for a second year student bear remarkable similarity to the descriptors for a low grade third year student, albeit with a clear further year of study between. However, grading of academic assessment was way in advance of grading of practice assessment, the processes of which will now be considered.

The development process of levels of attainment in practice

Ashworth *et al.* (1999) were one of the most recent in a line of investigators to grapple with levels of practice, using nurse educators to judge statements used to categorise diploma, degree

Box 16.1 Standards of education for specialist community public health programmes (NMC 2004b)

Standard	Guidance
Standard 1	Programmes are required to have an overall length of 52 weeks of which 45 are programmed weeks
Standard 2	Programmes will comprise practical and theoretical learning transferable to different settings, clients and areas of practice. Periods of theory and practice should be distributed throughout the programme
Standard 3	The balance between practice and theory will be 50% practice and 50% theory. A consolidating period of practice equivalent to at least ten weeks at the end of the programme is required
Standard 4	Where a particular practice route is required students must have completed their consolidated practice experience (minimum 10 weeks) and at least half the remaining practice time (minimum 6.3 weeks) in settings with clients that are central to the responsibilities for that defined area of practice
Standard 5	The minimum academic standard of specialist community public health programmes remains that of a first degree
Standard 6	The contents of the curricula should be that which will enable the achievement of standards of proficiency for safe and effective practice for entry to the third part of the register. Where a student intends to work in a particular area of practice, content must enable sufficient learning to take place within that area to ensure safe and effective practice
Standard 7	Students should be supported in both academic and practice learning environments by appropriately qualified teachers, who hold practice qualifications in the same area of practice as the qualification sought by the students they are supporting
Standard 8	The programme should be arranged so that teaching and learning of both core principles and those specific to particular practice routes are integrated through the whole programme at a level beyond initial registration as a nurse or midwife
Standard 9	In order to provide a knowledge base for practice, contemporary theoretical perspectives and public health standards should be explored
Standard 10	A range of assessment strategies should be used throughout the programme to test knowledge and standards of proficiency in all aspects of the specialist community public health nursing curriculum

and Masters' level practice. They made important observations on the form of knowing in nursing practice which is implicit, procedural knowledge and is difficult to assess because the usual assessment modes take practice out of context and create distortion of its subtleties. For this reason Ashworth *et al.* (1999) consider that the actual phenomena of nursing practice do not lend themselves to verbal categorisation so as to form discrete, reliable attainment levels. Ashworth *et al.* comment that the use of expert working

groups as a basis for delineating practice levels are initiatives that have not tested out the assumptions on which the original statements are derived. Earlier researchers, Elkan and Robinson (1993), White *et al.* (1993) and Wilson Barnett *et al.* (1995) all had similar problems in delineating diploma level practice and felt that this was due to the indeterminacy of practice.

Pioneers, in terms of grappling with social work education, Winter and Maisch (1992) used, as their expert group, external examiners to social work courses, drawing from their language, terms and phrases to distinguish between the competencies of social work students. In so doing, they formed a hierarchy of practice through descriptors that informed the criteria against which practitioners were assessed, and which, they felt, differentiated from lower level practitioners. Davis and Burnard (1992) explored the distinction between diplomas and different types of degrees using a Delphi technique with UK nurse educators and Dutch Masters' in Nursing students. The UK respondents reflected an 'academic' viewpoint whilst the Dutch nurses concentrated on practice. Davis and Burnard discuss the probability of transfer of skills learned at a lower level to a higher level of practice and postulate that as a person progresses they develop a whole range of learning skills that shorten the cycle of new learning. The important point made is that it may be distracting to talk of levels of expertise in terms of a hierarchy that suggests linear progression, whereas the process of developing knowledge and skills would appear to be a cyclical one.

Burns (1992) in early, influential work in grading practice approached the issue from three directions: that of identifying levels of competency; learning contracts to incorporate learning objectives, resources and strategies, evidence, and reflection and validation; grading profiles based on the three levels of reflection identified by Goodman (1984). These were concerned with techniques to reach given objectives, reflection on the relationship between principles and practice, reflection which also incorporates ethical and political concerns. The tool used by Burns (1992) was a learning contract which contained objectives for the practice module and these were validated by discussion between the student and mentor through reflective conversations. The student was asked to grade the component and then these grades were verified by the mentor and lecturer/practitioner.

Burns (1992) also commented on the need for the mentors/assessors to be well prepared for this approach to assessment, which was for nurses and midwives undertaking degree level, initial training and education.

Knowledge in practice

In an analysis of the conceptual and syntactical structure of nursing knowledge (Carper 1978) identified four patterns of knowing:

(1) Empirics, the science of nursing
(2) Aesthetics, the art of nursing
(3) The component of a personal knowledge in nursing
(4) Ethics, the component of moral knowledge in nursing

As in Medley's (1984) urgent search for a professionalism in teaching, so nursing in the 1970s began to develop a scientific structure through the development of a body of empirical knowledge specific to nursing. This rose from the need to identify nursing as a profession in its own right as opposed to a profession subsidiary to medicine. A number of models of nursing were developed which purported to be mechanisms whereby nursing effectiveness could be measured. McClymont *et al.* (1991) showed that models help practitioners to organise their thoughts and to justify how and what they do, and Fawcett (1992) showed a reciprocal relationship between conceptual models and practice – models guide practice while practice provides evidence for the credibility of the model.

Carper (1978) argues for empathy as an important mode in the pattern of aesthetic knowing and the more skilled a nurse becomes in the perception and empathy in the lives of others, the more knowledge and understanding is gained. In particular, the argument is carried into the recognition that what is done in part must be related to the whole. In other words, decision making in relation to what is appropriate and effective for the client must be chosen and guided to suit their circumstances. This requires the health care practitioner to interpret the felt experience of others and identify patterns and rhythms of lived life, in order to create a repertoire of choices for the client, based on the aesthetic.

Personal knowledge, Carper argues, is about knowing self and is based on the interpersonal transactions between professional and client. Carper argues for reciprocity between client/professional relationships and sees this as personal knowing which extends not only to other people but also to relations with oneself.

Knowledge in the moral component is what Carper (1978) considers to be the ethical dimension of modern health care. In health visiting, where the basis of intervention by health visitors is concerned with education, empowerment and partnership, difficulties arise where health care is impeded by deprivation, both psycho-social and economic-educative. Health visitors may plan health care pathways with clients in the full knowledge of the socio-economic inequity which may temper the choices available. In this sense the health visitor is forced down a moral pathway which, although embodying the concept of service to people and the respect for human life, nevertheless is aware of the dilemmas involved in Offering support which circumstances cause to be of poorer quality.

In using patterns of knowing, Carper considers that each must be conceived as necessary for achieving mastery in the nursing discipline. However, she also comments that none alone should be considered sufficient, neither are they mutually exclusive, and that each of these separate but interrelated and independent fundamental patterns of knowing should be taught and understood according to its distinctive logic.

Schön (1983) proposes that the professions are bound by a form of professional knowledge that fails to take into account the indeterminacy of practice. Schön argues that the dominant epistemology (a branch of science which deals with the nature and validity of knowledge) of practice is *technical rationality* which relies on the assumption that empirical science (based on positive facts and observable phenomena) is the only source of objective knowledge about the world. Schön suggests that there is an area in professional practice where practitioners can make use of research-based theory and technique, but equally there are other areas where there are uncertainties

and value conflicts which are incapable of technical solution. Benner (1984) also makes the point that not all knowledge embedded in expertise can be captured in theoretical propositions, or in analytical strategies that depend on identifying all the elements that go into a clinical decision.

Action in practice

An assumption can be made that action in practice is based on the use of knowledge. However, such is the nature of practice that situational factors may cause the practitioner to perform in a manner which may, seemingly, be divorced from a knowledge base. Schutz (1972) posited an idea of meaningful social action that he said was an adequate description of professional practice. Jarvis (1992) carried this idea further by suggesting that one had to understand action, and especially the sort of action that is not 'hands-on', such as health visiting action, in order to realise a theory of professional practice. Jarvis (1992) considered action to be dependent on levels of *conscious planning, conscious monitoring* and *conscious retrospection (reflection)*, see Box 16.2.

Taking categories of action, it can be seen that Jarvis has not described a category of action which reflects everyday professional practice, e.g. health visiting, that of 'doing the job'. This is because professional practice consists of several categories of action occurring at any one time, all of which may have varying levels of conscious planning, monitoring and retrospection. Looking at Box 16.2, of all the actions that Jarvis considered, experimental action is unique in being the only category that has to be performed with equally high levels of planning, monitoring and retrospection. This is because experimental action is dependent on the practitioner modifying practice, using all his/her theoretical knowledge and intuitive experience in the context of the situation (transferable skills).

Experimental action is exciting and creative but so also is repetitive action when carried out with high conscious levels of monitoring, planning and retrospection. In many ways repetitive

---

Box 16.2   A theoretical analysis of conscious action (Jarvis 1992). Reproduced by kind permission of Harcourt Publishers

Category of action	Level of consciousness Planning	Level of consciousness Monitoring	Level of consciousness Retrospecting
Non-action			
Anomic	None	None	High
Prohibited	Low-High	None	None-High
Non-response	None-High	None	None-High
Action			
Experimental	High	High	High
Repetitive	High-None	High-Low	High-None
Presumptive	None-Low	None-Low	None
Ritualistic	None	None-Low	None-High
Alienating	None	None-Low	None-High

---

action can be considered as 'doing the job', but doing a 'good' job. It is underpinned with theory, but this is tempered to meet the demands of the situation. Advising a mother how to cope with demanding toddler behaviour requires health visitors to suit the advice given to the contextual situation. This means relating guiding discipline to distractional handling that is necessary in, for example, a second-floor flat. It is important that in the conscious practitioner thinking processes, high levels of planning, monitoring and reflection are achieved.

The latter three action categories identified in Box 16.2 should have little part to play in sensitive and effective practice. A health visitor using presumption in practice may antagonise and alienate. No effective practice can be undertaken without good communication with the client to assess, in partnership, client need. Therefore high levels of planning, monitoring and retrospection would exclude the three categories – presumptive, ritualistic and alien-ating, and safeguard against their use. The practice teacher plays a big part in identifying and articulating these three categories with students.

Turning to categories of non-action (Box 16.2), the immediate response could be that non-action cannot be measured or assessed. Yet it is the 'art' of specialist community public health care nursing because the nature of

'science' in nursing is that it is measurable, through visible planning with clearly identi-fied outcomes. Thus this 'art' of non-action, rather than being seen as negative practice, is more likely to be an intuitive response to the circumstances of the situation. As all activities between client and practitioner should, mainly, be client-led then there may be anomic non-action by the practitioner because it is not part of the client agenda. For example, a practitioner goes to a client's home on a pre-arranged visit in order to discuss with the mother, her devel-oping infant's sleep problem, and finds the client in tears. Anomic non-action will take place because client distress leads to alternative practice of listening and discussing/counselling about the concerning matter. Subsequent de-briefing by the practice teacher will enable the student to articulate high levels of con-scious planning prior to the visit, but new high levels of monitoring and retrospection after the anomic non-action, with its causal reasons.

Prohibited does not necessarily mean illegal non-action and might be an action that is unprofessional. For instance, a client may complain about a treatment/advice suggested by another practitioner. The colleague had failed to find out the client's situation and the 'prohibited action', i.e. unprofessional approach would be to denounce the colleague to the client. The alternative positive action will be experimental and in discussion with the client, the practitioner might build on, or modify the proposal suggested by the colleague. The client then has the opportunity to see how the basic treatment/advice can still be used but in a modified way. It is up to the practitioner what is later said to the colleague, but at least client confidence in professional practice is not undermined.

Non-response action can be articulated by practitioner to client, e.g. the practitioner does not have the means or knowledge to respond to client need. This example suggests that there is a high conscious level of planning and an equally high level of retrospection, because the practitioner will seek out answers to the client need. The other aspect of non-response action without attendant conscious levels of planning and retrospection is more likely to occur when a non-alert practitioner fails to perceive a 'hidden' (covert) message from the client. Thus the client becomes ill-served by a stressed or inattentive practitioner. During debriefing with the practice teacher, the anomic or prohibited action categories can easily be articulated. The high conscious level of planning and retrospection in non-response category can also be articulated. However, the assessor/practice teacher can only identify non-response action which has no conscious levels if s/he is there at the time, and sometimes two persons attending might inhibit the client.

It can be seen that if competence and proficiency in practice are to be assessed to the same degree of penetration as theory, then action and non-action must be recognised.

A consideration of competence and proficiency in practice

Competence

The challenge set for specialist community health courses in the late 1990s was that practice was to be 50% of the course. The academic world was beginning to recognise that it was difficult to award an honours classification to a one-year top-up course, unless the whole of that year was assessed by grading, and not only the theoretical 50%, as the other 50% was mainly pass/fail. Thus we needed to learn how to grade practice, but we also needed to make sure that the practice was safe and effective and the term 'competence' became widely used.

In the nursing profession, Benner (1984) used the Dreyfus model of skill acquisition by chess players and airline pilots, to show how a student passes through five levels of proficiency: novice, advanced beginner, competent, proficient and expert. She argued that the different levels reflect changes in three general aspects of skilled performance. One is a movement from reliance on abstract principles to the use of past concrete experience as paradigms. The second is a change in the learner's perception of the demand situation, in which the situation is seen less and less as a compilation of equally relevant bits, and more and more as a complete whole in which only certain parts are relevant. The third is a passage from detached observer to involved performer engaged in the situation. The methodology used was a consensus approach using expert nurses to identify situations and the interpretative strategy was based on Heideggerian (1962) phenomenology which fits the description of constant comparative method (Glaser & Strauss 1967), to identify meanings and content. Eraut (1994) applauds Benner's use of the Dreyfus model of skill acquisition but challenges the assumption that how clinical decisions are made by experts is also how clinical decisions ought to be made.

Cameron-Jones (1988) uses Medley's (1984) work in attempting to determine competency in the teaching profession. Medley used four terms as basic clarification – competency, competence, performance and effectiveness. Competency he defined as a single knowledge, skill or professional value that a teacher might be said to possess; competence as the repertoire of competencies that a teacher possesses and which is regarded as sufficient in principle for the teacher to practice safely; performance as what the teacher does on the job; and effectiveness as the effect the teacher's performance has on the learners. Medley's work is important in that it begins to worry at what a competent profession might show, and it is interesting that Medley considered the last characteristic – that of effectiveness – as the bottom line. Cameron-Jones then raised the question of whether the most competent professional is the one with the greater collection of competencies or the one who is most effective in terms of performance outcomes.

The two approaches outlined above in the teaching and nursing professions illustrate early approaches and attempts to articulate the concept of competency. Cameron-Jones (1988) comments that Medley's work was the result of a paper written at a time when there was a crisis of confidence among the public at large as to education's productivity and its claim to the status of professionalism. Benner's work was a remarkable piece of research using a methodology that had little to do with the nursing profession but demonstrated the value of critical incident analysis to articulate clinical excellence in nursing. The approaches differ considerably because Medley looked at the teacher and the abilities possessed whereas Benner was more concerned about the experience-in-context of the nurse. Interestingly, neither author looked to the outcome as an expression of competence.

The problem with some of Medley's early thinking is that if a practitioner possesses a competency or competencies, then it is likely that these will be task-based or behaviourist. Gonczi (1994) points out that the possession of individual competencies can be seen as 'positivist, reductionist, ignores underlying attributes, ignores group processes and their effect on performance, is conservative, atheoretical, ignores the complexity of performance in the real world and ignores the role of professional judgement in intelligent performance' (p. 28). Gonczi suggests that this model of competence was originally adopted by training programmes with specified competency standards based on behaviours or tasks. Indeed the NVQ system developed by Jessup (1991), appears to have the first two levels following a behaviourist/task-based pattern.

Gonczi puts together the complex combinations of attributes such as knowledge, attitudes, values and skills, and sees the practitioner using them within a specific situation, using professional judgement. He argues that these show that competence is relational, bringing together disparate things, such as the abilities (attributes) of individuals, the appropriate professional situation and the need for intelligent performance.

Returning to Medley's (1984) suggestions of four basics of competence, there arises an interesting question about a *guarantee of competence* rather than a *guarantee of effectiveness* or a *guarantee of performance*. Medley points out that professionals are not expected to guarantee results, rather they offer the best effort to use competence in the best interests of clients/patients. He, therefore, sees effectiveness and performance as being lesser than competencies (attributes). Miller *et al.* (1988) suggested two senses in which competence can be defined: competence equating to performance, referring descriptively to an activity, and competence as a quality or state of being of an individual. Girot (1993) linked the suggestion of a state of being with Runciman's (1990) work which also considered competence as a state of being, but Runciman struggled with the difficulty in observing this 'state of being' and decided that it would be seen as competent performance. Thus competence and performance united in this way returns the thinking to Medley's (1984) basic characteristics of competence – competency, competence, performance and effectiveness.

Girot's (1993) assessment of competence in clinical practice used clinical ward sisters to make judgements on students' competence and a number of responses from the assessors bears out the discussions of other writers above. For instance, one comment suggested that students' performance deteriorated when out of familiar contexts – despite the student's apparent theoretical competence. Another student was criticised for an apparently uncaring attitude and was thus deemed to be incompetent although caring was not a criteria of competence. Girot's work shows that competence and performance are not necessarily correlated, depending to a great extent on the constructs of the assessors as to what is deemed to be competent.

McMullan *et al.* (2003) in examining the literature on assessing competence looked at three approaches, behavioural, generic and holistic and the assessment of these. The behavioural approach suggested that simple, objective levels of competence are distinguishable. Successful performance demonstrates underlying knowledge and understanding, but competencies are fragmented and non-transferable and ignore the context. In the generic approach assessment incorporates underlying knowledge, understanding and skills but there is the assumption that competencies are transferable and then assessment becomes difficult. In the holistic approach this incorporates context, ethics, and the need for reflective practice and is therefore difficult to assess.

Proficiency

In their various recent publications NMC (2002, 2003, 2004a) concentrated on proposals for standards using principles, domains and competencies. The discussion above has highlighted the difficulty writers had in articulating competence as a measurable phenomenon. Now however, the definitive document on standards (NMC 2004b) has changed terminology to require proficiency in practice articulated as principles and domains. In expounding on the background to these new standards NMC simply take a broad view:

'The standards of proficiency must, therefore, reflect a breadth of practice and learning, at a level commensurate with the specialist nature of community public health nursing practice. This requires an ability to assess risk in complex situations; to develop effective relationships based on trust and openness; to work flexibly with other services in a range of settings; to deal with conflicting priorities and ambiguous situations; and knowing when to use different and sometimes contradictory theories and perspectives.'

In the light of the statement above it is therefore necessary to consider whether the mechanisms for assessing proficiency differ from assessing competence.

Returning to Benner's (1984) original work, she made some interesting statements in her descriptor of proficient (p. 27) as related to nurses in practice in the acute field:

'Characteristically, the proficient performer perceives situations as wholes rather than in terms of aspects, and performance is guided by maxims. Perception is a key word here. The perspective is *not* thought out but presents itself based upon experience and recent events. Proficient nurses understand the situation as a whole because they perceive its meaning in terms of long-term goals.'

Benner makes useful recommendations on teaching a proficient performer by suggesting teaching by case studies and that proficiency is enhanced if the student is required to cite experience and exemplars for perspective.

Eraut (1994) approves Benner's use of the Dreyfus model and recognises that proficiency takes quite a different approach to the job: normal behaviour is not just routinised but semi-automatic; situations are apprehended more deeply and the abnormal is quickly spotted and given attention. Thus progress beyond competence depends on a more holistic approach to situational understanding.

Girot (1993) considers that in assessing competence a holistic approach is likely to be more valid than an individual fragmented competencies approach, and thus this would appear to be closer to the descriptor of a proficient performer '... perceives situations as wholes rather than in terms of aspects'.

Chambers (1998) also considers that a holistic approach to assessment is important in order to obviate the perspective and training of the assessor and considers that the use of reflective practice assessment is the most helpful in assessing holistically.

It would seem therefore that if it is possible to gain an accurate assessment of practitioner proficiency then a method of assessing reflection must be part of the process.

In developing a theory of reflection and teacher education Goodman (1984) was concerned that the meaning of the term reflection is clarified and his argument focuses on the need to recognise that reflection is not just a quiet rumination. If reflection is to be a worthwhile goal within teacher education then our notion of it must be comprehensive. First, reflection suggests a need to focus on the substantive, rather than utilitarian concerns. Second, a theory of reflection must be legitimate and integrate both intuitive and rational thinking. Finally, certain underlying attitudes are necessary in order to be truly reflective.

Dewey (1933) referred to *routine thought* which is a process of thinking and may lead to problem solving, but is in direct opposition to that of reflection. Routine thought is about how we confront, manage and deal with immediate situations, it does not allow time to reflect because it lacks the patience necessary to work through one's doubts and perplexity. Goodman (1984) identifies *rational thought* which is clearly distinguishable from routine thought, and which some observers equate to reflection. However, Goodman argues that rational thought does not encompass *intuitive thought* which is associated with the spark of creative ideas, insight and empathy. He thus posits reflective thinking as occurring with the integration of rational and intuitive thought processes.

Drawing again on Dewey (1933), Goodman identifies three attitudes as prerequisites for reflective teaching:

- *Open-mindedness* – an active desire to listen to more sides than one
- *Responsibility* – there must be a desire to synthesise ideas, to make sense out of nonsense and to apply information in an aspired direction. This attitude fosters consideration of the consequences and implications beyond questions of immediate utility
- *Wholeheartedness* – the internal strength necessary for genuine reflection and the ability to work through fears and insecurities

Goodman's levels of reflection (1984)

- 1st level   *Reflection to reach given objectives*: Criteria for reflection are limited to technocratic issues of efficiency, effectiveness and accountability
- 2nd level   *Reflection on the relationship between principles and practice*: There is an assessment of the implications and consequences of actions and beliefs as well as the underlying rationale for practice
- 3rd level   *Reflection which besides the above incorporates ethical and political concerns*: Issues of justice and emancipation enter deliberations over the value of professional goals and practice and the practitioner makes links between the setting of everyday practice and broader social structure and forces

Figure 16.1 and Box 16.3 show models of reflection recommended to the students.

Tools for assessment of proficiency in practice

Reflective journal analysis

The discussion above suggests that an assessor may use a student's reflective journal to gain some insight into the maturing processes of reflection shown by the student when gaining practice experience.

Guidelines for keeping a reflective journal (Johns 1994):

(1)   Use an A4 notebook
(2)   Split each page
(3)   Write up diary events on left side
(4)   Use right hand side for further reflection
(5)   Write up experience the same day if possible
(6)   Use actual dialogue wherever possible to capture the situation
(7)   Make a habit of writing up at least one experience per day
(8)   Balance problematic experiences with a satisfying experience

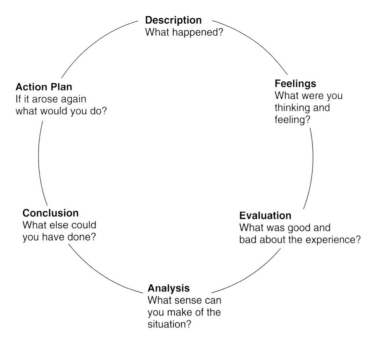

Figure 16.1 The reflective cycle (Gibbs 1988)

(9) Challenge yourself at least once a day about something that you normally do without thought/take for granted – ask yourself – 'why did I do that?' (i.e. make the normal problematic)

(10) Always endeavour to be open and honest with yourself – find the 'authentic you' to do the writing

The community practice teacher plays an important part in unpacking the reflective journal jointly with the student. Language and metaphor use in the journal requires exploration and checking back with student conceptualisation of the experience articulated. Initially, of course, this process is a shared process during the period of shadowing of the community practice teacher by the student. However, later, when the student is practising alone and articulating the content of the practice intervention, it is essential to explore the meaning of language and metaphor used. This entire process should be normalised to the extent that it becomes totally integrated into the student's subsequent qualified practice. Good specialist community public health practice

should always be managed in such a way that the practitioner deliberately allows time for reflection and this may need to be written rather than just mused upon.

It is suggested that the use of the term journal mitigates against a privacy factor, but nevertheless it is important that the journal is private to the student and practice teacher, in order for it to be both a formative and a summative tool.

Portfolio

The second type of tool to enable the assessment of practice proficiency is a portfolio which, in nurse education, is used for both professional and personal development. In the UK portfolios have been part of nursing for many years, particularly as an assessment strategy to integrate theory and practice. Students acquire knowledge and skills, such as problem-solving and critical thinking from academics, however, they acquire and develop equally important practical skills and experiences from clinicians.

The content of a portfolio should contain carefully selected examples of the achievements of

---

Box 16.3   A model of structured reflection (Carper 1978; Johns 1992)

(1) *Description of the experience*

    (1) Phenomenon – describe the here and now experience
    (2) Causal – what essential factors contributed to the experience
    (3) Context – what/who are the significant background actors to the experience
    (4) Clarifying – what are the key processes (for reflection) in this experience

(2) *Reflection*

    (1) What was I trying to achieve?
    (2) Why did I intervene as I did?
    (3) What are the consequences of my action for:
      — myself
      — the client/family
      — the people I work with?
    (4) How did I feel about this experience when it was happening?
    (5) How did the client feel about it?
    (6) How do I know how the client felt about it?

(3) *Influencing factors*

    (1) What internal factors influenced my decision making?
    (2) What external factors influenced my decision making?
    (3) What sources of knowledge did/should have influence(d) my decision making?

(4) *Could I have dealt better with the situation?*

    (1) What other choices did I have?
    (2) What would be the consequences of those choices?

(5) *Learning*

    (1) How do I now feel about this experience?
    (2) How have I made sense of this experience in the light of past experience and future practices?
    (3) How has this experience changed my ways of knowing?
      — empirics
      — aesthetics
      — ethics
      — personal

---

learning outcomes. The selection depends on the proficiency and creativity level of the student, applicability of past experiences, depth of self-reflection and purpose of the portfolio. Reflective processes have to be used, in the sense that the student needs to reflect on how the item selected will demonstrate to the assessor, theory/practice integration and development. For example, a student may have been asked to prepare a discussion session for a new group. The session plan could be used subsequently for the portfolio with an attached rationale for the content items selected for the session, as well as evidence of the effectiveness of the project.

Too much information in a portfolio creates an unwieldy collection of documents with possibly too fine an analysis of learning; too little information is a sterile exercise. It is important that a portfolio is not just a collection of items in a folder, but that it shows how reflection on these items by the student demonstrates learning (McMullan *et al.* 2003).

In reality it is difficult to grade the contents of a portfolio as a sole example of practice grading, but the portfolio and the reflective journal can be part of the total practice grading process.

Practice assessment document

Discussion in the preceding sections on competence and proficiency suggests that in both instances there is an indeterminancy of true definition and possible assessment. Nevertheless it is possible to build on previous approaches to practice assessment. In time, and with sufficient data an interpretive strategy based on Heideggerian (1962) phenomenology which fits the description of constant comparative method by Glaser and Strauss (Glaser, 1978; Glaser & Strauss, 1967), it can be proved that practice can be effectively assessed. This was shown to be possible by Robotham (2001).

Unpublished work by Robotham (1994) suggested that professional practitioners work with two general capabilities – a technical capability and a knowledge based capability. A *technical capability* consists of the personal professional resources, skills and strategies used by a practitioner e.g. listening skills, good articulation, true empathy, ability to challenge, assertiveness and so forth. *Knowledge capability* is the cognition skill to use valid knowledge to underpin practice, conceptualise links between complexities of practice and a multiplicity of theories, and see the boundaries between professionalism and the broader social structure.

Assessment of fieldwork practice can become an emotionally charged activity where there is resistance and challenge in terms of subjectivity or objectivity.

The position of the community practice teacher as assessor becomes fraught with difficulties when set within the above contexts. In gaining her own experience a community practice teacher will have developed a personal set of skills that will work most effectively in the situations of giving and receiving, negotiating and compromising. Indeed it may take several years to become experienced and effective, and yet the community practice teacher assessor is making a judgement on the abilities of a student to show effectiveness in the early days of practice.

Subjectivity, in the light of the above, would seem to be about the values and beliefs of the assessor and could lead to prejudging of issues within the intervention process between student and client which do not fit the community practice teacher's expectations of how the intervention should be performed. Jarvis and Gibson (1985) make the important observation that the emotion of subjectivity is considerably reduced where it is made very clear that it is the practice that is being commented on, and not the practitioner as an individual. Nevertheless, Jarvis and Gibson also show how using Rowntree's (1977) use of the term descriptive assessment, which is objective assessment, viz. – the student implemented an interaction with the client in a specific way – must be coupled with a judgement on the effectiveness of the intervention. This intervention may not have been carried out in a way that the community practice teacher might have used, but if the outcome was effective then the subjectivity becomes softened towards objectivity bound up in the outcome observed.

The grading assessment of fieldwork practice will be set against the following criteria for technical capability and the practice teacher, having selected the category then has to consider where the student's capabilities lie within the three options for each grade.

Technical capabilities

This section of the tool asks both practice teacher and student to look at the personal resources and abilities of the student. It is completed twice, first at the end of the first semester and then at the end of the second semester. It is primarily a subjective assessment by the practice teacher but the student should fully participate in the discussions surrounding the student's abilities and *may* determine the grade in partnership with the practice teacher. The grading criteria descriptors were based on a terminology that was appropriate for practice but was also recognised as linking closely to academic descriptors.

Box 16.4 shows grading criteria for technical capabilities. It is important to note that there is no scientific absolute when practising specialist community public health nursing and that it is likely that assessors will struggle not to use norm referencing when they make their judgements.

Box 16.5 shows the aspects of technical capability appropriate for specialist community public health practice.

Knowledge capabilities

In the first edition of this book knowledge capabilities were based on a health visiting programme of practice. Scrutiny of the new standards of proficiency for specialist community public health nurses shows that they lend themselves to a similar assessment of knowledge capability. It is argued that the grading criteria are appropriate for proficiency as the language used is commensurate with that of the NMC standards (2004b). (Box 16.6 shows the grading for knowledge capabilities. Box 16.7 shows knowledge capabilities for standards of proficiency for specialist community public health nursing. Figure 16.2 is an example of the design of the recording tool for knowledge capability.)

The assessment document should be designed in order to allow the student to provide evidence to satisfy the learning outcomes of major aspects of their fieldwork experience. At least two examples should be given for each outcome

---

Box 16.4   Grading criteria for technical capabilities (Robotham 2000)

A16 A15 A14
An articulate, enthusiastic and dynamic practitioner with highly developed communication skills using appropriate language and interaction relationships within the social context. Confident use of intervention strategies embracing a wide variety of techniques. Capability to deal effectively with contingency and with organisational characteristics of a superior rather than adequate performance. A creative practitioner drawing on well functioning cognitive skills and tacit knowledge.

B13 B12 B11
Well motivated, articulate and empathetic practitioner who occasionally requires time to establish appropriate interaction relationships. Well developed problem solving skills and good organisational strategies. Strong evidence of good use of cognition skills and tacit knowledge. A confident effective practitioner.

C10 C9 C8
Mainly good use of communication skills and with the ability to set up good relationships. Sometimes lacks confidence in problem solving skills but work processes and work outcomes are clearly visible. A good adequate job performance.

D7 D6 D5
Limitations in communication skills sometimes evident. Tendency to lack confidence and organisational abilities are somewhat restricted. Lacks flair or initiative and there is little evidence of effective use of technical capabilities. Recording and report writing of an indifferent standard. Nevertheless is safe to practice.

E4 E3 Marginal fail
Ineffective practice due to weak communication skills and lack of sensitivity both in client relationships and within social context. Poor organisation and shows incompetence in new situations.

F2 F1 Fail
Unacceptable performance.

Box 16.5   Aspects of technical capability used to assess specialist community public health nurses

(1)	Response to preventive work	Concept of primary prevention Grasp of opportunities to discuss health needs Effective use of resources to promote primary prevention
(2)	Competence in new situations	Assessment of confidence Enterprise Initiative Persistence Creativity Use of resources
(3)	Organisational capacity	Organisation of self Ability to prioritise effectively Management skills — workload — time — organisation and running of clinics — other team members
(4)	Capacity to make relationships	Manner with clients Non-judgmental interest in clients Empathy skills in assessment of client knowledge and attitudes Ability to develop partnerships Professional relationships with all levels of staff
(5)	Communication skills	Verbal and non-verbal communication Advanced communication — reflection — listening — interpreting Assessment — perceptual — psychological — emotional Adult management — relationships — attitude modification techniques Child interaction — language — non-verbal communication — sensitivity — listening Inter-agency liaison
(6)	Recording and report writing	Conciseness Spelling and grammar in writing Accuracy Contemporaneousness in recording

Box 16.5 (Continued)	
(7) Observational skills	Perception of relationships
	Family dynamics
	Class
	Culture and racial awareness
	Clinical observation
	'Hidden messages'
(8) Special aptitudes present	Strengths and weaknesses
	Present state of capability and potential

Box 16.6 Grading criteria for knowledge capability in relation to practice domains (Robotham 2000)

A16 A15 A14

Presenting a very high standard of practice evidenced by client feedback, reflective journal analysis and articulation of the use of models and theories within practice at debriefing sessions with CPTs. Reflects on own beliefs and values and the nature of moral and ethical issues in relation to health visiting practice. Uses predominantly research-based knowledge and demonstrates ability to transfer and modify this in different situations using, in addition, valuable personal knowledge where appropriate. Clearly demonstrates that knowledge is not static.

B13 B12 B11

Sound, careful and effective practice using appropriate theoretical perspectives evidenced by client feedback, reflective journal analysis and articulation at debriefing sessions with CPT. Clearly using research-based knowledge and shows ability to seek this out. Demonstrate effectiveness in all aspects of health visiting practice.

C10 C9 C8

Occasionally is not able to make clear links between knowledge sources and the stuff of practice. Is somewhat limited in ability to modify knowledge to suit practice situations but seeks guidance where unsure. Knowledge used is research-based but sometimes has difficulty in distinguishing between intuitive practice and research based practice as evidenced by reflective journal analysis.

D7 D6 D5

Has a knowledge base but often has difficulty in cognitive organisation of this in practical situations. Is aware of own weakness in some areas and avoids some aspects of a situation because cannot modify knowledge to solve problems. Reflective journal analysis shows inability to critically appreciate own knowledge levels.

E4 E3 Marginal fail

Is weak in areas of knowledge application and modification for practice. Practice is ineffective and evidence of client feedback and reflective journal analysis shows limited ability to correlate use of knowledge and practical abilities.

F2 F1 Fail

Fails to meet criteria for E. Unacceptable.

---

required. The technical capabilities and theories used at the time should be identified. Please note that *actual* capabilities and theories used should be shown, *not* espoused capabilities and theories. The practiceteacher comments should concentrate on the effectiveness of the student's performance in each example given.

Research (Robotham 2001) using both quantitative and qualitative data and document analysis over four cohorts (circa 120) students showed

Box 16.7   Knowledge capabilities for standards of proficiency for specialist community public health nursing

Domain	Outcome required
Search for health needs	Collect and structure data and information on health and well-being and related needs of a defined population
	Analyse, interpret and communicate data and information on the health and well-being and related needs of a defined population
	Develop and sustain relationships with groups and individuals with the aim of improving health and social well-being
	Identify individuals, families and groups who are at risk and in need of further support
	Undertake screening of individuals and populations and respond appropriately to findings
Stimulation of awareness of health needs	Raise awareness about health and social well-being and related factors, services and resources
	Develop, sustain and evaluate collaborative work
	Communicate with individuals, groups and communities about promoting their health and well-being
	Raise awareness about the actions that groups and individuals can take to improve their health and well-being
	Develop capacity and confidence of individuals and groups, including families and communities, to influence and use available resources, information and skills, acting as an advocate where appropriate
	Work with others to protect the public's health and well-being from specific risks
Influence on policies affecting health	Work with others to plan, implement and evaluate programmes and projects to improve health and well-being
	Identify and evaluate service provision and support network for individuals, families and groups in the local area or setting
	Appraise policies and recommend changes to improve health and well-being
	Interpret and apply health and safety legislation and approved codes of practice with regard to the environment, well-being and protection of those who work in the wider community
	Contribute to policy development
	Influence policies affecting health
	Develop, implement, evaluate and improve practice on the basis of research, evidence and evaluation
Facilitation of health-enhancing activities	Work in partnership with others to prevent the occurrence of needs and risks related to health and well-being
	Work in partnership with others to protect the public's health and well-being from specific risks
	Prevent, identify and minimise risk of interpersonal abuse and violence, safeguarding children and other vulnerable people, initiating the management of cases involving actual or potential abuse or violence where needed
	Apply leadership skills and manage projects to improve health and well-being
	Plan, deliver and evaluate programmes to improve the health and well-being of individuals and groups
	Manage teams, individuals and resources ethically and effectively

Plan, deliver and evaluate programmes to improve the health and well-being of individuals and groups	
Evidence from student of exemplars to satisfy the domain learning outcome	**Specific knowledge/theories used**
Technical capabilities used i.e. resources and strategies	**Observations made by CPT/mentor. Comments on evidence**
Agreed grade achieved	

Figure 16.2 Example of the design of the recording tool for knowledge capability

stability and reliability of the fieldwork tool. Content analysis of the technical grading capability section of the tool showed it to be sufficiently penetrative and comprehensive to summarise the professional and behavioural abilities of the students. Content analysis of the knowledge capabilities section showed that students were able to articulate, through written evidence and reflective processes, what knowledge they used in practice situations. A final comment on the value of the fieldwork assessment tool is that it can be used by a wide number of professions both within and outside the NHS, where professional and client group interaction is based on interpersonal processes.

Conclusion

The major evolution of the new register (NMC 2004b) has resulted in new standards of proficiency for the third part of the register. This chapter has explored how public health nurses, health visitors, midwives, occupational health nurses and school nurses must all aspire to the same standards of proficiency to enable them to be admitted to the third part of the register.

The chapter has looked at standards of education for specialist community public health programmes and it must be recognised that within these will also lie the specialist element of the course being undertaken. A brief exploration of grading within the education institution and practice has been presented, and practice itself has been analysed for knowledge and action in relation to academic levels. Finally, an exploration of competency and proficiency has been discussed and assessment tools for proficiency in practice have been considered.

References

Ashworth, P.D., Gerrish, K., Hargreaves, J. & McManus, M. (1999) 'Levels' of attainment in nursing practice: reality or illusion? *Journal of Advanced Nursing,* **30**(1), 159–168.

Benner, P. (1984) *From Novice to Expert. Excellence and Power in Clinical Nursing Practice.* Addison-Wesley, California.

Burns, S. (1992) Grading Practice. *Nursing Times,* **88**(1), 41–42.

Cameron-Jones, M. (1988) Looking for Quality and Competence in Teaching. In: *Professional Competence and quality assurance in the caring professions* (ed. R. Ellis) Chapman and Hall, London.

Carper, B. (1978) Fundamental ways of knowing in nursing. *Advances in Nursing Science,* **11**, 13–23.

Chalmers, K.I. (1992) Giving and receiving: an empirically derived theory on health visiting practice, *Journal of Advanced Nursing,* **17**, 1317–1325.

Chambers, M. (1998) Some issues in assessment of clinical practice: a review of the literature. *Journal of Clinical Nursing,* **7**(3), 201–208.

Davis, B.D. & Burnard, P. (1992) Academic levels in nursing, *Journal of Advanced Nursing,* **17**, 1395–1400.

Dewey, J. (1933) How we think. In: (1994) *Reflective Practice in Nursing: The Growth of the Professional Practitioner,* A. Palmer, S. Burns & C. Bulman, (eds). Blackwell Science: Oxford

Elkan, R. & Robinson, J. (1993) Project 2000: the gap between theory and practice. *Nurse Education Today,* **13**, 293–298.

Eraut, M. (1994) *Developing Professional Knowledge and Competence.* Falmer Press, London.

Fawcett, J. (1992) Conceptual models and nursing practice: the reciprocal relationship. *Journal of Advanced Nursing,* **17**: 224–228.

Gibbs, G. (1988) *Learning by Doing. A guide to teaching and learning methods.* Further Education Unit , Oxford Polytechnic, Oxford.

Girot, E.A. (1993) Assessment of competence in clinical practice: a phenomenological approach. *Journal of Advanced Nursing,* **18**, 114–119.

Glaser, B.G. (1978) *Theoretical Sensitivity. Advances in the Methodology of Grounded Theory.* Mill Valley CA: Sociology Press.

Glaser, B.G. & Strauss, A. (1967) *The Discovery of Grounded Theory.* Aldine Publishing Company, Chicago.

Gonczi, A. (1994) Competency Based Assessment in the Professions in Australia. *Assessment in Education,* **1**(1), 27–43.

Goodman, J. (1984) Reflection and Teacher Education: A Case Study and Theoretical Analysis. *Interchange* 15/3 © The Ontario Institue for Studies in Education: Ontario.

Heidegger, M. (1962) *Being and Time.* Harper and Row: New York.

Jarvis, P. (1992) Reflective practice and nursing, *Nurse Education Today,* **12**, 174–181.

Jarvis, P. & Gibson, S. (1985) *The Teacher Practitioner in Nursing, Midwifery and Health Visiting.* Croom Helm: London.

Jessup, G. (1991) *Outcomes: NVQ's and the Emerging Model of Education and Training.* The Falmer Press, London.

Johns, C. (1994) Guided Reflection. In: *Reflective Practice in Nursing* A. Palmer, S. Burns & C. Bulman (eds). Blackwell Science: Oxford.

McClymont, M., Thomas, S. & Denham, M.J. (1991) *Health Visiting and Elderly People. A health promotion challenge.* Churchill Livingstone: Edinburgh.

McMullan, M., Endacott, R., Gray, M., Jasper, M., Miller, C.M.L., Scholes, J. & Webb, C. (2003) Portfolios and assessment of competence: a review of the literature. *Journal of Advanced Nursing,* **41**(3), 283–294.

Medley, D. (1984) Teacher Competency Testing and the Teacher Educator. In: *Advances in Teacher Education Vol 1,* L.G. Katz & J.D. Raths (eds). Ablex: New Jersey.

Miller, C., Hoggan, J., Pringle, S. & West, G. (1988) *Credit where credit's due. The Report of the Accreditation of Work-Based Learning.* SCOTVEC (Scottish Vocational Educational Council): Glasgow.

NMC (2002) *Requirements for pre-registration health visitor programmes.* The Nursing and Midwifery Council, London.

NMC (2003) *Third part of the register: specialist community public health nursing. Proposed competency framework consultation document,* The Nursing and Midwifery Council, London.

NMC (2004a) *NMC News.* Nursing and Midwifery Council, July 2004 London.

NMC (2004b) *Standards of proficiency for specialist community public health nurses.* Nursing and Midwifery Council, London.

Robotham, A. (1994) *Are Academic Levels in Health Visiting Theory Discernible in Practice?* Unpublished dissertation for Masters in Education, University of Wolverhampton, Wolverhampton.

Robotham, A. (2000) Assessment of competence to practice. In: D. Sines, F. Appleby & E. Raymond (eds) *Community Health care Nursing 2nd edn.* Blackwell Science Oxford.

Robotham, A. (2001) *The Grading of Health Visitor Fieldwork Practice.* Unpublished thesis: University of Wolverhampton, Wolverhampton.

Rowntree, D. (1977) *Assessing students: how shall we know them.* Kogan Page: London.

Rowntree, D. (1992) *Assessing Students: how shall we know them.* 2nd ed. Kogan Page, London.

Runciman, P. (1990) *Competence-based Education and the Assessment and Accreditation of Work-based Learning in the Context of P2000 Programmes of Nurse Education: a Literature Review.* National Board for Nursing, Midwifery and Health Visiting for Scotland, Edinburgh.

Schön, D.A. (1983) *The Reflective practitioner.* Basic Books: New York.

Schutz, A. (1972) *The phenomenology of the social world.* Heinemann, London.

White, E., Riley, L., Davis, S. & Twinn, S. (1993) *A Detailed Study of the Relationships between Teaching, Support, Supervision and Role Modelling for Students in Clinical Areas Within the Context of Project 2000 Courses.* English National Board for Nursing, Midwifery and Health Visiting, London.

Wilson Barnett, J., Butterworth, T., White, E. *et al.* (1995) Clinical support and the Project 2000 student: factors influencing this process. *Journal of Advanced Nursing,* **21**, 1152–1158.

Winter, R. & Maisch, M. (1992) *Professionalism and Competence,* The Asset Programme, Chelmsford: Anglia Polytechnic University.

Chapter 17 **Inter-professional Practice and Teamwork**

Owen Barr

Introduction

The chapter commences with an overview of the range of professionals who work in community health services and considers the developments in service provision that have highlighted the need for increasing the effectiveness of teamwork between a wider range of professionals who provide community based health and social care services (DoH 2000a). The nature of teams is also explored to clarify the characteristics of effective teams and team working. Consideration is given to the factors that potentially reduce the outcomes of teamwork and steps that might be taken to facilitate effective team working.

Potential team members in community services

The majority of people who use health services receive support from community-based services. Community nursing services, such as those provided by district nursing and public health nursing/health visiting seek to provide services to the general population. Some other community nursing services have traditionally focused their work within specific settings such as schools or places of work, whilst other services have been focused on the health needs of people with learning disabilities, children with complex needs or people with mental health problems.

The services provided by staff within community health care nursing services include public health focused work with groups from local communities, including the provision of health advice aimed at maintaining the health of individuals, groups and communities. Community nurses are also involved in active health surveillance with members of the community ranging from young children to older people. Health surveillance is at the cornerstone of community practice and may be the point at which health needs are identified and further nursing responses identified to meet these needs. Community nurses are often involved in supporting people prior to their contact with acute hospitals services and they will usually be involved in providing ongoing support as part of a discharge plan for people with more complex health care needs. For other people their contact with community health care nursing services may only commence following the conclusion of treatment in an acute or mental health hospital.

Community nurses are one of a number of professional groups who are employed within statutory services to provide support for people with a range of health needs outwith hospital. Other professionals include nurses in specific posts such as diabetes nurses, stoma care nurses, those who provide palliative care services and general practice nurses. In providing services to clients and their families community nurses work together with general practitioners, pharmacists and members of the allied health professions including physiotherapists, speech and language therapists and occupational therapists. In addition, the services provided by social service departments, such as social work, domiciliary care, day services and residential care may play a considerable role in supporting some people with complex needs in the community.

Family carers usually provide the largest amount of support to relatives and members of the community health care team have a key role to play in providing effective support to family members. Family members may also access support from independent sector services, comprising those provided by private and not for profit organisations. For some people these services could include the provision of nursing care at home, or residential and nursing home provision, on an ongoing or respite care basis. The independent sector also has an important advocacy role in providing information to family carers and clients about health conditions and the availability of services and their entitlements to services. Clients and family members may contact independent services directly, or such services may be contracted by statutory service providers, for instance as part of a case management package.

The need for effective collaboration between individual professionals and the services they are part of has long been advocated as the most effective way to deliver community-based services (DoH 1989; DHSS 1991). More recently, several developments in the role expansion of nurses and others in community service personnel, as well as the reorganisation of services, has further emphasised the need for the provision of effective teamwork.

The continuing need for effective teamwork

The view that the development of effective teamwork is the only framework for providing co-ordinated 'seamless services' is well established in health services within the UK (DoH 1989; DHSS 1991; Hudson 1995; Towell & Beardshaw 1991). In addition to the health policy guidance on team working, the importance of working in collaboration with colleagues, clients and carers is stressed to nurses, midwives and health visitors in guidance relating to their professional practice (NMC 2002).

Team working has long been viewed as a strategy or conduit to co-ordinate the growing number of professionals who work within community services in order to encourage the delivery of more comprehensive services, bridge gaps in services and reduce duplication. The interest in teamwork within health and social care services had its origins in the health policy of the 1980s (DoH 1989). Since that time interest in providing effective team based services has intensified as the pressure has increased to find ways in which health and social service staff can

be encouraged to work more closely together than they did previously (Johnson *et al.* 2003).

The context in which health and social services operate is constantly changing as the expectations and needs of people using services and the structures within which services are provided alters (Thomas & Woods 2003). Five key changes in the context of community services have re-emphasised the need for effective teamwork within, and between, agencies. First, changes in service policy have emphasised the importance of people having the opportunity to live in their own home, complemented by the need to provide requisite support to clients and their families to facilitate this objective. The reconfiguration of hospital services that previously provided longer term care for older people, people with learning disability, and people with mental health problems, has also emphasised the need for increased opportunities to live in community settings, such as supported living arrangements that provide as much flexibility and choice as possible (SE 2000; DoH 2000a; DoH 2001). A move to providing support at home for people who are chronically ill or in need of palliative care has also been emphasised in the past few years (DoH 2000b). In addition, revised policy in the form of the National Service Framework for children has highlighted the need to increase the support made available to children and their families in order to promote their inclusion (and protection) within society (DoH 2004a).

Second, there is recognition of the increasing complexity of the needs of people who receive services in the community. People who may have previously been cared for in hospital settings are now being supported increasingly in their own home. This covers a wide range of people, including young children with complex health needs who live at home with the support of equipment only previously available in hospital settings. At the other end of the continuum are a growing number of older people, many of whom are healthy and yet need advice and support to remain so. There are also a growing number of people who present with complex health needs and require support from community services. Over the past few years there has been an increase in the number and range of services available for such persons.

Examples include the development of community children's nursing services, the provision of services that focus on people with specific health needs such as diabetes, epilepsy, behaviour support services and support for people with dementia.

Third, there has been a change in emphasis in the domains of practice for community nurses. The future of community nurses in primary care services has been identified as focusing on three key functions, namely:

- First contact/single case assessment, diagnosis, care, treatment and referral
- The provision of continuing care, rehabilitation, the management of longer-term conditions
- Public health/health protection and promotion programmes that improve health outcome and reduce inequalities (DoH 2001)

Alongside this, there have been developments in the role of nurses working in community settings, such as non-medical (nurse) prescribing. There has also been a growing emphasis on the need to bridge the perceived gap between community-based services and those provided within secondary, acute services. Recent developments in community-based services, for example, the evolving role of nurse practitioners has seen community-based nurses involved in closer involvement with the referral of people to hospital services (Price & Williams 2003). Such developments have altered the hierarchy that existed previously between nurses and other professionals working within community teams.

Fourth, the focus of many teamwork developments has been on the actions that might be taken to increase the extent that teamwork occurs between individual practitioners. However, there is now a clear recognition of the need to develop more effective inter-agency working practices and emphasis has been given to the need to review how agencies work effectively together. This is particularly important given the development of primary care trusts and their associated counterparts in Scotland, Wales and Northern Ireland, requiring the need to formalise structures in which health and social services can be effectively co-ordinated (DoH 2000a).

Finally, a series of national/judicial inquiries into 'gross failures' to support some of the most vulnerable people in society have highlighted that at times fatal consequences may arise as the consequence of ineffective teamwork (DoH 2003, 2004b). Difficult lessons have to be learnt quickly from the frequent failures highlighted in such reports regarding the need for individuals and agencies to communicate openly if effective interagency teamwork is to develop.

Given the complexity of the needs among people who require support from community-based health and social services, it is clear that no single professional group alone is able to provide comprehensive services to all people. Teamwork will therefore be an imperative that requires the co-ordination of complex community health and social service inputs. There continues to be an underlying assumption that teamwork is the most effective way to achieve this objective, and it has been argued that teamwork is essential between (and within) health and social services, if they are to remain intact and not become divisive, fragmented and profit-led (Leathard 1994). Such views have contributed to the current situation which assumes that teamwork is the most effective approach to provide maximum benefit to clients and team members (McLaughlin 2004).

However, despite the apparently clear rationale for developing teamwork in community health and social services, there is much less clarity about what constitutes a team and the form it should take. Malin *et al.* (1999) capture this in their observation that 'it seems easier to agree that teams are a "good" thing rather than to agree about what they are' (p. 189).

The nature of teams

The word 'team' is widely used in everyday language and it appears that there is a common understanding of the term. However, when exploring the nature of teams it becomes clear that the term may have a number of different meanings depending on the context in which the word is used. The meaning of the word may be clear when referring to one's favourite sports team, but when used within the context of health and social care the term is not so easily defined, nor its members listed. Indeed, it has been asserted that vagueness about exactly what constitutes a team within health and social care appears to have resulted in almost all forms of communication between colleagues and other professionals being described as multidisciplinary teamwork (Øvretveit 1986).

The variation in the structure of 'teams' within local community services may also have contributed to the lack of clarity as to what constitutes a team. It is recognised that the number and professional backgrounds of the people who comprise the membership of health and social care teams will differ depending on several factors, including the clients the team is seeking to support, the level of skills required of team members, the professionals available within that locality, and the other services available to the clients in that geographical area. The structure of teams working in community health and social services can include those developed to deliver individualised care packages to individual clients, such as those developed in case management. Equally so, more formal interdisciplinary teams may provide services to a number of people with a diverse range of health needs across a specific geographical area (Øvretveit 1993). There is no 'right' team structure as the organisation of a team will vary depending on the service the team is required to provide. Each team structure has advantages and disadvantages; therefore, it is important that decisions about team membership, processes and structures are made carefully. The team structure should be selected to meet identified client needs, both individually and across the locality the team serves.

Indeed, in acknowledging the vagueness around the word 'team', it has even been suggested that the term should be dropped and replaced with the term 'integrated care', in order to focus on the needs of clients, rather than the members of a team (NHS Executive 2000). Although a range of definitions for teams can be found to exist in the health and social care literature, there is some degree of consistency about the characteristics that are present among team members and the structures in which they work. West (2004), for example, states that in practice, teams have shared objectives among the team members in relation to their work and usually can be identified to belong to a 'team' by other members of their organisation. He also views teams as having a degree of autonomy and control to make decisions in order to achieve their corporate objectives and having responsibility and accountability for their work.

An important distinction has been made between 'teams' and what Hayes (1997) has referred to as a 'pseudo-team'. The former possesses the characteristics of teams as identified by West (2004). In contrast, some professionals or their managers may consider themselves, or a number of staff within their organisation to be a team. These people may well work in the same offices and be identified as a team within the local health and social care structures, but still lack the key characteristics of a team as identified by West. Although this collection of people may have the potential to become an effective team, if all they have in common is a location or collective name, then they do not possess the characteristics of a team. Hayes (1997) has referred to such groups as a 'pseudo-team', which she defines as 'a group of people who are called, or who call themselves, a team ... but don't actually try to co-ordinate what they are doing or establish collective responsibility ... in reality they act on a purely individual level and are concerned only with their own departments and responsibilities' (Hayes 1997, p. 129). In essence, such arrangements may have the structural attributes of a team, but in practice they lack the level of functional integration and interdependence required to work effectively (Johnson *et al.* 2003).

The distinction between teams and pseudo-teams is an important one, since the provision of effective support to clients is dependent upon the provision of a 'functioning' team. Conversely, it is important to identify and either facilitate enhanced teamwork or disband those groups of people that function as teams 'in name only'. People who work in teams and those who manage services that are team-based, need to remain alert to the emergence of factors that may limit the effectiveness of a team in order to ensure that these can be responded to promptly.

When teamwork is not effective

Teams may not always be the most effective way of meeting the needs of people who use services or in achieving the objectives set by service providers. The perceived wisdom that bringing several professions involved in the provision of health and social care into an integrated team would increase the quality of services has not always been witnessed in practice. For example, many professionals and people who use services are able to provide clear examples of how their experience with team members and team working did not result in the delivery of better services (Malin *et al.* 1999). Unfortunately, and in part due to the unquestioning assumption that teamwork is effective, shortcomings in teamwork are not often openly discussed until failures have occurred on a major scale, resulting in an investigation into the working practices of the team and its members (DoH 2003, 2004b; Hudson 2002). Such problems highlight the need to provide closer attention to the indicators of ineffective teamwork and to take preventative action before difficulties arise. Three key issues frequently commented upon in the literature are explored below.

Lack of investment in team development

In order to establish and maintain an effective level of functioning, teams require an investment of time. Managers of services seeking to develop teams need first to explore if a team is an appropriate way to achieve the identified objectives of care and then establish the nature of the team that may be required. Similarly, care must be taken to guard against pressure that may be placed on services to develop complex team structures when more simple solutions would suffice (Hudson 2002).

In reality it is all too easy to bring a group of people together, set them a task to achieve and call them a team. This limited approach to team development often results in the presence of a group of people forming a team 'in name only'

(a 'pseudo-team'). Such teams fail to lead to the provision of effective teamwork since the focus has been placed on the structural integration of the team, without providing adequate attention to the development of strong inter-professional working (Johnson *et al.* 2003). This in turn can result in the absence of positive leadership for team members, which may increase their uncertainty over their own roles and the professional contribution that they bring to the work of the team (Bateman *et al.* 2003).

'Teams' set up in this way usually fail to achieve the objectives set for them (West 2004). However, all too often managers tend to focus attention on lack of teamwork by attributing failure to team members' reluctance to work together, rather than on the lack of investment of time and energy provided by them to establish an effective foundation from which the team might develop. Whilst team members may have been provided with explicit objectives, the lack of discussion and opportunity to develop open communication between team members can result in people being reluctant to alter their previous ways of working and may strengthen their commitment to following their previous roles. This may be further complicated in larger teams by the emergence of contested leadership, when several leaders arise and groupings of team members around these people emerge within the team. Groupings may be formed on the basis of previous professional backgrounds; new allegiances may also develop as people seek to maintain or seek a favourable position within a team.

Teamwork may result in stress, tension and conflict for team members. This is particularly evident when members are asked to change their working arrangements/practices when they are largely unsupported. Such situations could result in team members experiencing mixed emotions of anxiety, confusion, frustration, anger, fear, excitement and anticipation. Some members may need support to realise that although their hierarchical position and power position has altered, they are still important and valued members of the team. On a more practical level the impact and frustration that may result from the need to relocate offices, travel further to work, or share offices with other professionals or people with whom they may have had limited contact for the first time, should not be underestimated.

This may be a particular challenge when people from diverse organisations (e.g. community nursing, social services, housing services, advocacy groups) who have limited actual experience of working with each other are brought together. In order to engage in open communication the people involved need time to build up a picture of the functions, ideologies and culture of the other agencies and how that agency views their role (Johnson *et al.* 2003).

Failure to promote opportunities for flexibility and creativity in providing services

Linked to the lack of investment in team development is the lack of flexibility and creativity within team working. When team members do not have the opportunity to reflect on their own professional contribution to the work of the team, they may seek 'security' by insisting on the development of rigid and complex decision making procedures, sometimes proffered in the name of effective teamwork. This situation can be further complicated when people outwith the team seek to influence the development of these procedures (Hudson 2002). Similar conflict can occur when managers outwith the team continue to exercise control over team members which may result in affected team members feeling that they are unable to make autonomous decisions, leading to frustration and a reduced commitment to the team. In reality the development of rigid procedures often has more to do with a desire to maintain previous hierarchical structures. Hence, the intensity with which some professional groups defend their perceived territory should not be minimised (Beattie 1995; Leathard 1994). Within such rigid structures the manner in which work is allocated to team members may have limited transparency and be perceived as originating from the assignation of roles based on one's position in the hierarchical structure, their previous status or perceived favouritism.

Inevitably, difficulties might arise when rigid procedures are imposed on team members, which

can be further compounded by the adoption of an authoritarian approach to leadership within which obedience to authority is the rule and those who comply are favoured within the team. From this viewpoint, there is no acceptance that conflict is an integral part of teamwork and any indicators of conflict among members are ignored, or suppressed. This situation has been referred to as 'groupthink' and has been widely recognised within other social groups and teams (Janis 1983; Moorhead *et al.* 1991) and continues to be highlighted as a potential problem within teams in health and social services (West 2004). This can result in team members considering few alternatives when making decisions, failure to re-examine alternatives in the light of new information, and the lack of attention to, or rejection of, available evidence. This can lead to a firm belief in the certainty of the decisions taken to the extent that no consideration is given to the development of alternative or contingency plans (Moorhead *et al.* 1991). With a team environment characterised by groupthink, individual team members become fearful of making autonomous decisions owing to the perceived or actual lack of support from other team members.

Lack of monitoring of team progress

Even when time and energy has been invested in facilitating the development of a team, ongoing support is necessary in order for the team to remain effective. New teams often emerge from the previous need to respond to changes in the needs of people who use the services, changing priorities in policy or the altering structures within organisations. As these factors continually evolve, there is a need for teams to monitor their success in remaining relevant to the services in which they operate.

Particular attention needs to be given to the operational culture and 'practice wisdom' as these evolve within teams. Operational culture has been described as 'the patterns of relationships and sets of assumptions which team members hold about themselves and their colleagues...the routine and often unspoken ways that members define their roles and their professional relationships' (Brown 1992, p. 372, 377). This comprises the tacit knowledge of how things are done in the team, the unwritten rules and procedures. The 'operational culture' of a team is as important to successful team functioning as appropriate team structures and agreed team operational policies. Practice wisdom is the product of informal rather than formal theory and seeks to address the everyday concerns and realities of practitioners' work. However, this is also rarely recorded, often not officially recognised and is therefore less often scrutinised (Hudson 2002).

A recognition of the importance of team culture requires managers and team members to invest time in open discussion about their perceptions/stereotypes of their own role and the role of other team members. Such discussions will provide opportunities for team members to get to know their colleagues as fellow professionals. Not doing so may lead to the situation outlined by Hattersly (1995) in which the failure to effectively monitor the performance of teams can result in a situation where they 'evolve gradually, without explicit review, and the resulting "monsters" can often establish their own demands for collaboration which exist only because of unnecessary division and barriers which have developed' (p. 261).

It is recognised that a number of problems can arise that will seriously impact on the effectiveness of a team in functioning to its full potential. These are not reasons for not pursuing teamwork, rather, they emphasise the need for service managers and team members to take active steps to facilitate effective teamwork.

When teams work well

Team development is facilitated
People do not always work effectively together, as evidenced in the continuing interest provided by government departments on how to enhance the effectiveness of teams to support people with increasingly complex needs and the poignant lessons that must be learnt from the consequences of failures in teamwork (DoH 2003, 2004b). The best opportunity to achieve successful teamwork is to build in and facilitate the growth of those factors that have been identified as contributing to effective teamwork.

Perhaps first among these is the need for prospective team members and their managers to accept that effective team working takes time to evolve (Tuckman & Jensen 1977). It is recognised that the collection of people who form the basis of a team need to work through the process of getting to know each other (forming) and agreeing initial core objectives and acknowledging the role of other team members (norming). These first two steps often occur without major difficulties and are usually assisted by the enthusiasm of people to make any new team a success. This process is assisted if the rationale for the team is clear to all involved and people have had the opportunity to shape the objectives of the team, rather then these being imposed on prospective team members (NHS Executive 2000). However, this apparent initial harmony and agreement is often disrupted for a period of time as team members start to provide services and face the challenges in doing so. Conflict is a key feature of this transition process to becoming a functioning team (Price & Williams 2003). These personal challenges often result in attempts to revise team objectives and roles. The core objectives of the team, as well as the role and value of team members may be directly and at times be forcibly questioned among team members (storming). If these periods of discussion, and on occasions open disagreement, among team members are facilitated, it usually results in further consensus developing among team members and this sets the scene for the team to provide effective services to clients (performing).

The initial stages of identifying the need for a team, be that a team to respond to the needs of one person, or a more formally structured team, require careful planning and attentive management. The formative stages of team working require the opportunity for staff to meet with other team members regularly. This has been reported as assisting in developing effective approaches to working together (Nancarrow 2004). It also provides opportunities to develop creative ways of thinking and make decisions according the situation in which they are working, but that are flexible enough to be amended as the situation changes (Molyneux 2001). Managers in services have an important role to play in creating the time and space for these initial stages of development to take place before team members are expected to manage large case/workloads (Øvretveit 1997).

People in the team want to be 'team members'

The personal qualities of team members also have a major influence on the rate at which team working develops, as well as the emergence of flexibility and creativity that influences how team members undertake their roles. In particular, the confidence of team members in their own role and their ability to undertake it is crucial to the willingness and ability of professionals to engage in open communication about their work with other professionals (Molyneux 2001). It is through this process of dialogue that a language that can be clearly understood among team members is established. The development of a common language code is an integral component of people successfully explaining their perceptions of their own role and understanding roles of other team members. This process of communication and the opportunity to more clearly understand the role of individual team members and getting to know more about people as individuals is important for team members to develop accurate knowledge about each other and to overcome stereotypes they may hold (Nancarrow 2004). This in turn facilitates the development of mutual trust and respect among team members and acknowledges the right of team members to make decisions based on mutual respect as well as professional and personal values or knowledge (although not all team members may agree with the decision made).

Teamwork requires people to work collaboratively, moving in the same direction and working with each other in order to achieve the objectives set for individual clients they are supporting and those of the overall team. Several of the factors noted above combine to form an environment in which collaborative working is possible. Such an approach is characterised by the sharing of power based on knowledge and expertise instead of role or title, and the provision of clear procedures for managing conflict within the team. Interaction between team members involves regular open and honest communication between all members, shared planning and decision making, and cooperative endeavour in which team members are interdependent on each other for the successful achievement of agreed goals (Hennemann *et al.* 1995).

Collaborative working develops and becomes consolidated over time as team members become less concerned about the specific boundaries of their previous roles and start to work more flexibly with other team members (Price & Williams 2003). However, for this process to commence and flourish a number of antecedents have been identified as necessary, namely: individual readiness of all (or at least the majority of) team members, understanding and acceptance of one's own role and expertise, confidence in one's own ability and recognition of the boundaries of one's own discipline. Furthermore, team members need to function within an environment that is appropriately managed to facilitate effective group dynamics (communication skills, respect and trust), a team orientation, organisational values of participation, interdependence and a leader supportive of autonomy (Hennemann *et al.* 1995).

The work of the team members is made positive and reinforcing

West (2004) outlined three key aspects that need to be addressed in order that the commitment of team members is maintained. First, he asserts that teams should have 'intrinsically interesting' tasks to perform and that individual team members should have 'intrinsically interesting' tasks to perform. Team members do not need to find every task they undertake to be of significant interest, but both at team and individual levels some aspects of their work should be of particular interest. The interest of team members in the success of the team can be enhanced by their active involvement in the development of team objectives and an understanding of where the team fits into and is valued by other components of the overall service (Nancarrow 2004).

In seeking to motivate individual team members and make their job intrinsically interesting, it is important to develop an understanding of what each team member may find interesting and perhaps has a particular ability for, or areas in which they wish to learn new skills. By doing so the team leader is in a better informed position to co-ordinate the use of members' knowledge and skills to meet client needs in a way that the team member will find motivating to them. It is important that the needs and interests of all team members, including the role of secretarial and other support staff, are considered in this process.

Second, not only should team members find their job (or at least some aspects of it) interesting, they should also feel that their individual contribution is important to the overall success of the team in achieving the agreed objectives. Whilst it is important that people know the role they play in achieving the overall success of the team and the interdependence on the contribution of individual team members, care needs to be taken to value equally the contribution of all team members. For this reason it is important to ensure that each team member has an aspect of their role which they feel is their particular contribution. Once the team member accepts the new role and is aware of the requirements of that role, they should be afforded a degree of autonomy in how they undertake these activities and receive encouragement to develop that area of their work.

Finally, feedback on progress towards agreed objectives should be provided to team members individually in relation to their role and to all members of the team in respect of the team's success and areas that might be considered for further development. Team members should also be made aware of the standards that will be used to evaluate both their individual role and that of the team. The involvement of team members in the negotiation of the areas to be focused upon can further reinforce their value as a team member and the importance of their contribution to the team.

The value of 'conflict' is acknowledged and appropriately channelled

An underlying premise of interdisciplinary team working is that by bringing together a group of people with differing knowledge, skills and perspectives more comprehensive solutions may emerge to meeting the needs of people who are supported by that service. It is through the process of sharing information and ideas that increased flexibility and creativity emerges in comparison to what the thoughts of an individual or a team of people from one professional background may have produced.

Inherent in this process is the need for some degree of discussion and at times the emergence and sharing of disagreements. This is to be encouraged and the creative energy that results should be channelled into the development of effective ways of working as a team. Disagreement is not a failing; indeed it is one of the few certainties the team will encounter as it evolves. Conversely, the absence of some level of disagreement from time to time may well reflect an unwillingness of team members to engage fully in the process of discussion and indicate the presence of some level of 'groupthink'. However, it is important that team members are aware of the limits of an acceptable disagreement and that clear procedures exist for dealing with differences between team members that cannot be resolved by discussion within the team. The presence of ground rules can enhance the development of trust and mutual respect among team members by providing a degree of certainty, predictability and fairness about how issues within the team are addressed. Such procedures need to acknowledge the need for discussion among team members and may vary between teams. However, procedures should be in place and agreed with team members shortly after the team is established, as it is likely to be more difficult to give adequate time and thought to develop the necessary procedures when a disagreement between team members has escalated at a later stage. As it is not possible to anticipate all eventualities, it is important that any strategies or procedures for dealing with conflict with the team are revised regularly.

Conclusion

The pressure to find more effective ways of co-ordinating health, social services and other agencies is set to continue. In recognition of the multitude of factors that can impact on the health of people and communities, community health care nurses will find themselves needing to collaborate effectively with people from a wider range of agencies and services than they have traditionally worked with. More attention now needs to be given to the development of teamwork and collaborative working practices between individuals in order to balance the present focus on collaborative working at policy level. If these inter-agency policies are to materialise for people in their local communities, it is important that those people who will deliver services have the opportunity to develop the necessary knowledge, skills and competence to work together effectively. Individual community nurses also need to take steps through their continuing professional development to develop the necessary knowledge and skills to master the challenges required for effective inter-agency and inter-organisational team working.

As discussed in this chapter the process of ensuring successful collaboration is complex, needs careful planning and ongoing attention from managers and team members. In addition to being aware of the factors that may facilitate effective teamwork, there is a need to remain vigilant and take action whenever dysfunctional team dynamics or practices are witnessed. Failure to address such issues may result in the insidious reduction of effective teamwork and an associated erosion of service quality to people who need the support of community nurses.

References

Bateman, H., Bailey, P., McLellan, H. (2003) Of rocks and safe channels: learning to navigate as an inter-professional team. *Journal of Interprofessional Care*, **17**(2), 141–150.

Beattie, A. (1995) War and Peace among the health tribes. In: *Interprofessional relations in health care*. K. Soothill, L. Mackay & C. Webb (eds.) pp. 11–30 Edward Arnold, London.

Brown, S. (1992) Profession in teams. In: *Standards and Mental Handicap, Keys to Competence*. T. Thompson & P. Mathais (p. 371–385) Bailliere Tindall, London.

Department of Health (1989) *Caring for People*. HMSO, London.

Department of Health (1997) *A First Class Service. Quality in the NHS*. DoH, London.

Department of Health (2000a) *The NHS Plan. The Government's response to the Royal Commission on Long Term Care*. CM 4818-II. DoH, London.

Department of Health (2000b) *The NHS Cancer Plan. A plan for investment. A plan for reform*. DoH, London.

Department of Health (2001) *Valuing People. A new strategy for learning disability for 21st century*. DoH, London.

Department of Health (2003) *The Victoria Climbie Inquiry*. DoH, London.

Department of Health (2004a) *Disabled Child Standard, National Service Framework for Children, Young People and Maternity Services*. Department of Health, London.

Department of Health (2004b) *Harold Shipman's clinical practice 1974–1998: a clinical audit commissioned by the Chief Medical Officer*. DoH, London.

Department of Health and Social Services (1991) *People First*. DHSS, Belfast.

Hattersly, J. (1995) The survival of collaboration and co-operation. In: *Services for people with learning disabilities*. N. Malin (ed.) (p. 260–273). Routledge, London.

Hayes, N. (1997) *Successful Team Management*. Thomson Business Press, London.

Hennemann, E.A., Lee, J.L. & Cohen, J.L. (1995) Collaboration: a concept analysis. *Journal of Advanced Nursing*, **21**(1): 103–109.

Hudson, B. (1995) A seamless service? Developing better relationships between the National Health Service and Social Services Departments. In: *Values and Visions. Changing ideas in services for people with learning difficulties* (eds T. Philpot & L. Ward) pp. 106–122. Butterworth Heinemann, Oxford.

Hudson, B. (2002) Interprofessionality in health and social care: the Achilles' heel of partnership. *Journal of Interprofessional Care*, **16**(1): 8–17.

Janis, I.L. (1983) *Groupthink*. 2nd ed. Houghton Mifflin, Boston.

Johnson, P., Wistow, G., Schulz, R. & Hardy, B. (2003) Interagency and interprofessional collaboration in community care: the interdependence of structures and values. *Journal of Interprofessional Care*, **17**(1): 69–83.

Leathard, A. (1994) *Going Interprofessional. Working together for health and welfare*. Routledge, London.

McLaughlin, H. (2004) Partnerships: panacea or pretence. *Journal of Interprofessional Care*, **18**(2): 103–113.

Malin, N. Manthorpe, J., Race, D. & Wilmot, S. (1999) *Community care for nurses and the caring professions.* Open University Press, Buckingham.

Molyneux, J. (2001) Interprofessional teamworking: what makes teams work well. *Journal of Interprofessional Care*, **15**(1): 29–35.

Moorhead, G., Ference, R. & Neck, C.P. (1991) Group decision fiascoes continue. Space shuttle Challenger and a revised groupthink framework. *Human Relations*, **44**(6): 539–550

Nancarrow, S. (2004) Dynamic role boundaries in intermediate care services. *Journal of Interprofessional Care*, **18**(2): 141–151.

NHS Executive (2000) *Making a difference: integrated working in Primary Care.* Nursing, Quality and Consumers Directorate, NHS Executive, London.

Nursing and Midwifery Council (2002) *Code of Professional Conduct.* 4th ed. NMC, London.

Øvretveit, J. (1986) *Organisation of Multidisciplinary Community Teams*, University of West London. A Health Services Centre Working Paper, Brunel, London.

Øvretveit, J. (1993) *Co-ordinating Community Care. Multidisciplinary Teams and Care Management.* Open University Press, Buckingham.

Øvretveit, J. (ed) (1997) *Interprofessional working for health and social care.* Macmillan, London.

Price, A. & Williams, A. (2003) Primary care nurse practitioners and the interface with secondary care: A qualitative study of referral practice. *Journal of Interprofessional Care*, **17**(3): 239–250.

Scottish Executive (2000) *The same as you? A review of the services for people with learning disabilities.* Scottish Executive, Edinburgh.

Thomas, D. & Woods, H. (2003) *Working with people with learning disabilities: Theory and Practice.* Jessica Kingsley Publishers, London.

Towell, D. & Beardshaw, V. (1991) *Enabling community integration.* King's College, London.

Tuckman, B. & Jensen, M. (1977) Stages of small group development revisited. *Group and organisational Studies*, **2**(3): 419–427.

West, M. (2004) *Effective Teamwork: Practical lessons from organisational research.* Blackwell Scientific Publications, London.

Chapter 18 **Measuring the Effectiveness of Community Health Care Nursing**

Elizabeth Porter

The measurement of effectiveness in the NHS

The measurement of effectiveness in the NHS is the business of all workers in the NHS and is linked to the political agendas of government. Since the 1980s there has been a growing concern amongst health professionals and the public about variations in clinical practice and the uptake of research evidence in health care. In addition, financial pressures within the NHS, the development of new health technologies, and increasing demands for more and better services, have led to an emphasis on improving both the cost-effectiveness and the quality of health services. The NHS reforms following the White Paper *Working for Patients* (DoH 1989) aimed to control costs and improve quality through a number of initiatives including the introduction of the internal market and managed competition, medical audit and the Patients Charter (Paton 1996). These, and subsequent policies (for example DoH 1992, 1996), emphasised the need for specific, measurable health outcomes. Such outcomes were intended to enable the health service and the public to know whether health care interventions actually maintain and improve health, and whether they do so with the best use of resources. This emphasis on measuring effectiveness and outcomes continued throughout the 1990s (NHSE 1996). The introduction of clinical governance, the new 'framework through which NHS organisations are accountable for continuously improving the quality of their services'(DoH 1998), means that there is now an obligation to examine the effectiveness and quality of services throughout the NHS, including primary and community care provision. In 1999 the Royal College of General Practitioners (RCGP) identified that clinical governance in primary care is about 'developing people, teams and systems within primary care while protecting patients' (RCGP 1999). Current developments in the NHS concerning quality and performance (DoH 2004a) indicate that this trend will continue. Current developments build upon existing activity such as professional regulation (NMC 2003) and continuing professional development (DoH 2001b); the development and implementation of guidelines and protocols (DoH 2002); clinical audit (Healthcare Commission 2004); and evidence-based practice (DoH 2003b). Nurses working in primary care trusts are already familiar with some or all of these activities. For example, clinical audit is often used by community health care nurses and specialist community public health nurses to examine their practice against agreed explicit standards and outcomes, and to modify practice where necessary. However, governance arrangements bring together all developments relating to clinical effectiveness and quality, with an emphasis on working inter-professionally with other practitioners and clinicians, and in partnership with users of the NHS (DoH 2004b; Donaldson 2001). Therefore, in the context of these developments, community health care nurses and health visitors must ensure that their practice is based on the best available evidence.

In order to achieve this objective, they must be able to measure the effectiveness of their interventions in conjunction with other members of both the primary health care team and public health team, patients, carers and service users. This involves various activities, which have been identified as stages in a 'clinical effectiveness process' (NHSE 1998a). These are:

- Questioning current practice and asking what evidence there is to support it

- Finding the evidence through searching the literature and using professional resources and networks
- Appraising and interpreting the evidence using critical appraisal skills
- Putting the evidence into practice and implementing changes where necessary
- Evaluating clinical change, for example through using audit
- Disseminating and sharing good practice

Community health care nurses and specialist community public health nurses therefore need to utilise skills such as literature searching, critical appraisal, audit and research. The arrangements for setting clear national quality standards through National Service Frameworks (DoH 2002) and developed from the National Institute for Clinical Excellence (DoH 1998), make this achievable by providing robust evidence and national guidelines upon which practice can be based at a local level. The National Electronic Library for Health (NHSE 1998b) provides a powerful medium for capturing and disseminating such evidence together with examples of good practice and methods of audit and evaluation.

The clinical effectiveness process, as described above, provides a systematic framework through which community health care nurses and health visitors can evaluate their contribution to health and health care. It provides an opportunity for them to demonstrate the value of their contribution to the health of the population by revealing the evidence base for practice and clearly identifying health outcomes. Problems are sometimes witnessed with this approach, however, when applying it to practice. In some areas there is robust research evidence to support specific interventions and guidelines for practice are clear, for example in pre-school vision surveillance by health visitors (Thorburn & Roland 2000) and for the development of a rapid assessment support service (Brooks 2002). However, sometimes the evidence to support practice is not available or does not provide clear guidance, such as with health screening programmes for older people (Iliffe & Drennan 2000). Additionally, health outcomes for community health care nursing and specialist community public health nurses' interventions are not always easily identifiable or measurable, so using audit to measure effectiveness can be difficult (Barriball & Mackenzie 1993). These problems are not unique to community health care nursing and can be explained by examining the underlying model of evaluation being used to measure effectiveness in health care.

A model of evaluation in health care

Campbell *et al.* (1995) suggest that the approach to clinical effectiveness and outcome measurement in the NHS, drawn from an industrial management model, offers a more predictable and objective context in industrial management than in health care. It may be possible to accurately measure inputs, outputs and end results in industry, but it is much more difficult in health care where the situation is complex, there are multiple influences on outcome and end results can be intangible. There has therefore been a tendency to over-emphasise outcomes in the assessment of the quality of health care (Martin & Henderson 2001). Campbell *et al.* (1995) see outcome measurement as crucially important, but only offering one part of an assessment of the quality of care. Seedhouse (2004) argues that the concentration on outcomes or end results means that much of the process (the complex activities and interactions involved in health care) is ignored. In fact, Donabedian's framework for the assessment of quality of health care, from which the concept of outcome measurement in health care is derived, does include measures of structure and process as well as outcome (Donabedian 1966). He proposed that a comprehensive evaluation of health care should include assessment of the environment and resources, and assessment of the intervention itself (what care is given and how), as well as the outcome.

Furthermore, some aspects and outcomes of health care are more easily quantifiable (such as survival rates or symptom relief) whilst others are more difficult to define and measure (such as raised self-esteem or quality of life). Seedhouse (2004), when looking at effectiveness in health care, concludes that there is therefore a tendency to concentrate on the more easily measurable outcomes, which leaves the effects of many aspects of health care hidden and untested. He also points out that there are often different ways of assessing even the most apparently simple quantifiable aspects of a service. He argues that the methods chosen to assess the effectiveness of an intervention tend to favour outcomes that can be 'objectively witnessed' (for example, numbers of children immunised) rather than those which are more subjective or descriptive (such as parental levels of knowledge and understanding about side effects, or alleviation of anxiety). However, unintended and unexpected consequences of health care interventions can be as valid and worthwhile as outcomes that are predetermined. For example, a nurse treating a diabetic patient at home may be able to improve the quality of life of the patient as well as treating the physical condition, through identifying social isolation and organising opportunities to meet other people (Holmes & Griffiths 2002).

This simplification of information regarding effectiveness in health care has resulted in a tendency to focus on outcomes which can be objectively defined and measured, such as death and illness rates. However, the use of mortality and morbidity data as health outcomes presents further problems, as this suggests a narrow view of health as a purely biological function, with illness resulting as a consequence of pathological abnormality. This reflects a biomedical model, where health is defined as the absence of disease. Bowling (1991) states that outcomes should be measured more comprehensively using a broad concept of 'positive health' which takes factors other than disease and disability into account, such as the ability to cope with stress; social support; morale; life satisfaction; and psychological well-being. Bowling reviews a number of 'quality of life' measurement scales which attempt to do this. Many of these methods involve the participation of patients or users of services in the assessment of health outcomes, yet the adoption of a biomedical model of outcome measurement militates against the involvement of service users in the evaluation of health care. Users' views do not fit neatly with the supposedly objective

measurement of medical outcomes. This reflects a view of professionals as 'experts' who hold the power to make health care decisions on behalf of patients and lay people. However, the increase in public demand for information about health and health care, suggests a widespread belief that people should make their own, informed decisions about their health (Naidoo & Wills 2001). There is an increasing interest in and commitment to user involvement in quality and evaluation in health care and evidence that users of care are contributing measurable outcomes of care they themselves see as relevant (HDA 2003a).

The domination of clinical effectiveness and outcome evaluation by a biomedical model has been further strengthened by the drive towards evidence-based practice, whereby individual expertise is integrated with the best available evidence from systematic research (Sackett *et al.* 1996). This may be accounted for by the fact that this approach began with evidence-based medicine, which is based upon a scientific, experimental model of research with a hierarchy of evidence which favours quantitative rather than qualitative methods of data collection. For example, randomised controlled trials (RCTs) are seen as 'gold standard' evidence, followed by other robust experimental or observational studies (NHSE 1996). Qualitative, descriptive studies may therefore be seen as less valuable or valid when considering the effectiveness of interventions. This poses problems, particularly for non-medical health professionals who often use qualitative methods of evaluation. For example, it is argued that nursing is not best served by such quantitative research methods, owing to the individualised nature of the therapeutic relationship between the nurse and the patient, and the complexity of nursing interventions and the social and health care context in which they take place (Rolfe 1998; Schutz 1994; Shih 1998). Although many research and evaluation studies have been undertaken looking at the effectiveness and outcomes of nursing interventions, there are relatively few RCTs specific to nursing (Cullum 1997). Therefore, for as long as the scientific, biomedical model remains the dominant model for evaluation in the NHS, the nursing profession remains exposed to criticism for lack of objective evidence of effectiveness and outcomes. This is particularly the case for nurses and health visitors working in primary care and the community.

Developments in research, in theory and in practice suggest an alternative model of evaluation which employs a variety of qualitative and quantitative methods, as appropriate. This model involves analysis of the process and quality of care delivery in addition to the measurement of health outcomes. Such an approach is reliant on the provision of user feedback and places all service users at the centre of the evaluation process.

The nursing literature demonstrates how the application of outcome measurement based on the scientific method has been inappropriate and unsuccessful in describing and explaining the effectiveness of nursing interventions (Griffiths 1995). Evidence suggests that outcome measurement should include an analysis of the process of care and should use qualitative as well as quantitative methods of evaluation. For example, Shih (1998) recommends the use of the qualitative approach in nursing research, but points out that many authors are recognising the benefits of a combined qualitative and quantitative approach. The use of combined methods is identified as enabling the nurse researcher to describe and conceptualise the 'multifaceted complexity of the human response to illness and various health care situations' (Shih 1998 p. 632).

The use of qualitative methods and concentration on process as well as outcome evaluation is also recommended in the field of health promotion. Macdonald *et al.* (1996) point to the unsuitability of quantitative methods to evaluate health promotion activities and suggest that traditional epidemiological indicators of health and behavioural outcomes are often inappropriate when appraising the effectiveness of health promotion. The authors criticise the use of the experimental research design and believe it is rarely possible or desirable to use such a design in the evaluation of health promotion. The rationale for this relates to the acknowledgement of the practical problems that exist when applying an experimental design in a complex, naturalistic setting and with

multifaceted programmes (such as experienced in community and primary care). They also point to the need for 'illumination' to gain insight into the processes involved in the implementation of health promotion programmes and the social and environmental context in which they take place. This involves a description in great detail of what occurs in the delivery of health promotion programmes, which enables reasoned judgements to be made about which particular features have been effective. Qualitative techniques are therefore needed to provide this 'thick, rich description' (Macdonald *et al.* 1996).

Macdonald *et al.* (1996) have therefore advocated that alternative approaches are needed which study programme development and process, including qualitative research, formative evaluation and naturalistic observation. Although such qualitative methods can be challenged as less robust by advocates of the experimental research design, there is evidence to suggest that the use of a number of different research methods and the combination and comparison of data from different sources, or 'triangulation', can provide robust checks on the validity of conclusions drawn about effectiveness. Naidoo and Wills (2001) also advocate process or illuminative evaluation, which employs a wide range of qualitative methods and takes into account different stakeholders' views. They consider the use of these methods to overcome the problem of attribution with health promotion activities, thus validating that the results are due to the health promotion input, rather than to other variables. In particular they point to the strength of the case study (where a health promotion programme is intensively studied using a variety of methods) for demonstrating that identified effects reliably result from a programme.

The problems associated with the use of biomedical health outcomes as indicators of success have also been identified in the field of health promotion. The use of 'indirect' and 'intermediate' indicators, such as the successful acquisition of teaching skills by health promotion workers (an indirect indicator) or changes in lifestyle (an intermediate indicator) is therefore recommended. Tones and Tilford (2001) describe outcome indicators, which can be used when measuring the effectiveness of health promotion programmes and suggest that the task of selecting indicators of effectiveness and efficiency is facilitated by the use of theories which not only suggest the appropriate strategies and methods to use in designing and running health promotion programmes but may also be employed to specify requirements for successful health promotion interventions.

Literature from the fields of nursing and health promotion combine to support the use of qualitative methods and the application of process indicators and intermediate outcomes in the evaluation of health care. This approach to evaluation can also take account of social and environmental influences on health and may be more suitable for studies aiming to investigate the effectiveness of long term interventions and interventions which are based on partnership with clients and have a community or public health focus. This method can therefore be seen to be more appropriate for community health care nurses and specialist community public health nurses (health visitors) than the scientific approach previously described in this chapter. Concerns remain regarding the reliability and validity of such qualitative evaluation methods and outcome measures, particularly if they are judged according to the 'rules' of the traditional scientific approach. However, the use of varied, rigorous methods in the development and measurement of outcome measures, the involvement of clients in the evaluation process, and the use of evidence to support the link between process, intermediate and final outcomes, can help to establish trustworthiness and rigour. The current policy context in the NHS appears to support this approach to evaluation, as evidenced by the emphasis placed on the involvement of service users and the examination of 'quality' issues, which include the effective delivery of, and fair access to appropriate health care (DoH 1998).

NHS policy developments

Of vital importance are current developments in government policy, which go some way towards changing the NHS's reliance on the use of quantifiable indicators of illness and disease and encouraging and validating qualitative approaches. This is seen in the current government policy focus which provides opportunities to establish a means of evaluating health care that is based on a broader, social model of health, and which involve users as well as health professionals in the process (Wanless 2004). Policies relating to quality and performance in the 'new NHS'(DoH 1998) propose a move away from 'counting numbers and measuring activity' and suggest an evaluation process which is based on a broader theory of health. This performance framework considers access to services; effective delivery of appropriate health care; and patient/carer experience, as well as efficiency and health outcomes. Health improvement is seen as reflecting social and environmental factors and individual behaviour as well as health and social care services.

The strategy for nursing (DoH 1999b) identifies the role for nurses, midwives and health visitors in contributing to, and leading the clinical governance/quality agenda, ensuring that it does not focus narrowly on medical interventions and outcomes.

Furthermore, policies relating to public health and to services for communities, families and individuals indicate a change in underlying philosophy away from a biomedical approach, towards a public health approach, which considers public health as the 'science and art of preventing disease, prolonging life and promoting health through the organised efforts of society and informed choices of society, organisations, public and private communities and individuals' (Wanless 2004, p. 3). This public health definition acknowledges the importance of those social aspects of health problems which are caused by lifestyles. This was proposed in *Saving Lives: Our Healthier Nation* (DoH 1999a), which recognised the influence of social and economic issues on health and proposed to improve the health of the population and reduce inequalities through promoting partnerships between government, local agencies, communities and individuals. This partnership theme is continued today in government policies designed to support families (DoH 2003b). Many of the new initiatives build on programmes within which community health care nurses and specialist community public health nurses are regularly engaged. For example, *Saving Lives: Our Healthier Nation* (DoH 1999a) specifically proposed modernising the role of health visitors and school nurses to respond effectively to the Government's new public health policies.

There is continued recognition of the problems involved in the evaluation of public health interventions. Furthermore, there is a need to widen the scope of research methods to establish the effectiveness of health programmes, thus reducing reliance on quantitative approaches to measuring health gain (HDA 2004). Evaluation of health care cannot be solely based on biomedical health outcomes; it has to encompass public health activity aimed at improving health gains. This focus offers community health care nurses and specialist community public health nurses the opportunity to demonstrate quality and effectiveness, through the development and use of more appropriate outcome measures based on a broad, holistic model of health and health care. Such measures relate, for example, to improving access to services, or to how they are delivered, and could be illustrated by the inclusion of subjective accounts of clients' experiences (Brooks & Barrett 2003; Dargie 2001; McHugh & Luker 2002).

However, the tension between different approaches and evaluative methodologies was and is still evident in policy documents and many of the indicative outcomes and targets continue to have a biomedical, quantitative focus. For example, performance indicators for the NHS include death and surgery rates, nurse contacts and vaccination rates (National Health Service Executive 1998) and the main targets in *Saving Lives: Our Healthier Nation* (DoH 1999a) are based on mortality rates. It is therefore important that community health care nurses and health visitors develop outcome methods of evaluation which reflect both the public health activity and broader concepts of health and health care, and which focus on the experience of service users. If they fail to do this there is a danger that policy developments will continue to be evaluated solely through the use of scientific, quantitative methods which have

dominated health care evaluation in the recent past. The evidence to support this view can be seen in the remit for the Audit Commission and in its review of primary care trusts (PCTs) (Audit Commission 2004a).

As an independent watchdog this organisation provides important information on the quality of public services. It is the driving force in the improvement of services and provides practical recommendations and spreads best practice. It is responsible for ensuring that public money is spent economically, efficiently and effectively, to achieve high quality local and national services for the public.

The Audit Commission review of primary care trusts' readiness to become proactive commissioners of primary care (2004a) identifies the three key elements of the GMS contract (British Medical Association & NHS Confederation 2003) supported by three funding streams:

- The global sum (funding for provision of essential primary medical services)
- The quality and outcomes framework (a proportion of practice income is generated by the achievement of quality standards)
- Enhanced services (to enable the expansion of work carried out in primary care)

The relevance of this to measuring effectiveness within primary care is that it identifies that a substantial proportion of practice income will be generated by achievement of quality standards, achievement which will be assessed against 146 evidence-based standards that generate 1050 points if all are achieved (Audit Commission 2004a). The standards are drawn from the National Service Frameworks (NSFs) and from other evidence, establishing systems for quality assurance, and an important role for PCTs in monitoring and supporting quality improvements. For the PCTs there is a strategic risk that value for money may not be achieved through an increase in expenditure and an operational risk in ensuring systems are in place to report quality achievements. Findings from a recent study by the Audit Commission show how service redesign benefits patients, but in many PCTs it is not a mainstream activity with sustainable outcomes (Audit Commission 2004b).

Both service users and providers of services have a vested interest in the quality of primary care. Users expect their needs to be addressed. Since the 1980s their needs have been commodified and converted into functions met through the operation of the NHS (Martin & Henderson 2001). Today NHS providers offer choice in services and enter into a partnership with users of the service to design the service options. Users of the health service demand a quality service alongside one that is delivered at a lower cost, with greater accessibility, accountability, efficiency and effectiveness. They require access to information to enable them to make informed choices about their health, a right to know about the quality of the services, and assurance that the investment of resources is leading to demonstrable improvements in health care provision.

The establishment of the Commission for Health Improvement (CHI) offered this opportunity. Following government legislation in 1997 (DoH 1997), CHI signalled a significant policy shift to prioritising the user experience as a central measure in the NHS assessment. CHI provided a balanced and independent mechanism for championing clinical governance. Its aim was to ensure that the user of the health services received the highest quality of NHS care possible. In informing the systems and processes within the NHS, CHI provided a mechanism for monitoring and improving services so that they could deliver a user centred approach which involved them in decisions about care and kept them informed. It also had a commitment to quality which ensured that health professionals were up to date in their practices and properly supervised where necessary and strove to promote continuous improvement to services and care within the NHS.

Following the Community Health and Standards Act 2003 this body was replaced in April 2004 by the Commission for Health Care Audit and Inspection (CHAI). Operational since April 2004, CHAI acts as an independent body encompassing the current work of CHI, the national NHS value for money work of the Audit Commission and the independent health care work of the National Care Standards Commission (NCSC).

A further tool is *The Essence of Care* (DoH 2003a), which offers patient-focused benchmarks for clinical governance and provides application guidance to practitioners. It enables health care professionals to work with users of the NHS to identify best practice and to develop action plans to improve care. A qualitative approach is adopted where patients, carers and the health professional work together to agree and describe good quality care and best practice. This is identified in eight areas of care relevant to all health and social care settings.

Measuring effectiveness in public health and primary care – established evidence

A few of the published examples of evaluation in practice outlined in this section reveal the application of a variety of qualitative and quantitative methods to measure a broad range of health gains and outcomes in public health and primary care. For example, Long *et al.* (2001) used standardised measures of clinical anxiety / depression, personality states and coping styles as part of a study to demonstrate the effectiveness of parenting programmes facilitated by health visitor interventions. Barnes (2000) describes how she used qualitative and quantitative evaluation methods to evaluate evidence-based disease management systems across a primary care group in order to develop a strategy for implementing clinically effective programmes in cerebrovascular disease and examine how nurses might evaluate practice innovations to the advantage of patients and professional support. Williams (2004) undertook a non-randomised mini-review to establish if cleaning, dressing and removing crusts from external fixator or skeletal pin sites affected the risk of infection. A multidisciplinary service evaluation project in the West Midlands used a range of outcome measures to evaluate the quality and cost effectiveness of community-based services for people with a learning disability across one health authority (Chamberlain *et al.* 1995). These included consumer outcome measures for Macmillan Nurses, health visitors and learning difficulties nurses, such as the achievement of improved relaxation and personal control of terminal illness, the detection rate of mental health problems in children, and the percentage of the working day engaged in meaningful activities.

School nurses have also used consumer outcome measures. 'Coping with Our Kids' is a school nurse led research-based programme designed to respond to an identified need to address the increasing numbers of children with behavioural problems, both at school and at home. It evolved in part as a result of a needs analysis and parental request and effectiveness is measured through the use of a pre- and post-course questionnaire given to parents (Health Development Agency (HDA) 2002).

An earlier qualitative study also considered the use of process indicators for health promotion in community health care nursing (Health Education Authority (HEA) 1997b). The project aimed to develop a series of process indicators to use as quality measures of health promotion activities undertaken by primary health care nurses. The quality indicators were developed as an exploratory exercise, which included observation, interviews and discussions with clients and with other stakeholders, including purchasers of primary health care nursing services, provider managers and primary health care nurses themselves. Six case studies were then used to refine and test these indicators in practice and to explore the relationship between quality indicators and health benefits or health gains for clients. Analysis of the case study data revealed many examples of primary health care nursing interventions which had made a difference to clients' lives, either in relation to short-term or intermediate improvements in health (health gain) or benefits which improved the way in which clients deal with health issues and problems (empowerment). This research study has provided evidence of the tangible relationship between the quality of primary health care nursing interactions and subsequent health benefits for service users and their families. It has demonstrated how qualitative research methods can illuminate positive health outcomes

through the examination of process and intermediate health indicators, and has emphasised the importance of involving the service user in the monitoring and measurement of quality and outcome. The authors conclude that gaining their view is essential in order to validate professional perceptions of whether health gain and quality care have actually been achieved. The indicators were operationalised into a 'guide to quality indicators for commissioners' (HEA 1997a) and included relevant research evidence to support the link between the indicators and outcomes.

In a review of district nursing services (Audit Commission 1999) the effectiveness of community nursing interventions was evaluated by examining some of the key processes that contribute to the quality of care, and outcomes in terms of users' experiences. Two specific conditions were selected to illustrate the process, leg ulcers and incontinence, owing to their high prevalence and prominence in district nursing caseloads, the high cost to the NHS and the existence of evidence-based clinical guidelines. As comprehensive, accurate assessment is acknowledged as a major determinant of patient outcomes in both these areas, assessment was taken as a key indicator of the quality of care. Once again, this study demonstrates the importance of determining the users' perspective in measuring effectiveness, as well as the need to ensure that reliable methods are employed to monitor practice outcomes. Of equal importance was the need to ensure that good practice was disseminated and implemented.

Evidence therefore exists to confirm that both qualitative and quantitative methods are being utilised in service evaluation.

Effectiveness in public health and primary care – emerging evidence

Additionally, new process and intermediate health outcome indicators are being developed to measure the effectiveness of public health interventions by community health care nurses and specialist community public health nurses, with service users. Increasingly studies are aggregating data about individual or family outcomes at a caseload, GP practice or community level, in order to examine the effectiveness of interventions which have a public health or population focus. For example, the effect of initiatives to promote breastfeeding or to increase the uptake of screening programmes may only be visible when information is collected from a large population (Prothero *et al.* 2003).

This was confirmed earlier by Kelsay who regarded the aggregation of data as a solution to the problems associated with outcome measurement in health visiting (Kelsay 2000). She described two approaches to collecting and using aggregated data. The first refers to a population approach, based on the compilation of an accurate and detailed community profile which is maintained and regularly updated. Community health care nurses and health visitors are increasingly using such profiles to identify needs and to plan and evaluate services (Mischenco *et al.* 2004; Rowland & Buckingham 2002).

The second approach involves the aggregation of outcomes which have been individually negotiated with clients, around issues such as nutrition, child behaviour, sleep, smoking, rest and recreation and family finances. In both cases, it is important that the information collected is accurate and comparable. For example, when collecting information about breastfeeding rates, the definition of breastfeeding and the schedule for data collection must be clearly stated and adhered to if comparisons are to be made locally, regionally and nationally (UNICEF 2003).

However, as Kelsay points out, there is a danger that standardisation of data collection may reduce sensitivity to local issues, therefore it is important to ensure that clients are actively engaged in the development and use of outcome measures. The Health Education Authority project (HEA 1997b) described earlier is an example where standardised indicators have been developed which can be adopted and applied to the local situation. Successful local adaptation is dependent on the provision of a qualitative approach that includes client participation and takes into account the complexity of practice in the community setting.

Ongoing issues for community nurses and specialist community public health nurses (health visitors)

The approach to clinical effectiveness and outcome measurement based on a scientific, biomedical model presents particular problems for community health care nurses and specialist community public health nurses. These problems are related to the context of practice as well as to the nature of nursing and health visiting itself. For example, public health and health promotion activities are often long-term and health gains may not be visible for many years. The social and environmental setting in the community is very complex, with numerous social, psychological and economic influences on health, and various different health and social care workers involved. This therefore creates difficulties isolating the contribution of community nurses and health visitors to health outcomes. Furthermore, the complexity of interventions creates problems with measuring outcomes. Community nurses and specialist community public health nurses often address multiple health and social care needs at an individual, family and community level, and practice is often client-led and unpredictable.

These problems have been widely documented, for example, Barriball and Mackenzie (1993) note that the outcome of preventative work may be more difficult to measure than other inputs, as results are often long-term and may also be influenced by social and environmental factors beyond the control of health professionals. They also identify the problem of isolating the contribution of nursing interventions to outcomes, as community nurses and health visitors practise within a multidisciplinary setting.

McKenna *et al.* (2004) identify barriers to evidence-based practice in primary care and Kelsay (1994) identifies problems associated with the different definitions of health and the current methods of measurement in relation to health visiting. She states that health visitors, adopting a broad concept of health, aim to maintain and improve health in the general population, therefore, changes in health status are more difficult to detect than, for example, health improvements for patients in hospital. Furthermore, tests are not always available to measure all the varied dimensions of health, and quantitative research methods may not be appropriate. Baseline measurements of health status are also difficult, as health visitors often first meet clients around the time of major life events (such as during the antenatal period). Kelsay (1995) also points to the risks of fragmenting practice and over-simplifying outcomes, as outcome measures do not always recognise the wide range of health visiting skills which may be needed to achieve a particular change in health status. Pressure to concentrate on simple, easily measurable outcomes, she believes, could result in health visitors focusing on one aspect of health, such as improving immunisation status, at the expense of trying to improve the overall health of their clients.

A recent study of approaches in decision making and child protection issues (Almond 2001) supports the view that the complexity of health visiting practice means that conventional measures of outcome could be and are often inappropriate. The author concludes that there is a dearth of literature on decision making in health visiting and it is possible that the gap exists because psychosocial situations do not lend themselves readily to rational approaches. The suggestion is made that rational approaches are more suited to structured situations where there is often a right or wrong answer and a phenomenological and ethical approach are more suited to exploring the nature of decision making in health visiting.

Current methods of monitoring and evaluating community nursing and specialist community public health nursing/health visiting performance therefore tend to concentrate on easily measurable outcomes and quantitative statistics such as activity numbers (number and 'type' of clients contacted). Community nurses and health visitors themselves have constantly argued that the data produced is meaningless and fails to describe the quality or effectiveness of their interventions (Cowley 1994; Macdonald *et al*. 1996). Additionally, the review of District Nursing services in England and Wales (Audit Commission 1999) found that services were generally commissioned using numbers of patient contacts or numbers of staff required by individual GP practices. Therefore in many cases, the award and design of contracts was not based on the needs of the local population or on the desired outcomes of care. They conclude that 'contact figures are inadequate for monitoring patient care . . . because they ignore the purpose, appropriateness and length of visit' (Audit Commission, 1999, p. 16).

This view is further supported by evidence produced by health visitors who noted that their service had come to focus almost entirely upon a mechanistic monitoring of child health and target achievement (HEA 1997b). This example indicates that using inappropriate statistics to monitor performance in community nursing actually may be influencing and changing practice, as activities become restricted to areas that can easily be measured.

A tension therefore appears to exist between the practice of community health care nursing and health visiting and the dominant approach to, and methods of, measuring effectiveness in health care. The scientific method, which emphasises the objective analysis of predictable phenomena, is not always able to capture the complexity of practice. It emphasises quantitative outcomes and does not value qualitative information which captures the 'processes' of care and consumer perspectives. Whilst community health care nurses and specialist community public health nurses are still required to collect information on biomedical health outcomes and are evaluated using quantitative statistics, only part of their role and perceived effectiveness is actually measured and recorded. However, current policy developments and developments in research and practice reveal opportunities, ideas and strategies that can be adopted and applied more appropriately to measure the effectiveness of community nursing and specialist community public health nurses practice.

Measuring health gain

Standards for Better Health (DoH 2004b) has introduced a series of key standards for the quality of care across the NHS. The aim is to set the foundations for a common high quality of health care throughout England; and to clarify what the

NHS can and should be reaching for in its ambitions for the public and health professionals. The standards fulfil a responsibility placed on the Secretary of State for Health under the Health and Social Care (Community Health and Standards) Act 2003. Taking a user friendly approach (written for the user) the standards are developed within two categories, 24 core standards, dealing with quality of care which can be expected by all users of the health service and 10 developmental standards. The developmental standards are aimed to enable the quality of health care to rise as additional resources invested in the NHS take effect. These core and developmental standards cover the entire spectrum of health work from measures to improve health through to primary care services and specialist care. The aim will be to address real issues; the standards are capable of assessment through criteria set by CHAI. The standards will set the framework for decentralising the management of the health service in order to shift the balance of power from central government to the NHS (DoH 2001b). It is anticipated that the adopted framework will consider the quality of health care in the future and provide a measurement of performance. It is anticipated that in 2004/2005 CHAI will develop assessment criteria for measuring how the standards should fit with performance ratings and how these performance ratings assessments can best draw on the standards set (DoH 2004b) and link into existing performance measures in the ratings system.

Conclusion

This chapter has focused on the particular issues that require consideration by community health care nurses and specialist community public health nurses/health visitors when measuring the effectiveness of their practice. The current emphasis on evidence-based practice and monitoring and improving the quality of health care through clinical governance provides opportunities for those working in primary care and community settings to demonstrate their positive contribution to the health of individuals, families and communities. However, the dominant, scientific approach to measuring effectiveness in the NHS is often inadequate and inappropriate for evaluating the complexity of nursing and health visiting interventions within the context of a dynamic social care environment.

Nevertheless, alternative methods of evaluation are being developed and used, which incorporate qualitative and quantitative techniques. Such combined approaches examine processes as well as outcomes of care and involve users and carers in the evaluation process. These evaluative methods complement and are supported by current government policies and strategic developments.

With appropriate education and support for this alternative approach to evaluation, community health care nurses and specialist community public health nurses/health visitors will be able to measure effectiveness in a more meaningful way, rather than relying exclusively on statistics and outcomes that measure only a small part of their work with clients, families and communities.

References

Almond, A. (2001) Approaches to decision making and child protection issues. *Community Practitioner*, **74**(3), 97–100.

Audit Commission (1999) *First assessmnent. A review of district nursing services in England and Wales.* Audit Commission, London.

Audit Commission (2004a) *Transforming Primary Care. The role of primary care trusts in shaping and supporting general practice.* Audit Commission, London.

Audit Commission (2004b) *Quicker treatment closer to home. Primary care trusts' success in redesigning care pathways.* Audit Commission, London.

Barnes, H. (2000) Implementing evidence based disease management systems across a Primary Care Group. *Primary Health Care*, **10**(9), 21–22.

Barriball, K.L. & Mackenzie, A. (1993) Measuring the impact of nursing interventions in the community: A selective review of the literature. *Journal of Advanced Nursing*, **18**: 401–407.

Bowling, A. (1991) *Measuring health. A review of quality of life measurement scales.* Open University Press, Buckingham.

British Medical Association & NHS Confederation (2003) *New GMS Contract: Investing in General practice.* BMA & NHS Confederation, London.

Brooks, N. (2002) Intermediate care rapid assessment support service: an evaluation, *British Journal of Community Nursing*, **7**(12), 623–633.

Brooks, N. & Barrett, A. (2003) Identifying nurse and health visitor priorities in a PCT using a Delphi technique. *British Journal of Community Nursing*, **8**(8), 376–380.

Campbell, F., Cowley, S. & Buttigieg, M. (1995) *Weights and Measures. Outcomes and evaluation in health visiting.* Health Visitors Association, London.

Chamberlain, P., Hipwell, R., Samuel, R. & Stevenson, J. (1995) Measuring the quality of service in the community. *Nursing Times*, **91**(16), 36–37.

Cowley, S. (1994) Counting practice: The impact of information systems on community nursing, *Journal of Nursing Management*, **1**: 273–278.

Cullum, N. (1997) Identification and analysis of randomised controlled trials in nursing: a preliminary study. *Quality in Health Care*, **6**, 2–6.

Dargie, L. (2001) Primary Care Trusts: An agenda for change. *Primary Health Care*, **11**(3), 16–18.

Department of Health (1989) *Working for Patients.* DoH, London.

Department of Health (1992) *The Health of the Nation: a strategy for health in England.* DoH, London.

Department of Health (1996) *The National Health Service: A service with ambitions.* Department of Health, London.

Department of Health (1997) *The New NHS: Modern, Dependable.* DoH, London.

Department of Health (1998) *A First Class Service. Quality in the new NHS.* Department of Health, London.

Department of Health (1999a) *Saving Lives: Our Healthier Nation.* DoH, London.

Department of Health (1999b) *Making a difference, strengthening the nursing, midwifery and health visiting contribution to health and health care.* DoH, London.

Department of Health (2000) *The NHS Plan.* DoH, London.

Department of Health (2001a) *Shifting the balance of power within the NHS. Securing delivery.* Department of Health, London.

Department of Health (2001b) *Investment and reform for NHS staff – taking forward the NHS Plan.* Department of Health, London.

Department of Health (2002) *National Service Frameworks: a practical aid to implementation in Primary Care.* DoH, London.

Department of Health (2003a) *Essence of Care: Patient-focused benchmarks for clinical governance.* Modernisation agency, Department of Health, London.

Department of Health (2003b) *Tackling Health Inequalities: A programme for action.* Department of Health, London.

Department of Health (2004a) *National Standards, Local Action, Health and social care standards and Planning Framework, 2005/6–2007/8.* Department of Health, London.

Department of Health (2004b) *Standards for Better Health: Health Care standards for services under the NHS, a consultation.* www.doh.gov.uk

Donabedian, A. (1966) Evaluating the quality of medical care, *Millbank Memorial Fund Quarterly*, **44**, 166–206.

Donaldson, D. (2001) *The report of the Chief Medical Officer's project to strengthen the public health function.* Stationery Office, London.

Griffiths, P. (1995) Progress in measuring nursing outcomes. *Journal of Advanced Nursing*, **21**, 1092–1100.

Healthcare Commission (2004) *Acute Trust performance indicators*, http//ratings2004.healthcommission.org. uk/Trust/results/indicatorresults.asp? indicatorId=1005

Health Development Agency (HDA) (2002) *National Healthy School Standard. School Nursing* p. 33. HAD, London.

Health Development Agency (HDA) (2003a) Influencing the decision making process through health impact assessment. HDA, London.

Health Development Agency (HDA) (2003b) *Public Health intervention research.* HDA, London.

Health Development Agency (HDA) (2004) Nine Steps to Health Development. *Community Practitioner*, **77**(2), 50.

Health Education Authority (HEA) (1997a) *Promoting health through primary care nursing. A guide to quality indicators for commissioners.* HEA, London.

Health Education Authority (HEA) (1997b) *The Developing Quality Indicators Project. Phase 2, final report.* HEA, London.

Holmes, V. & Griffiths, P. (2002) Self monitoring of glucose levels for people with type 2 diabetes. *British Journal of Community Nursing*, **7**(1), 41–46.

Illiffe, S. & Drennan, V. (2000) Primary care for older people: learning the lessons of history. *Community Practitioner*, **73**(5), 602–604

Kelsay, A. (1994) Measure for Measure, *Health Visitor*, **67**(11), 379.

Kelsay, A. (1995) Outcome measures: problems and opportunities for public health nursing, *Journal of Nursing Management*, **3**: 183–187.

Kelsay, A. (2000) The challenge for research. In: *The search for health needs*, J. Appleton & S. Cowley. Macmillan Press, London.

Long, A., McCarney, S., Smyth, G., Magorrian, N. & Dillon, A. (2001) The effectiveness of parenting programmes facilitated by health visitors, *Journal of Advanced Nursing*, **34**(5), 611–620.

Macdonald, G., Veen, C. & Tones, K. (1996) Evidence for success in health promotion: suggestions for improvement. *Health Education Research*, **11**(30), 367–376.

Martin, V. & Henderson, E. (2001) *Managing health and social care*. Routledge, London.

McHugh, G. & Luker, K. (2002) User perspectives of the health visiting service. *Community Practitioner*, **75**(2), 57–61.

McKenna, H., Ashton, S. & Keeney, S. (2004) Barriers to evidence based practice in primary care. *Journal of Advanced Nursing*, **45**(2), 178–189.

Mischenco, J., Cheater, F. & Street, J. (2004) NCAST: Tools to assess caregiver-child interaction. *Community Practitioner*, **77** (2), 57-60.

Naidoo, J. & Wills, J. (2001) *Health Promotion: Foundations for practice*. Bailliere Tindall, London.

National Health Service Executive (1996) *Promoting Clinical Effectiveness: A framework for action in and through the NHS*. NHS Executive, London.

National Health Service Executive (1998a) *The new NHS, Modern and Dependable: A national framework for assessing performance*. NHS Executive, London.

National Health Service Executive (1998b) *Achieving effective practice: a clinical effectiveness and research information pack for nurses, midwifes and health visitors*. NHS Executive, London.

Nursing and Midwifery Council (2003) Radical restructure: A new look register. *NMC News*, Autumn 2003, Number 3.

Paton, C. (1996) *Health Policy and management*. Chapman Hall, London.

Prothero, L., Dyson, L., Renfrew, M.J., Bull, J. & Mulvihill, C. (2003) *The effectiveness of public health interventions to promote the initiation of breast feeding*. Health Development Agency, London.

Rolfe, G. (1998) The theory practice gap in nursing: from research based practice to practitioner based research. *Journal of Advanced Nursing*, **28**(3), 672–679.

Rowland, L. & Buckingham, M. (2002) Developing an assessment device and service. *Community Practitioner*, **75**(6), 223–226.

Royal College of General Practitioners (RCGP) (1999) *Clinical governance: Practical advice for primary health care in England and Wales*. RCGP, London.

Sackett, D.L., Rosenberg, W.M., Gray, J.A., Haynes, R.B. & Richardson, W.S. (1996) Evidence based medicine: what it is and what it isn't (editorial) *British Medical Journal*, **312**(7023), 71–72.

Schutz, S.E. (1994) Exploring the benefits of a subjective approach in qualitative nursing research. *Journal of Advanced Nursing*, **20**, 412–417.

Seedhouse, D. (2004) *Health Promotion; philosophy, prejudice and practice*, 2nd edn. John Wiley, Sussex.

Shih, F. (1998) Triangulation in nursing research: issues of conceptual clarity and purpose. *Journal of Advanced Nursing*, **28**(3), 631–641.

Thorburn, R. & Roland, M. (2000) The effectiveness of pre-school vision screening by health visitors. *British Journal of Community Nursing*, **5**(1), 41–44.

Tones, K. & Tilford, S. (2001) *Health promotion: effectiveness, efficiency and equity*, 3rd edn. Nelson Thornes, Cheltenham.

UNICEF UK Baby Friendly Initiative (2003) *Public Health Strategies for breast feeding*. Unicef Baby Friendly Initiative. http://www.babyfriendly.org.uk/ph/index.asp

Wanless, D. (2004) *Securing good health for the whole population*. HMSO, London.

Warren, J.M., Henry, C.J.K., Lightowler, H.J., Bradshaw, S.M. & Perwaiz, S. (2003) Evaluation of a pilot school programme aimed at the prevention of obesity in children. *Health Promotion International*, **18**(4), 287–296.

Williams, H. (2004) The effectiveness of pin site care for patients with external fixators. *British Journal of Community Nursing*, **9**(5), 206–210.

Chapter 19 **Non-medical Prescribing**

Ann Clarridge and Dita Engová

Recent developments in the UK NHS have seen the emergence of new types of prescribing health care professionals, other than doctors and dentists, who traditionally undertook the prescribing roles. Prescribing by professionals other than doctors or dentists, including community nurses, is the focus of the following chapter and will be referred to as non-medical prescribing. The chapter is divided into three sections. Section one will consider development of non-medical prescribing within the framework of the NHS modernisation and within the context of various other existing forms of prescribing, administration and supply of medicines, and will introduce the new terminology created to describe the current prescribing arrangements. Section two relates to achieving and maintaining competence in prescribing and will discuss the education, training and continuing professional development of non-medical prescribers. Section three will review accountability and legal issues relevant to non-medical prescribing.

Medicines management and prescription, supply and administration of medicines

Modern management of illnesses often involves drug treatments. Consequently, health care professionals, including community nurses, contribute to the process referred to as 'medicines management'. Medicines management can be understood as a broad concept that encompasses a comprehensive range of activities and procedures from the development of new drugs through the choice of medicines by a prescriber to the use of medicines by a patient. The NHS health care professionals are closely involved in those parts of the process referred to as prescribing, supply and administration of medicines.

The terms prescribing, supply and administration of medicines all relate. However, they are not synonymous and the distinction should be understood. When prescribing, the prescriber makes a choice, based on the initial assessment of the patient and, ideally, in concordance with the patient, of medication to be taken or used by the patient. The prescriber then issues a prescription. A prescription is a legal order requesting supply of a medicine(s) and giving instructions on its administration (by a patient, carer or a health care professional). A health care professional involved in supply of medicines makes the prescribed medicine(s) available to a patient, carer or other health care professional so that the medicine(s) can be administered. Further distinction can be made between the supply and dispensing of medicines. Dispensing includes supply but also encompasses other activities aimed at ensuring safe and effective use of medicines. Administration means giving a medicine as intended to a patient either into the body (for example tablets, injections) or on the body (external preparations). Medicines can be administered by a health care professional, carer or a patient (self-administration). A health care professional who supplies and/or administers medicine(s) has to do so as instructed by a prescriber. The health care professional supplying or administering a medicine cannot change the drug, its formulation, dose or dose regimen; the medication has to be supplied or administered exactly as advised on the prescription.

Pharmacists have traditionally been involved in supply/dispensing of prescription-only medicines (POM). The role of a nurse would normally include administration of medicines (and supply in secondary care). However, since the late 1980s, these traditional roles of health care professionals in the UK have changed. Nurses were prescribing since the early 1990s and other non-medical health care professionals have joined them in the first years of the 21st century. New terms such as 'independent' and 'supplementary prescribing' and 'prescribers' have been introduced to name and describe the new roles.

Non-medical prescribing in the current health care agenda

The Government's strategy document *The NHS Plan* (Department of Health 2000d) integrated the main principles of the modernisation of the NHS, initiated in the late 1990s. The principal aim of the reform was to provide high quality, accessible health care, designed and delivered around the needs of its users. An important part of the reform, and one of the tools designed to achieve its aims, was the goal to redesign the NHS workforce and to develop and better utilise skills and abilities of the NHS staff. Major development of the roles of nurses and other allied health professionals was announced. Following *The NHS Plan*, the Department of Health (DoH), in collaboration with professional bodies, detailed changes to the NHS workforce in a range of specific documents (Department of Health 2000b, 2001a, 2002a); nurses, and other allied health professionals were encouraged to expand their clinical roles, particularly in chronic disease management, and were empowered to prescribe medicines (Department of Health 2000c). The Chief Nursing Officer defined ten key roles for the profession and these included prescribing (Department of Health 2000d).

Non-medical prescribing in community nursing

Independent prescribing: limited and extended nurse prescribers' formulary

In developing the non-medical prescribing agenda, the Government has built on the experience with prescribing by nurses who possessed the District Nurse (DN) and Health Visitor (HV) qualifications. DNs and HVs have been prescribing since 1994 (Department of Health 1992), following eight years of negotiations. 'The DHSS should agree a limited list of items and simple agents which may be prescribed by nurses as part of a nursing care programme, and issue guidelines to enable nurses to control drug dosage in well-defined

circumstances,' stated the Committee headed by Baroness Cumberlege in 1986 (Department of Health and Social Security 1986). Specific recommendations to the Government on prescribing by DNs and HVs were made by the Advisory Group on Nurse Prescribing in 1989 (Department of Health 1989, Crown Report I). The necessary legislation enabling nurse prescribing was provided in the Medicinal Products: Prescribing by Nurses etc. Act. The Act was passed in 1992 and was implemented in 1994. District nurses and HVs have since been able to prescribe a limited range of products approved by the DHSS/DoH and listed in the *British National Formulary* (BNF), Nurse Prescribers' Formulary (NPF) and Part XViiB(i) of the *Drug Tariff*. The products are suitable for management of patients in clinical areas such as wound care or head lice infestation (Department of Health 1997). The restrictiveness of this so called 'Nurse Prescribers' Formulary (NPF) for DNs and HVs' or 'limited' NPF has been criticised by nurse prescribers as well as doctors (Luker *et al.* 1997a) and these reactions led to the extension of prescribing rights; the Government later expanded the range of conditions that nurses were able to prescribe for and broadened the range of products they were able to prescribe (Department of Health 2000c). This is now referred to as Nurse Prescribers' Extended Formulary (NPEF) prescribing (see the BNF, NPF or Part XVIIBii of the Drug Tariff for the full list of conditions and preparations).

In the initial exploratory evaluation of the limited NPF pilot sites, doctors and patients supported nurse prescribing in the areas of their expertise (Luker *et al.* 1997a; Luker *et al.* 1998), although later research revealed some apprehension from general practitioners, with particular regard to autonomy of their role (Baird 2001). Although patients valued easier and faster access to prescriptions and medicines, some have also commented on the reverse effect of the limited NPF prescribing, leading to a more complicated access to medicines, for example because separate prescriptions were needed for general medicines and the nursing care items or because a prescription was left for patient's collection when, previously, the items were delivered by the nurse (Luker 1997a). Studies suggested that patients valued the approachability of nurses and frequency and time spent at consultations (Brooks *et al.* 2001; Luker 1997a; Luker *et al.* 1998).

However, the research also suggested that one in four nurses who completed a prescribing course did not prescribe (Luker 2002). The barriers included lack of confidence, sometimes linked to the lack of opportunity to prescribe. The lack of supportive infrastructures for prescribing nurses has been suggested as an important impeding factor in limited NPF prescribing. The difficulties reported by nurses who did prescribe included initial anxiety to correctly diagnose and to correctly complete a prescription (Baird 2001; Luker *et al.* 1998). The importance of preparatory education enabling nurses to prescribe has been emphasised (Baird 2002; Baird 2003; Campbell & Collins 2001; Courtenay 1999; Luker *et al.* 1997). Workforce development directorates, bodies within health authorities that are responsible for the professional development of NHS staff, now support higher education institutions (HEI) to provide continuing professional development (CPD) in prescribing to address some of these issues and to support nurses in prescribing roles.

Prescribing by nurses from the limited and extended NPF represents a form of 'independent prescribing'. The terms 'independent' and 'supplementary' (originally called 'dependent') prescribing were introduced by a review team headed by Dr June Crown in the final report from their *Review of Prescribing, Administration and Supply of Medicines* (Department of Health 1999). The aim of the review was to consider current, and make recommendations for future, arrangements in the prescribing, administration and supply of medicines. The report was fundamental in sponsoring new developments in prescribing; these are directly based on its recommendations.

The Crown review team defined 'independent prescribers' as 'professionals who are responsible for the initial assessment of the patient and for devising the broad treatment plan, with the authority to prescribe the medicines required as part of that plan' (Department of Health 1999).

Doctors and dentists are the traditional independent prescribers. Nurses with DN and HV qualifications have commenced working as independent prescribers using initially the limited NPF, and then the NPEF, in 1994 and 2002 respectively.

Supplementary prescribing

One of the most crucial recommendations in the Crown Report II was the recommendation to extend prescribing authority to new groups of health care professionals. For this purpose, the review team introduced the term 'dependent prescriber', later changed to the now used term 'supplementary prescriber'. According to the Crown review team, supplementary prescribers would be 'responsible for the continuing care of patients who have been clinically assessed by an independent prescriber. This continuing care may include prescribing, which will usually be informed by clinical guidelines and will be consistent with individual treatment plans; or continuing established treatments by issuing repeat prescriptions, with the authority to adjust the dose or dosage form according to the patient's needs. There should be provision for regular clinical review by the assessing clinician' (Department of Health 1999).

Following further discussions and developments in this area, the process of supplementary prescribing in the UK is now defined as 'a voluntary partnership between an independent prescriber (a doctor or dentist) and a supplementary prescriber to implement an agreed patient-specific Clinical Management Plan (CMP) with the patient's agreement' (Department of Health 2002b). Existence of a CMP is a prerequisite for initiation of any supplementary prescribing. Good communication between the independent and supplementary prescribers is perceived as necessary for successful supplementary prescribing as is sharing of common patient records. Communication and information sharing between health care professionals is gradually being made easier as a consequence to other NHS reforms, such as the introduction of electronic patient records and electronic prescribing. The independent and supplementary prescribers should also work according to the same evidence-based guidelines and review patient management plans regularly. The emphasis on patient involvement in their own management, embedded in the definition, should also be noted.

Supplementary prescribing allows those practitioners who can demonstrate the competencies required following successful completion of an accredited programme to prescribe from the whole of the BNF as identified within the CMP. Exceptions relate to the prescribing of controlled drugs, unlicensed drugs, unless the unlicensed drugs are used in clinical trials with clinical trials certificate or exemption, and other restrictions detailed in Schedules 10 and 11 of the NHS (General Medical Services) Regulations (Department of Health 2004a). The supplementary prescribers are not limited by law to management of certain conditions or therapeutic areas or to prescribe from a separate formulary. In this way the supplementary prescribers are able to improve patient care by reviewing and changing medication within the CMP in response to the patient's therapeutic requirements without necessarily referring the patient back to the independent prescriber at each visit made by the patient to the health care professional.

The Government announced the launch of supplementary prescribing by nurses and pharmacists in 2000 (Department of Health 2000c). Subsequently, s.63 of the Health and Social Care Act 2001 allowed Ministers to designate new types of prescribers. The amendments to the Medicines Orders 2003 and to the NHS regulations provided the legal basis for implementation of supplementary prescribing by non-medical health care professionals in practice. The changes to prescribing rights were to allow faster and more efficient access to medicines for patients, best use of the nurses' and pharmacists' skills and, in a longer term, reduction of doctors' workloads (Department of Health 2001b).

Preparation of nurse and pharmacist prescribers in England commenced in 2003. Scotland and Wales commenced the preparation of nurses and pharmacists in 2003 and 2004 respectively (Scottish Executive 2004; Task & Finish Group on Supplementary Prescribing 2003). By July 2004, England had more than 25 000 limited NPF nurse prescribers, around 2500 NPEF prescribers and 1700 nurses who have completed one of the accredited supplementary prescribing courses (personal communication, Department of Health, July 2004). Scotland had 382 nurses trained in May 2004 (Scottish Executive 2004). Wales planned a cohort of 250 nurses and pharmacists to complete the curriculum by 2004 (Task & Finish Group on Supplementary Prescribing 2003).

Further planned developments in non-medical prescribing currently include extension of prescribing powers to other allied health professionals, including physiotherapists, radiographers, chiropodists and optometrists in 2005 (Department of Health 2004b; Thyer & Robinson 2004) and commencement of discussions, in 2004, on independent prescribing by pharmacists and nurses that would include the full BNF and would be limited only by the scope of the prescribers' professional expertise (Department of Health 2003; Royal Pharmaceutical Society of Great Britain 2004).

Experience with supplementary prescribing to date

Supplementary prescribing is still very new. Those who have undertaken supplementary training to date represented nurses and pharmacists across disciplines, roles and settings. Supplementary prescribers have commenced work in both secondary and primary care sectors (Baird 2004; Bellingham 2002, 2004b; Erskine & Nuttan 2003; Green 2004; James 2004). For nurses this has been a continuation from their NPEF prescribing practice patterns (Green 2004). In secondary care, supplementary prescribing takes place in wards as well as outpatient clinics. In primary care, supplementary prescribers are prescribing in clinics attached to GP surgeries or prescribe from community pharmacies (pharmacists only) (Baird 2004; Bellingham 2002, 2004b; Erskine & Nuttan 2003; Green 2004; James 2004). In primary care, supplementary prescribers tend to undertake roles in chronic disease management (Baird 2004; Bellingham 2004b; Erskine & Nuttan 2003), in secondary care, their prescribing appears to be linked normally to their clinical speciality (Bellingham 2004a; Erskine & Nuttan 2003; Green 2004; James 2004). Although supplementary prescribing is implicitly suitable for the management of longer-term conditions, prescribing in acute situations in secondary care has also been described (Bellingham 2004a).

Those reporting about their supplementary prescribing practice tend to convey enthusiasm and report appreciation of their new professional role, improved interprofessional relationships and improved professional confidence (Baird 2004; Bellingham 2004a). Some prescribers commented on the positive acceptance of their role by patients (Bellingham 2004a; Hennell, Wood & Spark 2004) and perceived that supplementary prescribing improved patients' access to medicines (Bellingham 2004a). Positive response from other professionals in a hospital ward has also been reported (James 2004).

Supply and administration of medicines

As has been explained earlier, prescribing is only one part of the medicines management process. Health care professionals are also involved in the supply and administration of medicines. Apart from the supply and administration based on a patient-specific prescription or instructions (for example a patient chart in a hospital), nurses (including community nurses) are able to supply and administer POMs in accordance with Patient Group Directions (PGD).

Patient Group Directions

PGDs have been defined as 'written instructions for the supply or administration of medicines to groups of patients who may not be individually identified before presentation for treatment' (Department of Health 2000d). Therefore, there are important differences between prescribing, and supply and administration under PGDs.

As the term 'Patient Group Direction' suggests, PGDs are drawn up for groups of patients; these are normally patients with a common complaint (pain) or in a common clinical situation (vaccination, smoking cessation, emergency contraception). Individual patients, and their specific circumstances, are not known and cannot be considered when a PGD is formulated; PGDs deal with the situation, not the individual patient. PGDs would typically be used when a treatment needs to be initiated urgently, such as in intensive care, or where the risk of an interaction with other conditions or medicines is low (Department of Health 1999).

In contrast, CMPs in supplementary prescribing are compiled for an individual patient after the patient and his or her needs have been fully assessed by an independent prescriber. Independent prescribing also deals with individual patients and their individual situations and problems.

PGDs may be more restrictive in the choice of medication that can be supplied or administered by the non-medical professionals using them; PGDs are written for a medicine or a group of medicines that are exactly detailed within the PGD. Consequently, no other medicines, doses or dosing regimens can be used.

PGDs originally existed under the name 'group protocols'. The Crown review team in their interim report focused specifically on supply and administration of medicines under group protocols (Department of Health 1997). The team identified inconsistencies in the use of group protocols and concluded that some group protocols are 'merely general guidance' and that 'lines of accountability and responsibility are not always clear and documented'. The review team also suggested that group protocols may not meet the requirements in sections 55(1)(b) and 58(2)(b) of the Medicines Act 1968 for the supply and administration of medicines 'in accordance with the directions of a doctor' and that only a minimum discretion should be left to the health care professionals involved. The original reasons for the evolution of group protocols were: to provide timely access to treatment, reduce patient waiting times, speed patient discharge or avoid hospitalisation, make appropriate use of professional skills and maximise the effective use of resources. The review team concluded that these reasons are still applicable and that group protocols represent an important contribution to comprehensive health care. However, they recommended that legal aspects of their use have to be clarified and that the protocols need to be clear and comprehensive. The review team compiled guidance on their contents (Department of Health 1997).

The review team interim report was disseminated as part of the *Health Service Circular* (HSC) 1998/051. Subsequently, the instructions for the use of PGDs have been stipulated in the HSC 2000/026 (England; WHC (2000) 116 in Wales and HDL2001(7) in Scotland). HSC 2000/026 specified all aspects of the use of PGDs and also requested the use of the term 'patient group directions'. Modifications to the Medicines Act 1968 through Amendment Orders (Prescription Only Medicines (Human Use) Amendment Order 2000, Medicine (Pharmacy and General Sale – Exemption) Amendment Order 2000 and Medicine (Sale and Supply) (Miscellaneous Provisions) Amendment (No. 2) Regulations 2000) were also necessary to enable legal use of PGDs. These statutory instruments form the legislative framework for the use of PGDs in Great Britain.

Advice on and supply of general sales list (GSL) and pharmacy-only (P) medicines by a community pharmacist is a specific form of prescribing and supply of medication.

In the first part of the chapter, the context of non-medical prescribing, including an outline of the development of this role within the NHS, has been explained and the different forms of prescribing, supply and administration of medicines have been identified. It has also been explained that there currently are three categories of non-medical prescribers: district nurses and health visitors who prescribe from the limited NPF, nurses and midwives who prescribe from the NPEF, and nurse and pharmacist supplementary prescribers who can prescribe from the whole of the BNF (but within the constraints of the individual CMPs). The following text is a discussion on achieving and maintaining competence in prescribing through education and CPD.

Prescribing in practice: achieving and maintaining competence

A nurse can become a nurse prescriber by acquiring the necessary competence in prescribing.

Basford (2003) divides competence into three equally important strands: professional competence, occupational competence and behavioural competence. An educational programme governed by statutory legislation and regulations of a relevant professional body will equip a health care professional with professional competence. Clear criteria or benchmarks for practice have to be set in order to assess a professional's occupational competence. A range of skills, motives and personal traits showing commitment to work within the 'framework of moral obligation' (National Prescribing Centre 2001) defines one's behavioural competence. Achieving professional competence in prescribing through education is the focus of the next section.

Education

In order to prescribe, each category of prescribers (limited NPF, NPEF and supplementary) is required to undertake a specific course of education and training. The differences in the formularies from which each category can prescribe reflect the different needs of the practice of each group, although there is significant overlap between the three categories.

Education and training for limited NPF prescribers

In order to prepare the first wave of limited NPF prescribers, the former English National Board for Nursing, Midwifery and Health Visiting (ENB) developed a short course in nurse prescribing that comprised fifteen taught hours, an open learning pack and a final examination (English National Board 1992). This course was delivered by accredited HEIs and prepared the nurse prescribers in the eight limited NPF pilot sites. The content of the course included principles of nurse prescribing, practice and procedures of nurse prescribing, knowledge of drug reactions and interactions in relation to items in the limited NPF, roles of doctors and dentists, legislation, accountability and professional responsibility in relation to nurse prescribing and the economics of nurse prescribing (United Kingdom Central Council 1991). The examination tested knowledge of drugs and prescribing behaviour. The implementation of the course commenced in April 1993. Although, initially, the course to prepare DNs and HVs to prescribe from the limited NPF was a stand-alone module, preparation is now integrated into university-based specialist practitioner programmes for new DNs and HVs (Department of Health 2004a). Therefore, all newly qualified DNs and HVs who have had their qualification registered with the Nursing and Midwifery Council (NMC) and annotated 'Nurse Prescriber' are able to prescribe from the limited NPF. Some universities continue to offer the stand-alone module for DNs and HVs who are returning to practice.

Education and training for NPEF prescribers

On 25th October 2000 Lord Hunt announced proposals to extend prescribing powers for nurses following completion of an appropriate training and recognition by the NMC. This announcement followed a previous government announcement in March 2000 that it had accepted and would take forward the main recommendations of the Crown Report II to extend nurse prescribing (Department of Health 1999) (see Table 19.1). The intention was that, following specialised training, independent nurse prescribers under the extended scheme (NPEF) would be able to prescribe all GSL and P medicines prescribable by doctors, together with a defined list of POMs. The government recognised that the limited NPF was restrictive in the conditions that it covered and that there was a need to

allow nurses to prescribe a broader range of medicines for a broader range of medical conditions. The four clinical areas initially contained in the NPEF were: minor injuries such as burns, cuts or sprains, minor ailments such as hay fever or acne, health promotion and maintenance, and palliative care. This list has subsequently been extended; see the NPEF in the BNF, the NPF or Part XVIIBii of the *Drug Tariff* for the complete list of conditions and POMs.

The criteria for identifying nurses to be prepared for prescribing from the NPEF, and now also supplementary prescribing, are legal, educational and occupational. This means that they have to be registered with the relevant professional body, be able to study at degree level and able to utilise the NPEF items in their practice. The three key principles that should be used to prioritise potential nurses to undertake the extended and supplementary prescribing programmes are: patient safety, maximum benefit to patients in terms of quicker and more efficient access to medicines, and better use of nurses' skills (Department of Health 2004a). In order to undertake the NPEF programme, it is important that a nurse fulfils the criteria and is willing to undertake the programme. As required by the criteria, their subsequent prescribing practice must provide maximum benefit to patients. The items in the NPEF should be appropriate for their practice.

Examples of candidates who meet the occupational criteria include nurses who run their own clinics in accident and emergency departments,

Table 19.1 Current options for prescribing, supply and administration of medicines for various health care professional groups

	Nurses		Pharmacists	Doctors and dentists
Prescribing	Independent	Limited NPF	P and GSL medicines (exemption from the Medicines Act 1968)	Independent
		NPEF		
	Supplementary		Supplementary	
Supply	PGDs		P and GSL medicines	Dispensing GP practices
Administration	PGDs According to a patient-specific direction or prescription		(Rarely, when asked, for example to demonstrate)	Not usually but, for example, intravenous preparations

emergency care nurses and nurses working in family planning clinics. Additionally, those nurses who work with homeless or travelling families or in intermediate care also meet the criteria. Although palliative care is identified as one of the conditions covered by the NPEF, it has been recognised that the formulary is too limited for the use by palliative care nurses since they, currently, are unable to prescribe controlled drugs (CDs). The list of CDs is expected to be extended, subject to Home Office approval.

To prepare practitioners for this extended role, the former United Kingdom Central Council for Nursing, Midwifery and Health Visiting (UKCC) responded to the government's request to devise an educational programme to prepare nurses to prescribe with 'The Council's requirements for the standard, kind and content of educational programme for registered nurses, midwifes and health visitors to prescribe from the extended 'nurses prescribers' formulary' (United Kingdom Central Council 2001), and the former ENB prepared an outline curriculum based upon the UKCC requirements. This preparation is different from the preparation of DNs and HVs who prescribe from the limited NPF. DNs and HVs who are currently independent prescribers from the limited NPF, and who wish to extend their prescribing, are required to undertake the recognised preparation and training in order to prescribe from the NPEF.

The original NPEF prescribing programme consisted of twenty-five days of contact time for the theory component, plus twelve days of practice, during which the practitioner is supervised by a designated medical practitioner. Originally, the course took place over a period of three months. HEIs now have the option to extend the duration of the programme to six months and the programme is combined for the NPEF and supplementary prescribers (Department of Health 2004a). The National Prescribing Centre (NPC) produced the document *Maintaining Competency in Prescribing: an outline framework to help nurse prescribers* (National Prescribing Centre 2001) in order to support the training programme and as a tool for practitioners to reflect on their practice and to identify own CPD needs.

Education and training for supplementary prescribers

The preparation and training programme to prepare the third category of prescribers, supplementary prescribers (notwithstanding limited and NPEF nurse prescribers), has been clearly defined by the Government in cooperation with the NMC and the Royal Pharmaceutical Society of Great Britain (RPSGB). Simultaneously, the NMC (Nursing and Midwifery Council 2002a) agreed a set of standards for the preparation of nurses, midwives and health visitors, and the RPSGB (Royal Pharmaceutical Society of Great Britain 2002) endorsed a curriculum for pharmacists to become supplementary prescribers.

The criteria and the key principles for selection of applicants for the supplementary prescribing programme are the same as for the NPEF programme. However, the supplementary prescribing programme contains additional learning outcomes to ensure competency to practice as a supplementary prescriber. Consequently, the length of the programme has been extended by two days to accommodate these learning outcomes. As with the NPEF, future supplementary prescribers are supervised by a designated medical practitioner during the practice period.

Those nurses who completed the original education and training for the NPEF, and wish to become supplementary prescribers, are required to undertake one or two additional training days to achieve the added competencies (NMC 2002b).

Supervision in practice as part of education

Supervision in practice is an important part of the NPEF and supplementary prescribing education and training programmes. A crucial element in the process of completion of the prescribing programme is identification of and collaboration with a designated supervising medical practitioner (SMP), a doctor who will provide the student with supervision, support and opportunities to develop the appropriate competencies for prescribing practice and become a safe, effective and competent prescriber. The supervisor must be a registered medical practitioner who meets the Government's criteria for fulfilment of this role. The criteria include three years in the relevant field of practice and some experience or training in teaching and/or supervising in practice (Department of Health 2004d).

The extent of time spent with the SMP and the range of activities undertaken within the twelve days of practice vary, depending upon the student's experiences. However, time should be spent observing consultations with patients and their carers, where appropriate, and the development of a CMP. Time should also be spent in discussion and analysis of clinical management of patients using a case study approach.

Prescribers who have achieved professional competence through successful completion of an educational and training programme should aim to maintain this competence. The next section of the chapter considers maintaining competence in practice.

Maintaining competence in practice and CPD

Health care professionals should have an embedded moral motivation for competence, as they are responsible for the well-being of their patients. Furthermore, to ensure competence across the country and across professions and disciplines, the Government recently implemented the framework of clinical governance. Clinical governance is one of the tools the Government uses to achieve the aims of *The NHS Plan* (Department of Health 2000c) to provide safe and effective, high quality patient-centred care. The Government defines clinical governance as a 'system through which NHS organisations are accountable for continuously improving the quality of their services and safeguarding high standards of care, by creating an environment in which clinical excellence will flourish' (Department of Health 2004d). Organisations and their employees are responsible for ensuring that their work conforms to principles of clinical governance. The implications of this for non-medical prescribing are discussed below.

Non-medical prescribing has become an integral part of the practice of many NHS nurses. Therefore, in line with the current NHS policies, non-medical prescribing practice of these nurses has to be compliant with clinical governance. This can be achieved when non-medical prescribing practice is underpinned by high quality education and training, followed by CPD. Non-medical prescribing practice has to be subjected to regular audits and evaluations and be part of the risk-assessment procedures undertaken by the organisation employing the prescriber (Department of Health 2004a). In the definition of clinical governance, the Government uses the term 'clinical excellence'. Clinical excellence can only be achieved by a practitioner who is competent in the area of their practice and is able to achieve and maintain occupational and behavioural competence.

Employing NHS organisations are now obliged to support their staff in expanding and maintaining their competence. Nevertheless, equally, nurse prescribers are responsible for maintaining their competence, for example by proactive use of supporting structures and educational and training programmes that may be made available to them from their employing organisation.

Prescribing nurses' responsibility is to ensure that their practice is both clinically appropriate and effective. They have to be able to reflect upon and critique their prescribing practice, remain motivated to prescribe, develop a system of self-audit, and review regularly the status of their practice; the practitioners have to evaluate how current their practice is. Such evaluations should be a part of their CPD.

One tool that any prescriber can easily apply in their everyday practice is structured reflection. Reflection allows evaluation of own practice, identification of any insufficiencies in knowledge, and identification of areas for further development. There is a choice of different models of reflection and prescribers have an opportunity to identify and use the one that is most appropriate for their needs (Burns & Bulman 2004; Johns 2004). To support such reflections in prescribing, nurses can self-evaluate their competence against the NPC's competency framework for prescribing (National Prescribing Centre 2001).

Every practitioner has a range of options of how to keep their practice up-to-date. To keep their practice in line with new developments, prescribers should be aware of current research in the area of their practice. Professional journals publish research and thus make it available to large professional audiences. However, practitioners should evaluate validity of such research before implementing its findings in their practice; they should conduct critical appraisal of research. Although prescribers may find it difficult at first to conduct critical appraisal, this is an acquirable skill, crucial to ensuring effective and safe practice. For further reading on critical appraisal see, for example, Trinder & Reynolds (eds.) *Evidence-based Practice: a critical appraisal*, or Ajetunmobi *Making Sense of Critical Appraisal*. Practice will also help.

Prescribers can also use a range of existing evidence-based resources. The Government have been issuing national service frameworks (NSF) to support good practice. All prescribing nurses should be familiar with NSFs relevant to their practice. Prescribers should also use evidence-based guidelines produced by the National Institute for Clinical Excellence (NICE) and formularies, guidelines and protocols devised locally. All these documents are based on thorough evaluation of evidence. Prescribers are likely to work within health care teams and discussions with colleagues can be extremely useful as they will allow sharing of opinions and practical experiences. A pharmaceutical/prescribing advisor in a local PCT can also be a well of information on local prescribing issues. Economic data can be obtained in the form of Prescribing Analysis and CosT (PACT) data through the employing NHS organisation. Finally, the prescribers can seek help with their CPD needs from the NPC that has been commissioned by the Government to provide CPD support to the new prescribers.

One of the supporting structures for achieving and maintaining occupational and behavioural competence that may be provided by the employing NHS organisation is clinical supervision.

According to Winstanley (2000), clinical supervision should help practitioners to expand their knowledge base, clinical proficiency, and autonomy and self-esteem. The research studies exploring nurse prescribers' practice experiences suggested that workplace peer support, mentoring and clinical supervision were important factors in maintaining nurses' prescribing competence in practice (Basford 2003; Humphries & Green 2000; Otway 2001).

Transition to the new prescribing role may be difficult. One mechanism that could facilitate this process is development of a peer forum. A prescribers' forum would enable prescribers from different NHS organisations to gather together, share concerns and problems as well as successes of their prescribing practice, to seek solutions and discuss examples of good practice. Collins and George (2003) suggested a range of topics that could form an agenda for such a forum. This included discussions on critical incidents, identification of further training needs, sharing of and debate on local and specific concerns, consideration of national prescribing issues, contribution to development and implementation of local guidelines and policies relevant to prescribers' area of practice. The forum would also enable the nurse prescribers to identify and recommend additions to the limited NPF and NPEF.

Professional and legal accountability

With the extension of nurses' roles, the extent of their accountability has also broadened (Humphries & Green 2002). Following successful qualification, a nurse prescriber acquires the right to make prescribing decisions and is legally and professionally accountable for all aspects of this decision making process. The prescribing process includes the initial consultation, choice to prescribe or not, choice of treatment, advice given to the patient or carer, including information regarding the administration of medication, and subsequent treatment reviews. As in any other area of health care, prescribing nurses are accountable to the patient, the employing organisations, colleagues, the NMC and the law.

Professional accountability

The professional accountability is defined by the *Code of Professional Conduct* (Nursing and Midwifery Council 2002b). The code defines the criteria of appropriate nursing practice and serves as a benchmark against which any allegations of misconduct in practice are considered. According to the Code, registered nurses, midwives and health visitors are personally accountable for their practice (Nursing and Midwifery Council 2002b).

Professional accountability covers a range of issues, including respect for the patient as an individual, informed consent, confidentiality, cooperation with other professionals, the maintenance of professional knowledge and competence, and the identification and minimising of risk to patients and clients (Nursing and Midwifery Council 2002c).

Legal accountability

There are several statutory documents that define the framework of law for non-medical prescribing. All aspects of medicines handling in the UK, including 'manufacture, testing, research, distribution, sale, supply and administration of drugs' are defined in the Medicines Act 1968. Details of the legislation supporting specifically non-medical prescribing have been given in the first section of this chapter. In brief, The Medicinal Products: Prescribing by Nurses etc. Act 1992 enabled nurses to prescribe from the limited NPF. The prescribing rights were expanded by the Health and Social Care Act 2001 and the amendments to the Medicines Orders and the NHS regulations (all these are listed earlier in the chapter) that enabled prescribing from the NPEF and, subsequently, implementation of supplementary prescribing. Supplementary prescribing was further detailed in the Department of Health document *Extending Independent Nurse Prescribing within the NHS in England: A guide for implementation* (Department of Health 2004a) that provides a useful guide for nurses with regard to their prescribing practice and legal accountability. Any form of breach of the enactments of the Medicines Act 1968 and other relevant legislation makes the prescriber liable to prosecution.

The legal accountability also covers domains of practice such as scope of practice, consent, record keeping, vicarious liability and product liability (Preece 2002).

Scope of practice

Nurses, including prescribing nurses, are accountable to the civil law with regard to the scope of their practice. This means that they must maintain a reasonable standard of practice and they must not practise outwith their defined and assessed competence (Humphries & Green 2002). The same principles apply to medical practitioners (Preece 2002). Luker (1997b) suggested that, in the eight limited NPF pilot sites, the nurses were able to acknowledge their limitations and work only within the scope of their expertise.

Consent

Patient consent to treatment or care is a crucial element of health care practice and is based on the legal and ethical principle that a patient has the right to decide what will happen to their body (Department of Health 2001c, d). Prescribers who omit this patient right may face legal action from a patient or their professional body (Department of Health 2001c). Clarification of the consent process has been requested in *The NHS Plan* and consent policies should be a firm part of clinical governance agenda of all NHS organisations. Provision of information is core to the consent process and the prescribing practitioner is responsible for providing appropriate information to the patient. Specific issues, for example consent from children or people with mental health problems, can be found in the guidance documents published by the DoH (Department of Health 2001c, d). Prescribers should use 'safety netting' (Neighbour 1987) as an integral part of the consultation process. This means that they should confirm that patients know and understand what the treatment is for, how it will work and any risks or possible adverse reactions.

Record keeping

Nurse prescribers are required to adopt good record-keeping practice. Records should include details of the prescription as well as details of the consultation (Preece 2002; Department of Health 2004a). The nurse prescribers should comply with the requirements for record keeping specified by the NMC (Nursing and Midwifery Council 2002c).

Vicarious liability

Professional indemnity in health care means that health care professionals have legal exemption from liability for damages or claims made by patients and resulting from performing their NHS duties specified in their contract. Health care professionals are, for their NHS duties, indemnified by their employing NHS organisation (Preece 2002). Despite this, nurses should ensure that they also have personal professional indemnity insurance. For example, professional organisations such as the Royal College of Nursing, the Community and District Nurse Association and the Community Practitioner and Health Visitor Association usually provide indemnity as part of the membership fee (Caulfield 2004). The Medical Defence Union provides indemnity cover for members who are involved in prescribing. Although indemnity protects the prescriber in case of patients' claims, any such claims will also be reviewed with respect to contractual law. Contractual law demands that practitioners adhere to all policies and procedures of their employer. Practitioners must then accept responsibility for acting within the context of these policies and procedures and within the parameters of their employment contract and job description.

Product liability

Product liability refers to the fact that equipment and medicines should be used according to the manufacturers' specifications. Otherwise, the manufacturers may not be liable for failures in their products (Preece 2002).

Conclusion

Non-medical prescribing provides community nurses with significant professional opportunities on several levels. Competent nurse prescribers contribute to improving the effectiveness and efficiency of patient care in the NHS. This improves patients' experience with the NHS and thus plays an important part in achieving the aims of the NHS reform as stipulated in *The NHS Plan*. Non-medical prescribing also enables nurses to enhance their professional skills and competencies and thus to fundamentally change the ways they manage and care for their patients. Finally, prescribing transforms and strengthens nurses' roles within multidisciplinary health care teams and provides new prospects for the nurses to be assumed in their careers.

References

Ajetunmobi, O. (2002) *Making Sense of Critical Appraisal* Hodder Arnold, London.

Baird, A. (2001) Diagnosis and prescribing: the impact of nurse prescribing on professional roles, *Primary Health Care*, **11**(5), 24–26.

Baird, A. (2002) Supplementary prescribing: workable in practice?, *Practice Nursing*, **13**(6), 242–244.

Baird, A. (2003) Supplementary prescribing: a review of current policy, *Nurse Prescribing*, **1**(1), 32–36.

Baird, A. (2004) Supplementary prescribing: one general practice's experience of implementation, *Nurse Prescribing*, **2**(2), 72–75.

Basford, L. (2003) Maintaining nurse prescribing competence: experiences and challenges, *Nurse Prescribing*, **1**(1), 40–45.

Bellingham, C. (2002) Space, time and team working: issues for pharmacists who wish to prescribe, *Pharmaceutical Journal*, **268**(Apr), 562–563.

Bellingham, C. (2004a) How supplementary prescribing is working for pharmacists in practice, *Prescribing and Medicines Management*, July, 2–3.

Bellingham, C. (2004b) How supplementary prescribing helps in both acute and chronic hospital care, *Pharmaceutical Journal*, **272**(22 May), 640–641.

Brooks, N., Otway, C., Rashid, C., Kilty, E. & Maggs, C. (2001) The patients' view: the benefits and limitations of nurse prescribing, *British Journal of Community Nursing*, **6**(7), 342–348.

Burns, S. & Bulman, Ch. (2004) *Reflective Practice in Nursing*. Blackwell Publishing, Oxford.

Campbell, P. & Collins, G. (2001) Prescribing for community nurses, *Nursing Times*, **97**(28), 38.

Caulfield, H. (2004) Legal aspects, responsibility, accountability in nurse prescribing, *Prescribing Nurse*, **1**, Spring, 20–22.

Collins, G. & George, K. (2003) Development and support of community nurse prescribers, *Primary Health Care*, **13**(2), 38.

Courtenay, M. (1999) Nurse prescribing: implications for the life sciences in nursing curricula, *Nurse Education Today*, **22**(6), 502–506.

Department of Health (1989) *Report of the Advisory Group on Nurse Prescribing*. Department of Health, London.

Department of Health (1997) *A report on the supply and administration of medicines under Group protocols (Crown Report I)*. The Stationery Office, London.

Department of Health (1999) *Review of prescribing, administration and supply of medicines. Final Report (Crown Report II)*. The Stationery Office, London.

Department of Health (2000a) *The NHS Plan: a plan for investment, a plan for reform*. Deaprtment of Health, London.

Department of Health (2000b) *Pharmacy in the future: implementing the NHS Plan*. Department of Health, London.

Department of Health (2000c) *Lord Hunt announces proposals to extend prescribing powers for around 10 000 nurses. Press release 2000/0611*. Media Centre, Department of Health, London.

Department of Health (2000d) *Health Service Circular 2000/026*. Department of Health, London.

Department of Health (2001a) *The NHS Plan: an action guide for nurses, midwives and health visitors*. Department of Health, London.

Department of Health (2001b) *Primary care, general practice and the NHS Plan. Information for GPs, nurses, other health professionals and staff working in primary care in England*. Department of Health, London.

Department of Health (2001c) *Reference guide to consent for examination or treatment*. Department of Health, London.

Department of Health (2001d) *Good practice in consent implementation guide*. Department of Health, London.

Department of Health (2002a) *Liberating the Talents. Helping Primary Care Trusts and nurses to deliver The NHS Plan*. Department of Health, London.

Department of Health (2002b) *Extending independent nurse prescribing within the NHS in England: a guide for implementation*. DoH, London.

Department of Health (2003) *A vision for pharmacy in the new NHS*. Department of Health, London.

Department of Health (2004a) *Extending Independent nurse prescribing within the NHS in England. A guide for implementation*, 2nd Edition, Department of Health, London.

Department of Health (2004b) *More health professionals to be given power to prescribe. Press Release 2004/0179*. Department of Health, London.

Department of Health (2004c) *Supervision in practice for nurses and midwife independent prescribers and nurse and pharmacist supplementary prescribers*. Department of Health, London; www.dh.gov.uk.

Department of Health (2004d) *HSC 1999/065. Clinical Governance: in the new NHS*. Department of Health, London.

Department of Health and Social Security (1986) *Neighbourhood nursing: a focus for care (Cumberlege Report)*. HMSO, London.

English National Board (1992) *Nurse prescribing: Background briefing*. English National Board, London.

Erskine, D. & Nuttan, T. (2003) *Supplementary Prescribing: Models developing within the UK primary care setting*.

Green, H. (2004) Nurse prescribing: in the acute sector: one trust's experience, *Nurse Prescribing*, **2**(1), 9–14.

Hennell, S.L., Wood, B.B. & Spark, E.W. (2004) Competency and the use of clinical management plans in rheumatology practice, *Nurse Prescribing*, **2**(1), 26–30.

Humphries, J.L. & Green, E. (2000) Nurse prescribers: infrastructures required to support their role, *Nursing Standard*, **14**, 35–39.

Humphries, J.L. & Green, J. (2002) *Nurse prescribing*. 2nd edn. Palgrave, Basingstoke and New York.

James, J. (2004) Supplementary prescribing by a diabetes specialist nurse on a hospital ward, *Nurse Prescribing*, **2**(3), 112–116.

Johns, C. (2004) *Becoming a reflective practitioner*. 2nd edn. Blackwell Publishing, Oxford.

Luker, K. (1997a) Patients' views of nurse prescribing, *Nursing Times*, **93**(17), 51–54.

Luker, K. (1997b) *Evaluation of Nurse Prescribing. Final Report*. University of Liverpool, University of York, Liverpool, York.

Luker, K. (2002) Nurse prescribing from the community nurse's perspective, *International Journal of Pharmacy Practice*, **10**(4), 273–280.

Luker, K., Austin, L., Ferguson, B. & Smith, K. (1997) Nurses' and GPs' views of the nurse prescribers' formulary, *Nursing Standard*, **11**(22), 33–38.

Luker, K., Austin, L., Hogg, C., Ferguson, B. & Smith, K. (1998) Nurse–patient relationships: the context of nurse prescribing, *Journal of Advanced Nursing*, **28**(2), 235–242.

National Prescribing Centre (2001) *Maintaining competency in prescribing. An outline framework to help nurse prescribers*, 1st edn. National Prescribing Centre, Liverpool.

Neighbour, R. (1987) *The inner consultation. How to develop an effective and intuitive consultation style*. Libra Pharm Ltd., MTP Press, Lancaster.

Nursing and Midwifery Council (2002a) *The Council's requirements for 'Extended independent nurse prescribing' and 'supplementary prescribing'*. NMC Circular 25/2002, Nursing and Midwifery Council, London.

Nursing and Midwifery Council (2002b) *The NMC Code of Professional Conduct: standards for conduct, performance and ethics*. Nursing and Midwifery Council, London.

Nursing and Midwifery Council (2002c) *Guidelines for records and record keeping*. Nursing and Midwifery Council, London, 1998 UKCC Reprint.

Otway, C. (2001) Informal peer support: a key to success for nurse prescribers, *British Journal of Community Nursing*, **6**(11), 586–591.

Preece, S. (2002) Nurse prescribing: accountability and legal issues In: *Nurse Prescribing*, 2nd edn, J.L. Humphries & J. Green, (eds). Palgrave, Basingstoke and New York.

Royal Pharmaceutical Society of Great Britain (2002) *Outline Curriculum for training programmes to prepare Pharmacist Supplementary Prescribers*. RPSGB, London.

Royal Pharmaceutical Society of Great Britain (2004) *Supplementary prescribing by pharmacists*. RPSGB, London.

Scottish Executive (2004) *Scottish executive announcement: Supplementary prescribers extension*. Scottish Executive, Edinburgh.

Task & Finish Group on Supplementary Prescribing (2003) *Supplementary prescribing in Wales*. All Wales Medicines Strategy Group, Cardiff.

Thyer, A. & Robinson, P. (2004) *Proposals for supplementary prescribing by chiropodists, physiotherapists, radiographers, and optometrists and proposed amendments to the Prescription Only Medicines (Human Use) Order 1997*. Department of Health, London.

Trinder, L. & Reynolds, S. (2000) *Evidence-based Practice: A Critical Appraisal*. Blackwell Science, Oxford.

United Kingdom Central Council (1991) *The Council's response to the Department of Health invitation to establish the standard, kind and content of educational preparation for nurse prescribing*. MW/GM/8.107. United Kingdom Central Council, London.

United Kingdom Central Council (2001) *Registrar's letter 28/2001. The Council's requirements for the standard, kind and content of educational programme for registered nurses, midwifes and health visitors to prescribe from the extended 'nurses prescriber's' formulary*. United Kingdom Central Council, London.

Winstanley, J. (2000) Manchester clinical supervision scale, *Nursing Standard*, **14**(19), 31–32.

Chapter 20 **Public Health Nursing**

Marion Frost

Introduction

This chapter will explore the changing political philosophy that has placed public health at the centre of health care reforms and led to the development of a new part to the Nursing and Midwifery Council (NMC) register – specialist community public health nursing. In response to increased public expectations and demand, changes in the health and social needs of the population and the requirement to use limited resources more cost effectively, a programme of health service modernisation has been developed with the aim of improving the health of the population and reducing inequalities in health. A vital part of this modernisation programme is for nurses, midwives and health visitors to work in new ways across organisational boundaries and with local communities in order to support the developing public health strategy (DoH 1999a). Issues to be considered include the changing context of public health work and the modernisation agenda, the development of standards for specialist community public health nursing practice and the new roles that may emerge.

The context of public health work

The concept of public health – defining the parameters

There is a growing interest in improving the health and well-being of the population. The challenge for the government and health professionals is to provide a service that is responsive to the needs of service users, carers and populations and is designed around the journey that people take when using the health and social care system. The aim is to encourage individuals to engage in healthy lifestyles supported by a society that values and maintains healthy environments that promote and protect health, prevent disease and reduce inequalities in health. Nursing, midwifery and health visiting have a responsibility to improve health and reduce inequalities through the provision of public health programmes at both the individual and population level.

According to the Tripartite Steering Group, the purpose of public health is to:

- Improve the health and well-being of the population
- Prevent disease and minimise its consequences
- Prolong valued life
- Reduce inequalities in health

> (Prime Research & Development Ltd for Skills for Health 2003)

Evidence suggests that the opportunity for a healthy life is still linked to social and economic circumstances with inequalities in health status differing across geographical areas, social class, gender and ethnicity (DoH 2001). Whilst recognising that some differences in health status may be difficult to combat, for example the consequence of genetic factors, others are due to lack of opportunity such as material disadvantage, insecure employment and poor educational attainment. Nationally, the proportion of people living in poverty and in low-income families has increased since the 1970s. The risk of premature death from the major killers coronary heart disease and cancers remains unacceptably high and continues to reflect a social class gradient, whilst poor mental health and chronic diseases affect the quality of life for many people. A public health approach to practice therefore aims to improve the health of society through:

- Taking a population perspective
- Mobilising the organised efforts of society and acting as an advocate for the public's health
- Enabling people and communities to increase control over their own health and well-being

- Acting on the social, economic, environmental and biological determinants of health and well-being
- Protecting from and minimising the impact of health risks to the population
- Ensuring that preventive treatment and care services are of high quality, based on evidence and are of best value

(Skills for Health 2004, p. 6)

Wanless (2004, p. 3) further defines public health as 'the science and art of preventing disease, prolonging life and promoting health through the organised efforts and informed choices of society, organisations, public and private, communities and individuals'. Public health is therefore acknowledged to be the responsibility of both society and the individual. There may however be conflict between the views of government and individuals concerning which key public health issues should be targeted. Conflict may also arise depending on whether public health is defined from a medical perspective in terms of longevity of life and freedom from disease, from a social perspective that values the role of the state and social justice or from a liberal individualist viewpoint which favours protection of individual freedom (Baggott 2000).

Public health therefore reflects ideological debates about the rights and responsibilities of individuals and the state and the need for collective action in responding to identified issues that affect the health of the population. Evidence of civilisations taking collective action to promote health and prevent disease through such measures as urban planning, effective sanitation, quarantine methods and food inspection suggests that states have at various times intervened to protect the health of the population. The creation of the National Health Service in 1948 can be considered as a major public health achievement or conversely as the development of a 'treatment focused' service that lost sight of the underlying social and economic determinants of health and disease (Griffiths & Hunter 1999).

Whilst inequalities in health status and health care delivery remain a feature of modern society, the focus on a treatment oriented health care service coupled with market style reforms has fragmented public health services and, all too often, focused responsibility at the individual level. Lack of collaboration between central government departments and marginalisation of local governments have also thwarted the implementation of national health promotion strategies such as *Health of the Nation* (DoH 1992) which aimed to improve the nation's health in terms of life expectancy, reduction of premature death and improvement in the quality of life (Hunter 1999).

The Modernisation Agenda

Modernisation of the NHS – a changing public health agenda

More recently the Labour Government has demonstrated its commitment to public health with the appointment of the first ever Minister for Public Health for England with a cross-governmental role to ensure the health impact of policies is recognised by all relevant departments. The Government's key focus to date has been to improve access to high quality health services in response to public demands (DoH 2000). The consultation, *Choosing Health* (DoH 2004a), set out to determine the public's views on who should be involved in helping people to be healthier and has led to the development of a White Paper on public health. *Choosing Health: Making Healthy Choices Easier* (DoH 2004d) proposes significant changes aimed at improving the health of the population through enabling individuals to make informed healthy choices with personalised support services tailored to meet people's needs. The Government recognises that at a local level, primary care trusts, local government, business, the media, the voluntary sector and others need to work more closely with local communities in order to tackle the causes and consequences of health inequalities.

Making better use of staff skills is another key element of the Government's Modernisation Agency 'Changing Workforce Programme' proposals to improve health and tackle health inequalities (DoH 2002a). Primary and community care services are vital for promoting the health of local populations through taking a pro-active approach to smoking cessation, teenage pregnancy reduction and the development of healthy schools programmes for example. Redesigned roles and skill mix teams are doing much to improve service provision and facilitate NHS staff to respond to the changing public health agenda.

Furthermore, *Making a Difference* (DoH 1999a) recognised that the changes involved in modernising the health service required effective leadership at all levels. The need was identified for professionals who could inspire, motivate and empower their colleagues to achieve improvements in the quality of service delivery. This theme has been further reiterated within more recent government policy documents (DoH 2000, 2002b, 2004b). Specialist community public health nurses as part of the public health workforce must therefore harness this opportunity to take on a leadership role and be pro-active in leading change to improve the quality of service provision and the health of populations.

Overall, the public health workforce involves people from a wide variety of backgrounds from within the state, voluntary and private sectors (Wanless 2004). At the core of the service are consultants in public health medicine and specialists in public health, experts who work at a strategic level and may be medically qualified but may also come from other backgrounds. They work as consultants across the whole spectrum of public health. Secondly there are public health practitioners who spend a major part of their time working in public health or preventive practice such as health promotion specialists who have expertise in specific areas of public health work. Health professionals such as health visitors, occupational health nurses, school nurses and environmental health officers may combine aspects of public health work with other areas of work. Finally, there is a growing body of workers from a variety of sectors who contribute to the public health workforce such as community development workers from the voluntary sector, housing officers, educationalists and others.

Ten broad areas of work have been identified as those which enable the purpose of public health to be met:

(1) Surveillance and assessment of the population's health and well-being
(2) Promoting and protecting the population's health and well-being
(3) Developing quality and risk management within an evaluative culture
(4) Collaborative working for health and well-being
(5) Developing health programmes and services and reducing inequalities
(6) Policy and strategy development and implementation to improve health and well-being
(7) Working with and for communities to improve health and well-being
(8) Strategic leadership for health and well-being
(9) Research and development to improve health and well-being
(10) Ethically managing self, people and resources to improve health and well-being

(Skills for Health 2004, p. 6)

Public health is therefore composed of a number of activities including health promotion, health protection and illness prevention as well as creating healthy public policies plus empowering individuals and communities to take responsible action for their own health and the health of others. Efforts to improve health need to be aimed at all of the population with a specific focus on the most disadvantaged.

Public health and the policy agenda

From the 1970s onwards the Government came under increasing pressure from both the public and the medical profession to develop a national public health strategy. The Conservative Government's response in 1992, *The Health of the Nation*, in aiming to continue to improve the health of the population focused on mortality and morbidity ignoring underlying socio-economic causes of ill health (Baggott 2000).

A change of government in 1997 was followed by a new public health strategy, *Saving Lives: Our Healthier Nation* (DoH 1999b, p. 5), which proposed to 'improve the health of everyone and the health of the worst off in particular'. It incorporated a greater awareness that health inequality was widespread and that the most disadvantaged suffered most from poor health. Health improvement programmes were proposed and led by health authorities working in partnership with local authorities and others. These action plans would show how the national strategy was to be implemented at a local level. As well as identifying specific settings for health promoting initiatives (schools, the workplace and neighbourhoods) modern roles were planned for nurses and midwives, whilst health visitors and school nurses were specifically identified as public health practitioners.

Other developments included the setting up of the Health Development Agency whose purpose was to advise on standards for public health and health promotion practice and to improve the evidence base for public health (DoH 1999b). Public health observatories were planned for each region of the country forming a national network of knowledge, information and surveillance of public health activities, through monitoring health trends and evaluating the progress made by local agencies to improve health and reduce inequalities.

Following the implementation of the White Paper *Saving Lives: Our Healthier Nation*, the government then set about reforming the National Health Service with the publication of *The NHS Plan* (DoH 2000) which centred on modernising the health service around the needs of the patient. Crucially, in aiming to prevent ill health and reduce health inequalities, the Government recognised that good health depended on social, environmental and economic factors such as deprivation and housing. The development of local strategic partnerships aimed to strengthen the links between the statutory, voluntary and private sectors in order to reduce social exclusion. The plan proposed liberating and supporting the skills and potential of NHS staff through the breaking down of hierarchical barriers, the undertaking of a wider range of clinical tasks and reforming NHS education and training.

These new ways of working were reinforced in *Liberating the Talents* (DoH 2002b) which emphasised the importance of health care professionals responding to meet the changing expectations of the public and delivering services based on the needs of individuals and populations. This would include leading and delivering priority public health programmes that improved health and reduced health inequalities. All community practitioners and health visitors needed to start from a public health perspective assessing the health needs of populations in schools, the workplace and the community assessing priorities and reaching those with greatest needs (CPHVA/DoH 2003). As well as assessing health needs, other principles identified for public health work included ensuring accessibility of services, working with others from health and other sectors, involving local people, a readiness to respond to threats to health and the use of evidence-based practice.

The issue of health inequalities was further addressed by the Department of Health in *Tackling Health Inequalities: A Programme for Action* published in 2003 (DoH 2003). Health inequalities had been widening since the 1970s and were acknowledged as being difficult to change. The Government recognised a need for a co-ordinated programme of action to address the inequalities found across different geographical areas, between genders and differing ethnic communities, and between different social and economic groups. It laid the foundations for achieving the national health inequalities targets to ensure that those who gained most would be those in poorer circumstances (DoH 2001, p. 13).

- By 2010 to reduce inequalities in health outcomes by 10% as measured by infant mortality and life expectancy at birth

The target is underpinned by two objectives:

(1) Starting with children under one year, by 2010 to reduce by at least 10% the gap in mortality between routine and manual groups and the population as a whole
(2) Starting with local authorities, by 2010 to reduce by at least 10% the gap between the fifth of areas with the lowest life expectancy at birth and the population as a whole

Evidence reviewed in the *Independent Inquiry into Inequalities in Health* (Acheson 1998) indicated a need for policy developments across all government departments to tackle socio-economic determinants of health, inequalities in health across the lifecycle and inequalities in health related to gender and ethnicity. The report recognised whilst the previous twenty years had brought a marked increase in material prosperity and reduction in mortality rates to the population as a whole the gap between the top and bottom of the social class had widened. The need for partnerships and joined up working with a range of players, including government departments, local government, and the voluntary and community sectors was further reiterated in the cross-cutting review *Tackling Health Inequalities* (HM Treasury/DoH 2002).

As well as co-ordinated action the Wanless report (2004) suggested that for the Government to succeed in its plans, there needed to be a fundamental culture change from caring for the sick to promoting good health. As part of the 'fully engaged scenario' (see Box 20.1) health services would need to keep healthy people fit as well as manage chronic disease as actively as possible (Wanless 2002). Objectives to improve health outcomes and tackle risk factors such as obesity and smoking needed to be considered as important in terms of performance management as targets set for waiting times. The report also commented on the need for strengthening the cost-effectiveness evidence base on public health interventions. Whilst there have been successes such as the reduction of injury from accidents owing to the wearing of seat belts, there has been, for example, limited evaluation of the long-term impact of environmental policies on the health of the population.

The more recently published *NHS Improvement Plan: Putting People at the Heart of Public Services*

Box 20.1   Fully engaged scenario

Under the fully engaged scenario, the level of public engagement in relation to health is high, life expectancy goes beyond current forecasts, health status improves dramatically, use of resources is more efficient and the health service is responsive with high rates of technology uptake.

(Wanless 2002, p. 35)

(DoH 2004b) has set out plans to improve the health of the population and narrow the gap which exists when compared with other industrialised countries. By 2008, it intends that people should view the attainment of health as a shared responsibility between the state and themselves. Development of the public health agenda is considered to be a central element of the plan which suggests a need to strengthen the public health capacity and delivery of services so that health improvement, health protection and health inequalities are actively targeted. Early detection of public health issues and sharing of information are crucial to taking the agenda forward. To meet these demands the workforce will need to be more flexible and adaptable and supported by a modernised education and training system. Interprofessional education and work-based learning will become more widespread with an increased focus on electronic learning, although professional regulations will continue to ensure protection of the public.

Specialist community public health nursing

The new Nursing and Midwifery Council register

The primary function of the Nursing and Midwifery Council (NMC) which came into being on the 1st April 2002 is to protect the public (NMC 2002a). This is achieved in various ways through the registration of all nurses, midwives and health visitors, the setting of standards for education and training and the monitoring of professional conduct. The register, inherited from the United Kingdom Central Council for Nursing, Midwifery and Health Visiting, had 15 parts that reflected the historical development of differing levels and branches of the professions. Whilst an external review commissioned by the Government recommended replacement with a two part register (nursing and midwifery) the NMC advocated for a three part register with a separate part for public health practitioners. This was in response to the government agenda which placed public health work as a central element of its modernisation programme for health care.

Following consultation with individuals and organisations the NMC recommendation for a three part register for nursing, midwifery and specialist community public health nursing (SCPHN) was accepted (NMC 2004a). Council agreed that the SCPHN part of the register would include all health visitors registered on part 11 of the existing register. Future access to this part of the register would be based on nursing or midwifery registration, thus eliminating the possibility of direct entry candidates. Practitioners would be required to show that that they could meet the public health competencies at specialist level. Council also agreed to work collaboratively with employers to seek to restrict the use of titles to those that the Council regulate. Users and carers should be confident that a registered practitioner who claims to be a specialist in a particular field of practice is able to demonstrate that achievement of the standard set by the NMC.

The new three part register opened on 1st August 2004 with a new set of standards for specialist community public health nurses agreed at the June Council meeting (NMC 2004d). All registered health visitors, with or without a specialist practitioner level qualification, will automatically transfer to the SCPHN part of the register. Following a mapping exercise, it was also agreed that school nurses and occupational health nurses who hold a recordable specialist practitioner qualification will move to the third part of the register, along with family health nurses in Scotland. The first 52 week programmes of education based on these standards are expected to be available from September 2005.

Standards for Specialist Community Public Health Nursing

The NMC has confirmed the view of the Standing Nursing and Midwifery Advisory Committee (SNMAC 1995) which reported on the contribution, role and development of nurses, midwives and health visitors to public health, that all nurses and midwives have an important contribution to make to the public health agenda. However, the NMC is of the view that there is a distinction between practice focused on the provision of clinical nursing care to individuals and public

health nursing practice related to working with populations as well as individuals. This may involve making decisions on behalf of populations without having direct contact with every individual (NMC 2004b).

Guiding principles of proficiency for entry to the register include:

- Preparation: fitness for practice
- Service: fitness for purpose
- Recognition: fitness for award
- Responsibility: fitness for professional standing

The practitioner is expected to 'assess risk in complex situations, develop effective relationships based on trust and ownership, to work in a range of settings acting flexibly with other services and to deal with conflicting priorities and ambiguous situations, knowing when to use different, sometimes contradictory theories and perspectives' (NMC 2004c p. 3).

The framework for SCPHN practice has been developed from the principles of health visiting (CETHV 1977), the standards for community specialist practice (UKCC 1994), the health visiting competencies (NMC 2002b) and the public health standards (Prime Research and Development Ltd for Skills for Health 2003). This new part of the register offers the opportunity to meet the changing requirements of primary care trusts. Public health will need to be a prime consideration when planning services and setting objectives. In the future, the provision of health care services will be based on the skills required to meet the assessed needs of individuals and populations (DoH 2002b). Programmes for education must prepare practitioners not only to work in rapidly changing environments but to influence and lead change. Practitioners must be able to adapt to new systems of service delivery through participating in continuing professional development and extending their scope of practice.

This specialist workforce will be a small but important part of a wider public health function, working for different organisations within the state, voluntary and private sector. The challenge is to harness the resources of contributors across all sectors using the principles of public health practice to ensure delivery of a quality service

---

Box 20.2   Principles of good public health practice. (Source: Prime Research and Development Ltd for Skills for Health – Approval Version – November 2003)

(1) Balance people's rights with their responsibilities to others and to wider society challenging those who affect the rights of others

(2) Promote the values of equality and diversity, acknowledging the personal beliefs and preference of others and promoting anti-discriminatory practice

(3) Promote and welcome community and individual diversity by working with agencies to reduce social exclusion

(4) Balance the need to share information between agencies to improve health and well-being with the need to maintain confidentiality and manage risk

(5) Recognise the effect of the wider social, political and economic context on health and well-being and on people's development

(6) Enable people to develop to their full potential, to be as autonomous and self-managing as possible and to have a voice and be heard

(7) Recognise and promote health and well-being as a positive concept

(8) Develop and maintain effective relationships with people and maintain the integrity of these relationships through setting appropriate role boundaries

(9) Work in ways which are sustainable and based on evidence of effectiveness

(10) Develop oneself and one's own practice to improve the quality of services offered

(11) Work within statutory and agency frameworks

---

that is responsive to the needs of the population (Box 20.2).

New roles for specialist community public health nurses

A changing philosophy of care

Working effectively in public health at the population level will require the development of a different way of working that may not have been part of traditional nursing training (see Table 20.1). The notion of a profession that focuses on caring for patients in a reactive manner, constrained by professional boundaries needs to change (DoH 2002b). The Government's determination to break down the barriers between health and social care not only require government departments to work more closely together but also practitioners to work across boundaries with a variety of agencies to organise care that is responsive to the needs of clients. The development of government flagship initiatives such as Sure Start programmes and extended schools provide public health nursing expertise for children, families and communities making a real difference to their lives (DoH 2004c). Allowing clients to set the

agenda, encouraging the team of workers to take risks, persevering despite setbacks and challenging workers' own prejudices are all part of the new ways of working (Rehal & Langley 2004).

Cowley (2003) suggests that rather than focusing on roles specific to occupational groups, the planning of services is now to be based on the following three questions:

- What needs doing?
- How should it be done?
- Who should do it?

These three questions need to be located within the context of the *Code of Professional Conduct* (NMC 2002c, p. 3) which sets the standard of conduct expected of registered practitioners and demands that a registered nurse or midwife must:

- Protect and support the health of individual patients and clients
- Protect and support the health of the wider community
- Act in such a way that justifies the trust and confidence that the public have in you
- Uphold and enhance the good reputation of the professions

Table 20.1   Developing a public health culture

Public health practice	Traditional nursing practice
Population focus	Individual focus
Leadership model	Servant model
Empowering communities	Controlling clients
Service user led	Professional led
Assertive and challenging	Submissive and respectful
Flexible professional boundaries	Rigid professional boundaries
Collaboration across health and social care	Liaise across health and social care
Community health needs assessment	Individual and caseload health needs assessment
Pro-active approach	Reactive approach
Reflective time	Busy 'doing'
Think creatively	Follow traditions
Take into account health inequalities	Treat everyone equally
Localised budgets	Centralised budgets
Devolved decision making	Hierarchical managerial decision making
Influenced by a variety of government departmental policies	Influenced by Department of Health policy
Supportive clinical supervision	Lack of clinical supervision
No blame culture, risk taking encouraged	Blame culture, risk taking stifled
Evaluation of long-term outcomes	Evaluation of short-term outcomes
Evidence-based practice	Custom and practice
Development of a research culture	Lack of a research culture

Practitioners are personally accountable for their actions and omissions and clients have the right to safe and competent care. It is therefore the responsibility of individual practitioners to identify areas of professional competence and areas of practice that require further professional development as part of their personal development planning. In relation to the new standards for specialist community public health nursing, concerns were expressed as to whether it would be possible for students to become safe and effective practitioners across all areas of practice within the 52 week training course agreed. Whilst it is assumed that students will continue to be sponsored by employers to follow a particular practice route such as health visiting, school nursing or occupational health nursing the standards allow for flexibility and the possibility of alternative approaches to be built into the programme (NMC 2004d).

Professional education needs to respond to the changing agenda, equipping practitioners to work with and empower clients, their carers and the wider population. Programmes must be practice centred, recognising that:

- Evidence should inform practice through the integration of relevant knowledge
- Students are actively involved in the delivery of community public health under supervision
- *The Code of Professional Conduct* applies to all practice interventions
- Skills and knowledge are transferable
- Research underpins practice
- The importance of lifelong learning and continuing professional development is recognised

On qualification, specialist community public nurses must be able to function to the standards required by the professional body and the employer contributing safely and effectively to maintaining and improving the health of communities, and as part of accountability, recognising areas of competence and limitations of practice. Developing a strategic leadership role and managing projects to improve health and well-being is also a requirement for practice. Continuing professional development as part of lifelong learning is therefore a central requirement for those working in health care. For the public health practitioner, assessing the health needs of populations, promoting and protecting health, managing risk, influencing and developing policy, leading and managing change, collaborative working and community development will be fundamental to reducing inequalities in health.

The following example illustrates how specialist community public health nurses could develop their role to promote the health of a population building on the Skills for Health scenario (2004 p. 26).

A case study

'A team of primary care staff identify the need to form a breastfeeding steering group, working together to improve the breastfeeding rates in a deprived community in line with government policy (DoH 2002c) and the local health improvement programme. Service users and interested members of the public are invited to join the group. The project is supported by a public health research lead whose role is to advise the group on data collection methods, analysis of findings, presentation and dissemination of results. Specialist community public health nurses with expert knowledge and skills in breastfeeding, midwives and a health promotion specialist, collect, organise and analyse available data on breastfeeding rates between birth and eight months recognising the need for more rigorous data collection.

Alongside this, they develop an information pack and a newsletter to inform the public of the project. Attendance and satisfaction rates of clients are collected at antenatal, postnatal and breastfeeding groups facilitated by community staff nurses and nursery nurses as well as midwives and community specialist public health nurses. The purpose of the groups is to encourage clients to develop their knowledge and skills of how to improve health during pregnancy and of the importance of breastfeeding

for long-term health gains. Breastfeeding mothers volunteer to facilitate some of the client centred sessions and also support antenatal mothers. With support from the nurse manager and other members of the skill mix team, specialist community public health nurses, midwives and clients hold a fair to celebrate the success of the groups, inviting the public (including local schools and youth groups) to attend.

Furthermore, the specialist community public health nurses and midwives supported by clients, the local branch of the National Childbirth Trust and the local Member of Parliament promote the development of breastfeeding friendly locations (including shops, restaurants and pubs) in the neighbourhood. All those involved in the project keep up to date through attending courses and sharing information to ensure evidence-based practice. They also feel more confident to tackle professional colleagues and family members or friends who are inappropriately advising the use of top up formula feeds to women who are breastfeeding. The manager takes responsibility for disseminating the results of the project to Sure Start teams and feeds the results into the local health plan.

All members of the Steering Group become champions of breastfeeding, ensuring that a group representative attends local, regional and national meetings about breastfeeding and develops networks wherever relevant. Future plans are made to collaborate with other specialist community public health nurses working in schools to promote breastfeeding with local school children as part of the Personal, Social and Health Education programme.

Concerns are also expressed by a member of the steering group that some of the local employers are not supporting breastfeeding women in the workplace and suggests that the group consults with a specialist community public health nurse with expertise in occupational health.'

The elements of public health work can be clearly seen within this scenario. Working with service users in this manner may prove challenging for some professionals but will be essential for empowering individuals and society to take responsibility for health and health care.

Conclusion

This chapter has considered the changing context of public health practice and the challenge this presents for public health practitioners. The government has given clear directives that the public health workforce must work with both individuals and populations to promote health and prevent ill health. The way forward is for specialist community public health nurses to respond positively to change, using the opportunities that arise to influence and develop innovative ways of working, designing, leading and delivering services that empower service users and carers and the wider population. However, protection of the public is of paramount importance and needs to be reflected both in the quality of the professional learning programmes leading to qualification and in the way practitioners take responsibility for their own professional development and accountability in practice. Finally, the importance of developing a better evidence base for practice is essential so that specialist community public health nurses can determine what works well and makes a difference to people's lives.

References

Acheson, D. (1998) *Independent inquiry into inequalities in health*. The Stationery Office, London.

Baggott, R. (2000) *Public Health: Policy and Politics*. Macmillan Press, London.

CETHV (1977) *An investigation into the principles of health visiting*. CETHV, London.

Cowley, S. (2003) Modernising health visiting education: potential problems and progress. *Community Practitioner*, **76**(11), 418–422.

CPHVA/DoH (2003) *Liberating the Talents of Community Practitioners and Health Visitors*. Department of Health, London.

DoH (1992) *The Health of the Nation*. DoH, London.

DoH (1999a) *Making a Difference: Strengthening the nursing, midwifery and health visiting contribution to health and healthcare*. DoH, London.

DoH (1999b) *Saving Lives: Our Healthier Nation*. DoH, London.

DoH (2000) *The NHS Plan: A plan for investment, a plan for reform*. DoH, London.

DoH (2001) *Tackling Health Inequalities: Consultation on a plan for delivery*. DoH, London.

DoH (2002a) *Workforce Matters: A guide to role design in primary care*. www.modern.nhs.uk.

DoH (2002b) *Liberating the Talents: Helping Primary Care Trusts and Nurses to deliver The NHS Plan*. DoH, London.

DoH (2002c) *Improvement, expansion and reform: The next 3 years priorities and planning framework 2003–2006*. www.doh.gov.uk/planning2003-2006.

DoH (2003) *Tackling Health Inequalities: A Programme for Action*. DoH, London.

DoH (2004a) *Choosing Health: A consultation on action to improve people's health*. www.dh.gov.uk.

DoH (2004b) *The NHS Improvement Plan*. DoH, London.

DoH (2004c) *The Chief Nursing Officer's review of the nursing, midwifery and health visiting contribution to vulnerable children and young people*. DoH, London.

DoH (2004d) *Choosing Health: Making Healthy Choices Easier*. www.dh.gov.uk.

Griffiths, S. & Hunter, D.J. (1999) Introduction. In: *Perspectives in Public Health* (eds S. Griffiths & D.J. Hunter). Radcliffe Medical Press, Oxford.

HM Treasury/DoH (2002) *Tackling Health Inequalities Summary of the 2002 Cross Cutting Review*. Department of Health, London.

Hunter, D.J. (1999) Public Health Policies. In: *Perspectives in Public Health*, S. Griffiths & D.J. Hunter (eds). Radcliffe Medical Press, Oxford.

NMC (2002a) *NMC News Autumn 2002 Number 3*. Nursing and Midwifery Council, London.

NMC (2002b) *Requirements for pre-registration health visitor programmes*. NMC, London.

NMC (2002c) *Code of Professional Conduct*. Nursing and Midwifery Council, London.

NMC (2004a) *NMC News April 2004 Number 7*. Nursing and Midwifery Council, London.

NMC (2004b) *NMC News July 2004 Number 8*. Nursing and Midwifery Council, London.

NMC (2004c) *Standards for Specialist Community Public Health Nursing* (C/04/57). NMC, London.

NMC (2004d) *Standards of proficiency for specialist community public health nurses*. Nursing and Midwifery Council, London.

Prime Research and Development Ltd for Skills for Public Health Work (2003) *Functional map for the practice of public health*. November 2003.

Rehal, F. & Langley, H. (2004) Ensuring a Sure Start. *Community Practitioner*, **77**(5), 168–171.

Skills for Health (2004) *National occupational standards for the practice of public health guide.* Skills for Health, Bristol.

SNMAC (1995) *Making it happen: Public Health – the contribution, role and development of nurse, midwives and health visitors.* Department of Health, London.

UKCC (1994) *The future of professional practice – the Council's standards for education and practice following regulation.* United Kingdom Central Council, London.

Wanless, D. (2002) *Securing Our Future Health: Taking a Long-Term View.* United Kingdom Central Council, London.

Wanless, D. (2004) *Securing good health for the whole population.* HM Treasury, London.

Chapter 21 **Modernisation in the Primary Care Workforce**

Stephanie Stanwick and Ami David

Introduction

The NHS Plan (DoH 2000a) clearly highlighted the need for all health service employers to develop new ways of working by introducing new roles, skill mix and the expansion and deepening of existing jobs. Trusts across the NHS have responded to the modernisation agenda introduced by the Labour Government. The resulting changes are having an impact across the entire health care workforce as traditional barriers are broken down and old demarcations are eroded. Throughout the NHS, roles are being refashioned on the overriding principle that the responsibilities of clinical teams should be based on the needs of the patient and the competencies of the health care professional, not merely on their discipline or job title. Building on the progress of the *NHS Plan*, in 2004 the Government outlined new priorities in *The NHS Improvement Plan* (DoH 2004c). The new priorities with fewer targets include continuing to speed up access to services, ensuring better quality care, greater efforts to improve the quality of life for people with long-term conditions and promoting healthy living. It is clear that in meeting these goals, more care will be provided out of hospital and closer to people's homes. This chapter will explore a wide range of issues including the changes in the workforce profiles brought about by changing roles and work patterns of key primary health care professionals.

The case for change

The NHS Plan was first presented to Parliament in July 2000 and since then policies produced and published by the Department of Health have been focused on the development, implementation and monitoring of this major plan for

change in the NHS. It has impacted significantly on the culture and improvement in the NHS; it was responsible for setting a new vision, securing new investment and developing standards for improvement. In its wake the NHS saw the development of the Modernisation Agency and performance improvement; the Commission for Health Improvement (the Health Commission as it is today) and 'Star Ratings', measuring a wide range of standards in health care. Alongside that there have been significant changes in the structure and organisation of the NHS with the establishment of primary care groups, followed by primary care trusts; new strategic health authorities were established covering larger geographical areas and focusing on strategic development and performance management of local NHS organisations, and currently 'high performing' acute trusts are eligible to become foundation trusts.

The NHS was encouraged to become the 'model employer' with accreditation processes for improving the working lives of staff (IWL) which included personnel policies, communication, staff care, incentives and working times together with a systematic reform of working hours and pay; including junior doctors' working hours, European working times directions, consultants and their contracts and hours of work, new contracts and service conditions for general practitioners and, currently, the total job evaluation and pay reform for all other groups of staff under *Agenda for Change* (DoH 2002a).

There isn't a corner of the NHS that remains unchallenged or untouched by these changes. *The NHS Plan* argued that the NHS had delivered major improvements in health since inception but fell short of the standards patients expected and staff wanted to provide. The public were expecting:

- More and better paid staff using new ways of working
- Reduced waiting times and high quality care centred on patients
- Improvements in local hospitals and surgeries

The NHS Plan argued that the NHS was a 1940s system operating in a 21st century world. It went on to promise:

- Extra beds for hospitals and intermediate care
- 100 new hospitals (by 2010), 500 new one-stop primary care centres
- 3000 modernised GP premises
- Clean wards overseen by 'modern matrons'
- Modern IT systems in every hospital and GP surgery
- 7500 more consultants, 2000 more GPs, 20000 extra nurses and 6500 extra therapists
- 1000 more medical school placements
- Child care support for NHS staff with 100 on-site nurseries

There were key themes identified for the NHS around preventive care and primary care with more screening to minimise risks in health, being at the forefront in the use of medicines ensuring that they were implemented rapidly, helping people adopt healthier lifestyles, keeping down blood pressure and cholesterol levels. The concept of NHS Direct was introduced as a means to help provide advice and support to people as well as self-care being seen as the frontline for care at home. For primary care, NHS Direct was seen as the NHS gateway to health care to provide information in accessing health care services. *The NHS Plan* described many GPs working in teams in modern multi-purpose facilities alongside nurses, pharmacists, dentists, therapists, opticians and social care staff. The concept of GPs specialising in treating different conditions was introduced, the consulting room described as the place where appointments for diagnostic tests, for outpatients and for operations were booked, tests results received and more diagnosis carried out using video- and tele-links to specialists. It was proposed that more care would take place in these settings to support the changes in hospital care. A new

range of intermediate care services would be created to build a bridge between hospitals and home, helping people to recover more quickly and resume independent living, speeding up discharge from hospital and establishing new services for older people living at home as an alternative to being forced to choose a nursing or residential care home. The concepts of rapid response teams, intensive home support, better rehabilitation after strokes – all working on an integrated basis with social services, was also described. The consequences of all these service changes on the primary and community services workforce are described later in this chapter.

The NHS Plan was seen as a ten-year plan with these improvements developing over that time frame. Another document which emerged in December 2000 – *The NHS Plan Implementation Programme* (DoH 2000b), set out a timetable and planning process for implementation and review at both a local and a national level, with a new modernisation board, bringing stakeholders together to advise the Secretary of State and the Chief Executive of the NHS (DoH 2000b). This document set out a series of stepped targets for 2001/02 until 2004. At a national level, implementation of *The NHS Plan* was divided into 10 functional areas with a task group set up for each to drive things forward, these included: access, cancer, capacity including IT, coronary heart disease, children, mental health, older people, public health, quality and workforce.

The work programme of the workforce task group included the following: the increase in staff numbers, improving working lives, modernising pay and contracts, modernising education, training and development, implementing new ways of working, and modernising workforce planning. These objectives worked through the national level to a local level where workforce confederations were established as arm's length organisations charged with taking this forward. Today workforce confederations are integral parts of strategic health authorities but still responsible for the management and implementation of these elements of the NHS Plan.

In 2002, another document produced by the Department of Health (*Delivering the NHS Plan,*

Next Steps on Investment, Next Steps on Reform, 2002d) heralded a new era for pay reform, including liberating the talent and skills of all the members of the workforce so that every patient gets the right care in the right place at the right time. In 2003 *The NHS Plan Progress Report*, set out in the National NHS Modernisation Board's Annual Report (DoH 2003b), described the progress achievements so far and made clear the recognition that the strength, diversity and creativity of staff in the NHS is fundamental to driving forward changes and that these are making a visible difference to patient care and creating greater opportunities at all levels for staff to develop their full potential.

The most recent document, published in June 2004, outlines the overall progress in NHS improvement and sets priorities for the NHS between now and 2008 (*The NHS Improvement Plan – Putting People at the Heart of Public Services*) (DoH 2004b). Its key message is that the drive for a responsive, convenient and personalised service takes 'root across the whole NHS', and that for the millions of people who have illnesses such as diabetes, asthma or heart disease, they receive closer personal attention and support in the community and at home. This document goes on to describe the right service for patients at three levels:

- Level 1 as 'self-management' where people are supported to manage their own chronic disease
- Level 2 is described as 'disease management'. With proper tailored support in primary care and tailored packages of care for individuals for health and social care services, these can make a real impact on slowing the progression of these diseases
- Level 3 is described as 'case management' and is where people often have three or more complex problems and the NHS needs to personalise packages for more complex care

Some of the examples referred to in this document are also described in this chapter where staff are working differently and making best use of their skills, using a 'skills escalator' and developing through a career through the NHS.

Modernising primary and community health care nursing

Never before in the history of the NHS has primary and community care nursing taken such a centre stage position. Professionals working in primary care settings are now required to deliver care through the acquisition of higher level clinical and technical skills because of a 'quicker and sicker' throughput of patients from acute settings.

At the same time a sophisticated focus on prevention and public health places primary care professionals in a vantage position to provide both targeted and opportunistic preventative care.

Improving access to health care is an important service improvement goal for the NHS. The expressed view from all quarters is that care must be widely available and delivered where it is convenient for patients in the community.

The four key areas of work identified in the Public Service Agreement for 2004–2008, all indicate a need for active contributions from the primary and community nursing workforce (see Fig. 21.1).

Ensuring a responsive workforce

Responding to the national priorities requires an assessment to be made of the capacity and

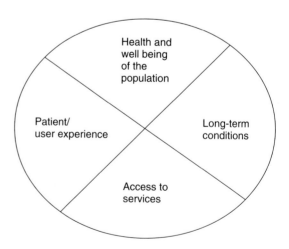

Figure 21.1   National priority areas as set out in the DoH Public Service Agreement 2005/06–2007/08. (Source: The NHS Improvement Plan (DoH 2004c)).

capability of the current workforce in primary and community care settings and a move towards redesigning the way services are delivered.

The primary care nursing workforce forms 17% of nurses, midwives and health visitors employed in the NHS in England (DoH Workforce Statistics 2002c; Office of Manpower Economics 2003). A recent study into flexible entry to primary care nursing (Drennan *et al.* 2004) has revealed whilst the health visiting and district nursing workforce have remained static over ten years the real growth within primary care nursing has been of registered nurses in posts not designated as requiring specialist community nursing qualifications. It is, however, also clear that demographic trends within the nursing profession and specifically within the community nursing workforce has resulted in an ageing workforce (DoH 2002a).

To achieve the goals a key policy document allied to *The NHS Plan* (*Liberating the Talents* DoH 2002b) set the direction for nursing in primary care by offering a framework to:

- Redesign services around the changing needs of the population and the rapid changes in acute in-patient care
- Provide nurses in primary care greater freedoms to develop new approaches to patient care
- Move from the tendency to place too much emphasis on rigidly defined roles in primary and community nursing towards providing the services patients want

The three key foci of this report are presented at Figure 21.2.

Policy documents such as *Working Together, Learning Together* (DoH 2001) and the introduction of primary care service models, including for example non-medical prescribing; effective chronic disease management; the development of first contact practitioners and practitioners with special interests (DoH 2003a,c, 2004b) have also signalled a renewed focus on the preparation of practitioners.

In addition the new General Medical Services Contract (2004c) presents primary care organisations with new challenges including emerging new

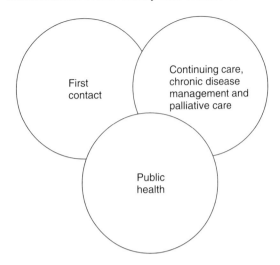

Figure 21.2 *Liberating the Talents* framework – a redesign model for primary and community nursing in the twenty-first century (DoH 2002b)

roles for nurses and a demand for an integrated system of 24-hour care.

Policy shifts have forced boundaries between acute/primary/continuing care to become blurred. Whilst unique 'core' functions of agencies and professional groups can be clearly identified, increasingly generic functions across traditional boundaries are also being acknowledged and introduced. This pattern of service development raises questions on the need for generic multidisciplinary education for practitioners that addresses the needs of patient groups in care pathways rather than focus on the location of care delivery.

The modernisation agenda has also introduced a comprehensive framework for quality including mechanisms to set standards and assess/inspect both individuals and organisations performance in the delivery of care. With the advent of clinical governance it is clear that the quality of care delivered to patients depends crucially on the calibre of staff working in the NHS. Within a modernised NHS that promotes lifelong learning and learning through significant events, and in order that the focus on quality is facilitated, there is recognition within primary care organisations of the need to create high quality working environments that support work-based learning and e-learning.

Constraints and challenges to workforce redesign in primary and community nursing

The reduction in the number of trained primary and community nurses across the country, together with an ageing workforce has, of necessity, resulted in primary care trusts employing a range of team members to support the trained community nurses.

Whilst there has been an increase in health care assistants in teams, the real growth has been amongst the numbers of registered nurses at staff nurse levels D, E and F grades (see for example evidence gathered by the DoH commissioned group on flexible entry to primary care nursing (Drennan *et al.* 2004).

This significant group of the workforce – composed of staff nurse grades – is currently delivering care in community settings with very little or no additional training.

Existing qualified specialist practitioners, it would appear, also demonstrate variable levels of knowledge and skills. This has led to a situation of, on the one hand, evidence of pioneering innovators in community nursing, and on the other, apathy and failure to grasp opportunities to develop practice. This is a pattern replicated across the country.

The pattern that is emerging is therefore inconsistent and does not offer a cohesive response to new patient care needs in the community. Other constraints include those listed in Box 21.1.

The vision for redesign

The following vision for change is offered in order to assure the delivery of a service based on need rather than the current preoccupation with professional titles.

The new vision for nursing in primary care therefore must stem from:

Organisational redesign

- Breakdown of the rigid boundaries that currently exist between practitioners working in acute/primary and social care
- Enable easier movement for nurses, particularly staff nurses, between hospital and primary care
- Services planned on the basis of need rather than professional title
- Direct access to services for patients through the use of first contact practitioners operating across traditional boundaries

Workforce redesign

- Shift in the shape of the workforce in primary care
- Shift in how nurses will be rewarded from remuneration based on qualification towards a more flexible approach that rewards the acquisition of skills and knowledge relevant to the role as part of a managed career pathway
- Supporting specialisation at junior levels of the workforce as well as the development of high-level generalists

---

Box 21.1   Constraints on patient care needs in the community

- A perceived reluctance to give up 'traditional community nursing turf' to other practitioners specifically to staff nurses, nursery nurses and health care assistants
- A perceived inability to work across traditional organisational boundaries (in part assumed to be due to the constraining titles that confine practitioners to a location-based service rather than one which is centred on patient care needs)
- The current preparation of specialist practitioners does not address sufficiently the demands of a modernised NHS (e.g. access issues; patient and public involvement; choice; chronic disease management and leadership at all levels)
- Very little movement within universities towards preparing current specialist practice students for the three domains of practice elaborated in *Liberating the Talents* i.e. first contact; chronic disease management, rehabilitation, continuing care and public health, health protection

---

Professional practice and development redesign

- Prepared to work across traditional boundaries at all levels
- Moving away from a professional title focused service to one that offers practitioners preparation in all three domains of practice in *Liberating the Talents* (public health; first contact and chronic disease management/ continuing care)
- A flexible career structure that enables progression through continuous development at all levels rather that a set series of steps.

The matrix table (Table 21.1) plots the potential contribution of primary and community nurses using the key public service agreement targets and the principles espoused in *Liberating the Talents*.

Ensuring the 'right' mix of skills

The modernisation and redesign of the qualified nurse role cannot take place in isolation. Therefore, to ensure the provision of an adequately skilled workforce to meet the aspirations of *The NHS Plan*, the redesign/re-skill programme must of necessity address the need to prepare differently

Table 21.1 Potential contribution of primary and community nurses using the key public service agreement targets and the principles espoused in *Liberating the Talents*

| **Public Service Agreement Targets** | **New Community and Primary Care Nursing Practice and Education Redesign Challenges** | | | | |
	Leadership and teamwork	*New roles*	*Clinical excellence*	*Patient and public involvement*	*Partnership working*
Health and well-being of the population	Nurse-led models which include public health approaches	Role re-design for all team members	Evidence-based care health protection	Proactive case finding Self care management/ enabling choice	Power sharing/ cross boundary working
Long-term conditions	Effective clinical leadership and advanced practice competencies/ ability to make direct referrals	Use existing DNs skilled to be 'community matrons'	Robust clinical indicators based on new standards framework	Choice and satisfaction Admission avoidance/ shorter stays	Joint goals/ multi-agency core standards
Access to services	First contact care involving a range of practitioners	Walk-in-centre approaches	Advanced physical assessment/ history taking	Working with expert patients Utilise the Wagner (2000) framework for chronic disease management	Effective whole system/ reflected in local plans
Patient and user experience	Integrated teams focused on patient needs – not title	Reward for new roles via patient satisfaction and AFC	Clinical governance credibility with the public	Range of service models Attractive to patients	Integrated care via managed clinical networks

Note: Targets based on the 2004–2008 NHS Improvement Plan.

all staff in the skills escalator to work in multi-disciplinary teams/multi-agency settings.

Primary care organisations (PCOs) experiencing recruitment and retention challenges have, of necessity, begun to take a skills escalator approach introducing health care assistants, rehabilitation assistants and nursery nurses.

These essential members of the workforce have begun – through NVQ and skills based learning – to undertake a number of clinical tasks hitherto only seen as the province of a trained nurse. The clinical components of such programmes have been developed locally with little or no involvement of education institutions. However, the emergence of new foundation degrees for assistant practitioners, prepared to work competently in primary and social care, has recently been witnessed as a welcome addition. Despite a lack of national recognition and regulation for this workforce group (e.g. health care assistants) they have been introduced successfully into the primary care workplace, including general practice across the country. However, the long awaited regulation of the health care assistant/support workforce is now planned for implementation by 2007.

In primary care, re-skilling of the workforce has been also extended to the development of staff nurses in the community. This group of nurses (currently in D, E and F grades) have entered primary care settings with 1–3 years post-registration experience in acute settings. On entry they have often been de-skilled and compelled to work 'below their competency levels' owing to a perceived view in primary care that only specialist practitioners can offer care based on higher level skills. This approach disregards recent initiatives such as *Making a Difference* (DoH 1999) and the changes made in pre-registration education and training. One other key change has been the announcement of at least one university (London South Bank University) to adapt the adult nursing branch programme to meet the outcome competencies required by PCTs to prepare a 'fit for purpose' primary care nurse at the point of qualification.

A number of PCOs have attempted to overcome this hierarchical structure by developing appropriate programmes in partnership with higher education institutes (HEIs) to prepare staff nurses to undertake a wider range of tasks in primary care. This in turn has meant that specialist practitioners in primary care can now be freed to undertake more leadership, special interests, prescribing and other higher-level tasks.

The challenge to engage all practitioners in new ways of learning and development is one that many organisations find difficult to address. In primary care it is acknowledged that much of this can be achieved through a shift in emphasis towards work-based learning and e-learning. However, its success is dependent on the development and implementation of a shared philosophy between HEIs and PCOs.

People at the centre of new approaches to care

The case studies shown in Box 21.2 provide some examples of service models that reflect the principles of new roles for staff, better access for patients, with improved outcomes.

These case studies demonstrate how important it has become to challenge the demarcation lines that exist between different professional groups – one of the key NHS Plan targets. This is vital if patients are to receive a timely and responsive service.

The combined impact of challenging and changing traditional working patterns in the NHS is beginning to lead to the development of a range of new and innovative roles for nurses in primary and community care. The case studies demonstrate the new models emerging that span traditional professional boundaries, underpinned by the concept of a skills escalator approach. The skills escalator enables professionals functioning at different levels to acquire new skills responsive to patient needs and thus maximising the capacity and capability of individual professionals.

The skills escalator approach is further expanded on in the next section, which outlines a model in action in one PCT.

Box 21.2 Case studies

Case study 1 – patient experience
'I was nearly at the end of my tether, I didn't know how to cope with my son at home, he kept throwing tantrums and swearing ... was difficult at school. The teachers say he has been seen bullying other children and they have had complaints. I went to see the GP and he got the specialist health visitor to call. She worked with me for six weeks helping me understand how to set behaviour targets with my son and to structure his home time. Some of the time she visited us at home but other times we went to a group with other mums and children it was nice to see other mums with the same problem. I made some new friends.'

Responsive service delivery – new way of working
Service re-design: This supports the issues surrounding child and adolescent mental health services. Developing parenting skills – helping manage child behaviour
Roles re-design: Re-focusing health visitor or school nurse skills to provide this targeted service
Outcomes: Early identification of children with problems and providing support to parents does improve access, prevents problems getting entrenched and children get on better in school. Meets NHS improvement plan objective to provide a comprehensive child & adolescent mental health service

Case study 2 – patient experience
'My wife had a stroke just before our golden wedding anniversary. We called the GP and he came to visit and asked the stroke co-ordinator nurse to call. She arranged for her to go to hospital to have some tests as an outpatient and she came home that same day. Then she arranged for the stroke team to look after my wife at home. There was a generic worker who came and helped get her up and in a chair, she also encouraged my wife to do her exercises that the physiotherapist and occupational therapist has set her. It took her six weeks but in that time she slowly regained her strength. I am not too strong myself so was worried we would have to be split up.'

Responsive service delivery – new ways of working
Service re-design: This supports service for coronary heart disease and stroke with early interventions maximising rehabilitation for patients
Role re-design: The stroke co-coordinator – a nurse or therapist with special interest in stroke care authorises access to diagnostic tests and ensures the right supporting package of care is in place. Generic rehabilitation workers support the multi-disciplinary care and have developed skills working under the supervision of the physiotherapist and occupational therapist. She works closely with a care manager who as part of the team ensures comprehensive home support
Outcomes: Early intervention and follow-up through a team approach resulting in effective health care valued by patients cared for in their own home setting

Case study 3 – patient experience
'I have diabetes and used to be a smoker so I have a bad chest. Over the last couple or years I have been in hospital two or three times in the course of the year. I go in, have some tests and some antibiotics and have my diabetes sorted out. However, this year it's different; I have my own special nurse who calls and monitors my progress, she checks my diabetes and listens to my chest, she spotted an early infection and I'm convinced the treatment prevented my last admission.'

Responsive service delivery – new way of working
Service re-design: The NHS improvement plan describes the benefits of these service developments in preventing repeated admissions
Role re-design: Community nurses and practice nurses with additional skills in case finding, history taking, physical assessment, differential diagnosis and supplementary prescribing, authorise tests to support the diagnosis and refer on to others including consultants in acute care and are ideally placed to deliver this. They would need to be able to help patients navigate the system and manage their condition better
Outcomes: Research evidence indicates a targeted approach and more effective management can prevent inappropriate admissions and improve patient experiences

---

Box 21.2 (Continued)

Case study 4 – patient experience
'My young son had been niggly and irritable all day, I sent him to nursery school but he didn't settle. I decided to wait and see how he went; he had a temperature but I didn't know what else was wrong. He has had a couple of wheezy illnesses so I do worry. By 10pm I was really concerned. I phoned the out of hours service and they told me to bring him into the centre. I saw the nurse who checked him over and gave us some medicine to take home. She also told us what to look out for and who to contact if we needed further help.'

Responsive service delivery – new ways of working
Service re-design: Out of hours services are being developed to support the changes introduced by the new GP Contract (the new General Medical Services Contract) Many out of hours calls can be dealt with by a skilled nurse or other first contact practitioners working in a primary care walk-in centre/out of hours service centre
Role re-design: Nurses working in the community with advanced practice skills and the ability to see and treat patients with undifferentiated conditions using diagnostic, prescribing and caring skills to effect
Outcomes: Patients can access skilled practitioners out of hours with effective and timely responses

---

Case study 5 – patient experience
'My husband has had a bad chest, he's quite frail and normally gets up and dresses himself but does need looking after. With his chest, he has been quite unwell and off his food and he has also been a bit incontinent which upsets him. I'm not as fit as I was and it is wearing me down. I rang the doctor and the nurse came to our house and arranged admission to the community hospital not far from us. The nurse in charge assessed that he needed some intravenous fluids and some antibiotics. He was back on his feet in few days and had some physiotherapy and now he's home.

Responsive service delivery – new ways of working
Service re-design: The provision of community hospitals nurse-led intermediate care services supported by a range of specialists. Community hospitals play a key role in providing services for older people
Roles re-design: Enabling nurses to act autonomously using advanced practice skills and exercising the CNO 10 key roles outlined in the NHS Plan. Initiating nurse led admission and discharge with support from a doctor
Outcomes: Skilled nurses provide interventions which support the patient without admission to an acute bed

---

A local framework for redesign in community nursing

In response to policy imperatives and socio-demographic changes impacting on the local population and the workforce, a skills escalator framework entitled the 'Dartford, Gravesham, Swanley (DGS) PCT step up model' was developed in the authors' PCT. This model, developed in close partnership with London South Bank University colleagues, was further endorsed by the PCT Executive Committee and the PCT Board.

Staff ownership and understanding was fostered across the PCT.

The key objectives underpinning the framework are:

- To respond to service developments in primary care, health improvement initiatives, intermediate care and the National Service Framework standards by ensuring the provision of an appropriately skilled workforce
- To demonstrate improvements in access to care in modernised care settings

- To redesign our services based on the needs of patients and not just on previous practice
- To meet anticipated fall in recruitment of primary care professionals compounded further by an 'ageing' workforce

The DGS PCT 'step up' framework for redesign

To facilitate the step up framework a model known as the DGS PCT '4 Rs process' has been established across primary and community services. This is shown in Box 21.3.

New roles, new competencies

As nurses are being empowered to undertake a wider range of clinical tasks, working to implement the Chief Nursing Officer's ten key roles for nurses outlined in *The NHS Plan* (DoH 2000a) – for example, running clinics, admitting, referring and discharging patients, diagnostic testing and prescribing – the potential impact of the profession in improving the standard of care

is increasingly being realised. It is therefore essential that competency frameworks are put in place in all extended roles and specialities to ensure that a consistent quality of care is achieved and allow for the professional development of all team members to continue through education, training and support.

This will in turn encourage confidence and shared working processes to develop within and between teams. Additionally, the continual auditing and monitoring of these competencies will be vital to assure nurses and their employers that they are working to the best of their abilities and improving care for patients. Advanced autonomous practice brings into sharp focus the need for clear lines of accountability and the need to ensure robust risk management systems are in place. Many of the new ways of working are, however, not currently reflected in how services are measured. In time we will see patient experiences and evidence-based outcomes used to assess the performance of staff

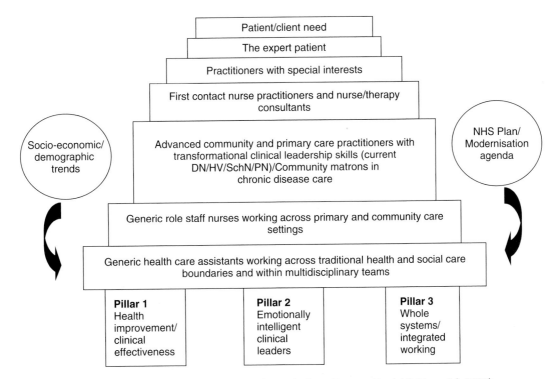

Figure 21.3 The DGS PCT 'Step up' framework for redesign. (Source: David & Stanwick 2003)

Box 21.3   The 4 Rs process

Stage 1

Review and reconsider the vacant post in the light of local health care needs/health improvement priorities to determine if the same post should be re-established or if a new set of skills and provision is required.

Stage 2

Refocus potential care delivery and the skill mix required in consultation with the team.

Stage 3

Redesign the post by identifying specific knowledge, skills and experience required to meet the emerging health care needs and population profile.

Stage 4

Re-skill both new and existing practitioners to meet identified skills deficit in conjunction with education providers and the Workforce Confederation.

and services (*National Standards, Local Action* DoH 2004d).

Conclusion

The NHS Plan and the subsequent Improvement Plan have created an environment in which change can take place ensuring better patient experiences. Many of the improvements that patients want to see relate to their everyday interaction with services. This in turn requires not only supporting environments, but also change at the front line and in service redesign. For nurses working in primary and community care the significant opportunities that exist for role redesign are unprecedented offering a range of models to ensure both patient and professional satisfaction.

References

Dartford, Gravesham & Swanley PCT (2002) *A Force for Positive Change – a strategic plan to enhance the contribution of therapists, nurses and health visitors.* DGS, PCT.

Dartford, Gravesham & Swanley PCT (2003) *Improving Access to Services: establishing the PCT workforce 'step up' projects.* http://www.dh.gov.uk/assetRoot/04/07/92/94/04079294.PDF

Department of Health (1999) *Making a Difference: Strengthening the Nursing, Midwifery and Health Visiting Contribution to Health and Health Care.* The Stationery Office, London.

Department of Health (2000a) The NHS plan, A Plan for Investment, A Plan for Reform. The Stationery Office, London.

Department of Health (2000b) *NHS Plan Implementation Programme.* The Stationery Office, London.

Department of Health (2001) *Working together, Learning together: a framework for lifelong learning for the NHS.* DoH, London.

Department of Health (2002a) *Agenda for Change.* DoH, London.

Department of Health (2002b) *Liberating the Talents – helping Primary Care Trusts and nurses to deliver The NHS Plan.* DoH, London.

Department of Health (2002c) Non Medical Workforce Census. DoH, London.

Department of Health (2002d) *Delivering the NHS Plan, Next Steps on Investment, Next Steps on Reform,* DoH, London.

Department of Health (2003a) *Practitioners with special interest in primary care: implementing a scheme for nurses with special interests in primary care.* DoH, London.

Department of Health (2003b) *The NHS Plan Progress Report* – the National NHS Modernisation Board's Annual Report, London.

Department of Health (2003c) *Nurse prescribing and Preparation: extended formulary nurse prescribing.* DoH, London.

Department of Health (2004a) *Chronic Disease Compendium.* DoH, London.

Department of Health (2004b) *Chronic Disease Management Strategy.* DoH, London.

Department Of Health (2004c) *The NHS Improvement Plan – Putting People at the Heart of Public Services.* DoH, London.

Department of Health (2004d) *National Standards, Local Action Health and Social Care Standards and Planning Framework.* DoH, London.

Department of Health Workforce Statistics (2002) Healthcare: Workforce. The Stationery Office, London.

Drennan, V., Andrews, S. & Sidhu, R. (2004) *Flexible Entry to Primary Care Nursing,* Project Final Report. Primary Care Nursing Research Unit, University College London.

Office of Manpower Economics (2003) *Workforce Survey Results for Nursing Staff, Midwives and Health Visitors.* Office of Manpower Economics, London.

Index